CURRICULUM DEVELOPMENT FOR MEDICAL EDUCATION

CURRICULUM DEVELOPMENT FOR MEDICAL EDUCATION

A SIX-STEP APPROACH

Third Edition

Edited by

Patricia A. Thomas, MD

David E. Kern, MD, MPH

Mark T. Hughes, MD, MA

Belinda Y. Chen, MD

The Johns Hopkins Faculty Development Program
The Johns Hopkins University School of Medicine
Baltimore, Maryland

JOHNS HOPKINS UNIVERSITY PRESS | BALTIMORE

Johns Hopkins University Press
2715 North Charles Street
Baltimore, Maryland 21218-4363
www.press.jhu.edu

Library of Congress Cataloging-in-Publication Data

Curriculum development for medical education : a six-step approach /
edited by Patricia A. Thomas, David E. Kern, Mark T. Hughes, Belinda Y. Chen. — Third edition.
p. ; cm.
Includes bibliographical references and index.
ISBN 978-1-4214-1851-3 (hardcover : alk. paper) — ISBN 1-4214-1851-7 (hardcover : alk. paper) —
ISBN 978-1-4214-1852-0 (pbk. : alk. paper) — ISBN 1-4214-1852-5 (pbk. : alk. paper) —
ISBN 978-1-4214-1853-7 (electronic) — ISBN 1-4214-1853-3 (electronic)
I. Thomas, Patricia A. (Patricia Ann), 1950– , editor. II. Kern, David E., editor.
III. Hughes, Mark T., editor. IV. Chen, Belinda Y., 1966– , editor.
[DNLM: 1. Curriculum. 2. Education, Medical—methods. W 18]
R834
610.71'173—dc23   2015008459

A catalog record for this book is available from the British Library.

*Special discounts are available for bulk purchases of this book. For more information,
please contact Special Sales at 410-516-6936 or specialsales@press.jhu.edu.*

Johns Hopkins University Press uses environmentally friendly book
materials, including recycled text paper that is composed of at least 30 percent
post-consumer waste, whenever possible.

To the many faculty members
who strive to improve medical education
by developing, implementing, and evaluating
curricula in the health sciences

Contents

Preface

Curriculum Development for Medical Education: A Six-Step Approach has been widely used by educators in the health professions for the past 17 years. Since its publication, the editors have presented the model to medical educators in North America, as well as in Africa, Asia, the Middle East, and South America. The book has been translated into both Chinese and Japanese. Our assumption that medical educators would "benefit from learning a practical, generic, and timeless approach to curriculum development that can address today's as well as tomorrow's needs" has been supported by the book's readership and requests for related courses and workshops.

Readers may question why a new edition was needed within five years of the second edition. Unbeknownst to the editors at the time, the second edition was published at the dawn of a turbulent era in medical education. The past five years have seen a wave of calls for reform, new accreditation standards, and regulatory guidelines, which are noted in the Introduction and are cited repeatedly in the third edition. The century-old paradigm of "2 + 2" basic science and clinical clerkship predoctoral model, the hospital-based residency model, and even discipline-based (e.g., medicine, nursing, and pharmacy) education have been challenged. As health care delivery is rapidly changing, there is wide consensus that medical education needs to adapt. In the United States, the triple aims of the Affordable Care Act—better health care access, higher quality, and lower cost—have become the goals of new competency-based frameworks. The science of learning has further matured with the partnering of cognitive science and neuroscience; the implications of this understanding of learning have modified approaches to education. Technology, in addition to its impact in health care delivery, has made information and learning more accessible worldwide with innovations such as massive open online courses (MOOCs) and the Kahn Academy. High-fidelity simulation and virtual reality for education and training have also become more robust and efficacious. These are just some of the changes driving unprecedented curriculum development and renewal across the medical education continuum.

The editors chose three themes to emphasize in the latest revision of the book: competency-based education, including milestones and the entrustable professional activities (EPAs) as an assessment tool; interprofessional education; and educational technology. We have emphasized these themes within the presentation of the six steps as well as in the examples used to apply the concepts. Acknowledging the tremendous growth in medical education publication and dissemination, we especially researched the published literature for examples. References have been extensively updated.

Several chapters deserve specific mention. Chapter 2, Problem Identification and General Needs Assessment, incorporates the contemporary demands for change discussed above. Chapter 3, Targeted Needs Assessment, includes more detail on how to increase response rates to surveys. Chapter 4, Goals and Objectives, has an elaborated discussion of competency-based education and integrates the concept of competency as a higher-level and integrated (knowledge, attitude, and skill) objective. Chapter 5, Educational Strategies, incorporates science of learning as a driver for design of educational strategies and has a new section on educational technology and online learning. Chapter 6, Implementation, provides more information on considerations of time and resources, particularly how to reward faculty for teaching or educational administration. Chapter 7, Evaluation and Feedback, incorporates increased emphasis on competencies, milestones, and EPAs. Table 9.3 in Chapter 9, Dissemination, which lists peer-reviewed journals that are likely to publish curriculum-related work, now includes data on the number and percentage of articles in each journal that are curriculum-related, as well as journal impact factors and rank. An entirely new chapter, Chapter 10, Curriculum Development for Larger Programs, discusses the additional issues of curriculum development for large, long, and integrated programs. Appendix A, which demonstrates how all six steps organize into curricula for undergraduate (UME), graduate (GME), and continuing medical education (CME), includes an update of the CME example and two entirely new examples: a simulation example for UME and a geriatric education example for GME.

We welcome Belinda Chen as a new editor and new coauthor for this edition. Our other new authors are Chadia Abras, who provides expertise in educational technology for Chapter 5; Brenessa Lindeman as coauthor for Chapter 7; Julianna Jung and Nicole Shilkofski as authors of the UME example in Appendix A; and Nancy Schoenborn and Matthew McNabney as authors of the GME example in Appendix A. David Kern has stepped down as lead editor but has been deeply involved in all chapters and revisions to this edition, in addition to remaining an active author for several chapters. As with previous editions, the editors reviewed every chapter in detail, in addition to serving as chapter and appendix authors.

We wish to thank the wonderful faculty with whom we have worked for so many years in the Faculty Development programs in Curriculum Development. We have learned much from watching the application of the Six-Step model to a variety of curricula. Many of these faculty have generously shared their unpublished curricula as examples in the book.

We also acknowledge the expert guidance of our external reviewers, Joseph Carrese and Ken Kolodner for Chapter 7 and Sanjay Desai, Colleen O'Connor Grochowski, and John Mahoney for Chapter 10.

Contributors

Chadia N. Abras, PhD, Assistant Professor, Johns Hopkins University School of Education, and Program Director for Distance Education, Johns Hopkins University School of Education, Center for Technology in Education, Baltimore, Maryland

Eric B. Bass, MD, MPH, Professor, Departments of Medicine, Epidemiology, and Health Policy and Management, Director, Foundations of Public Health Course, and Director, Evidence-based Practice Center, Johns Hopkins University School of Medicine and Bloomberg School of Public Health, Baltimore, Maryland

Belinda Y. Chen, MD, Instructor in Medicine (part-time), Department of Medicine, Division of General Internal Medicine, Johns Hopkins University School of Medicine, and Director, Programs in Curriculum Development, Johns Hopkins Faculty Development Program, Baltimore, Maryland

Mark T. Hughes, MD, MA, Assistant Professor, Department of Medicine, Division of General Internal Medicine and Palliative Care Medicine, and Core Faculty, Johns Hopkins Berman Institute of Bioethics, Johns Hopkins University School of Medicine, Baltimore, Maryland

Julianna Jung, MD, Assistant Professor and Director of Undergraduate Medical Education, Department of Emergency Medicine, Johns Hopkins University School of Medicine, Associate Director, Johns Hopkins Medicine Simulation Center, and Faculty, Curriculum Development Course, Master of Education for the Health Professions, Johns Hopkins University School of Education, Baltimore, Maryland

David E. Kern, MD, MPH, Emeritus Professor of Medicine, Johns Hopkins University School of Medicine, Past Director, Division of General Internal Medicine, Johns Hopkins Bayview Medical Center, and Past Director, Programs in Curriculum Development, Johns Hopkins Faculty Development Program, Baltimore, Maryland

Brenessa M. Lindeman, MD, MEHP, Resident Physician in General Surgery, Department of Surgery, Johns Hopkins University School of Medicine, Baltimore, Maryland

Pamela A. Lipsett, MD, MHPE, Warfield M. Firor Endowed Professorship, Professor, Departments of Surgery, Anesthesiology, and Critical Care Medicine, and School of Nursing, Program Director, General Surgery Residency Program, and Surgical Critical Care Fellowship Program, and Co-Director, Surgical Intensive Care Units, Johns Hopkins University School of Medicine, Baltimore, Maryland

Matthew K. McNabney, MD, Associate Professor of Medicine, Department of Medicine, Division of Geriatric Medicine and Gerontology, and Fellowship Program Director, Johns Hopkins University School of Medicine, Baltimore, Maryland

Nancy L. Schoenborn, MD, Assistant Professor, Department of Medicine, Division of Geriatric Medicine and Gerontology, Johns Hopkins University School of Medicine, Baltimore, Maryland

Nicole A. Shilkofski, MD, MEd, Assistant Professor, Departments of Pediatrics and Anesthesiology/Critical Care Medicine, Johns Hopkins University School of Medicine, Baltimore, Maryland

Patricia A. Thomas, MD, Professor of Medicine, Vice Dean for Medical Education, Case Western Reserve University School of Medicine, Cleveland, Ohio

Introduction

Patricia A. Thomas, MD, and David E. Kern, MD, MPH

PURPOSE

The purpose of this book is to provide a practical, theoretically sound approach to developing, implementing, evaluating, and continually improving educational experiences in medicine.

TARGET AUDIENCE

This book is designed for use by curriculum developers and others who are responsible for the educational experiences of students, residents, fellows, faculty, and clinical practitioners. Although written from the perspective of physician education, the approach has been used effectively in other health professions education. It should be particularly helpful to those who are planning to develop or are in the midst of developing a curriculum.

DEFINITION OF CURRICULUM

In this book, a curriculum is defined as *a planned educational experience*. This definition encompasses a breadth of educational experiences, from one or more sessions on a specific subject to a year-long course, from a clinical rotation or clerkship to an entire training program.

RATIONALE FOR THE BOOK

Faculty in the health professions often have responsibility for planning educational experiences, frequently without having received training or acquired experience in such endeavors, and usually in the presence of limited resources and significant institutional constraints. Accreditation bodies for each level of medical education in the United States, however, require *written* curricula with fully developed educational objectives, educational methods, and evaluation (1–3).

Ideally, medical education should change as our knowledge base changes and as the needs, or the perceived needs, of patients, medical practitioners, and society change. Some contemporary demands for change and curriculum development are listed in Table I.1. This book assumes that medical educators will benefit from learning a practical, generic, and timeless approach to curriculum development that can address today's as well as tomorrow's needs.

Table I.1.   Some Contemporary Demands for Medical Education

Outcomes
Educational programs should graduate health professionals who:
- Practice patient-centered care (4, 5).
- Promote patient safety and quality (6-9).
- Use effective communication, patient and family education, and behavioral change strategies (10).
- Access and assess the best scientific evidence and apply it to clinical practice (evidence-based medicine, or EBM) (8, 9).
- Use diagnostic and therapeutic resources cost-effectively, i.e., practice high-value care (6, 11).
- Routinely assess and improve their own practice (practice-based learning and improvement, or PBLI) (8, 9).
- Understand, navigate, advocate for, and participate in improving health care systems (systems-based practice, or SBP).
- Work collaboratively in interprofessional teams (8, 9, 12).
- Use population- and community-centered approaches to providing health care.
- Use technology effectively to assist in accomplishing all of the above (6).

Content Areas
Educational programs should improve instruction and learning in:
- Professional identity formation (13).
- Professionalism, values, and ethics (14).
- Major societal health issues, such as chronic disease and disability, nutrition and obesity, and preventive care.
- Genomics and the use of genomics to individualize care.

Methods
Educational programs should modify current methods to:
- Individualize the learning process (8, 13).
- Integrate education across the continuum of health professional training programs (15).
- Train the number of primary care physicians and specialty physicians required to meet societal needs (6, 7).
- Increase the quantity and quality of clinical training in ambulatory, subacute, and chronic care settings, while reducing the amount of training on inpatient services of acute care hospitals, as necessary to meet training needs (7).
- Construct educational interventions based on the best evidence available (8, 9, 16, 17).
- Integrate formal knowledge with clinical experience (13).
- Address the informal and hidden curricula of an institution that can promote or extinguish what is taught in the formal curricula (5, 18).
- Harness the power of sociocultural learning to develop learning communities within educational programs (19).
- Effectively integrate advancing technologies into health professional curricula, such as simulation and interactive electronic interfaces (8, 9).
- Develop faculty to meet contemporary demands.

Assessment
Educational programs across the continuum should:
- Move to outcomes-defined rather than time-defined criteria for promotion and graduation (13).

- Develop and use reliable and valid tools for assessing the cognitive, skill, and behavioral competencies of trainees.
- Certify competence in the domains of patient care, knowledge for practice, practice-based learning and improvement, systems-based practice, interprofessional collaboration, and personal and professional development (20).
- Evaluate the efficacy of educational interventions (8, 15, 16).

BACKGROUND INFORMATION

The approach described in this book has evolved over the past 28 years, during which time the authors have taught curriculum development and evaluation skills to more than 1,000 participants in continuing education courses and the Johns Hopkins Faculty Development Program (JHFDP). The more than 300 participants in the JHFDP's 10-month Longitudinal Program in Curriculum Development have developed and implemented more than 130 medical curricula in topics as diverse as preclerkship skills building, clinical reasoning and shared decision making, musculoskeletal disorders, office gynecology for the generalist, chronic illness and disability, transitions of patient care, surgical skills assessment, laparoscopic surgical skills, cultural competence, professionalism and social media, and medical ethics (see Appendix A). The authors have also developed and facilitated the development of numerous curricula in their educational and administrative roles.

AN OVERVIEW OF THE BOOK

Chapter 1 presents an overview of a six-step approach to curriculum development. *Chapters 2 through 7* describe each step in detail. *Chapter 8* discusses how to maintain and improve curricula over time. *Chapter 9* discusses how to disseminate curricula and curricular products within and beyond institutions. *Chapter 10* discusses additional issues related to larger, longer, and integrated curricula.

Throughout the book, *examples* are provided to illustrate major points. Most examples come from the real-life curricular experiences of the authors or their colleagues, although they may have been adapted for the sake of brevity or clarity. Recognizing that the literature in medical education has flourished in the past decade, the authors have purposefully included, as much as possible, published examples. Those examples that are fictitious were designed to be realistic and to demonstrate an important concept or principle.

Chapters 2 through 10 end with *questions* that encourage the reader to review the principles discussed in each chapter and apply them to a desired, intended, or existing curriculum. In addition to lists of *specific references* that are cited in the text, these chapters include annotated lists of *general references* that can guide the reader who is interested in pursuing a particular topic in greater depth.

Appendix A provides examples of curricula that have progressed through all six steps and that range from newly developed curricula to curricula that have matured through repetitive cycles of implementation. The three curricula in Appendix A include examples from undergraduate (medical student), postgraduate (resident), and continuing medical education. *Appendix B* supplements the chapter references by providing the reader with a selected list of published and online resources for curricular development, faculty development, and funding of curricular work.

REFERENCES

1. Liaison Committee on Medical Education. Function and Structure of a Medical School [Internet]. Available at www.lcme.org.
2. Accreditation Council for Graduate Medical Education. Common Program Requirements [Internet]. Available at www.acgme.org.
3. Accreditation Council for Continuing Medical Education. Accreditation Standards [Internet]. Available at www.accme.org.
4. Hemmer PA, Busing N, Boulet JR, et al. AMEE 2010 Symposium: medical education in the 21st century—a new Flexnerian era? *Med Teach*. 2011;33:541–46.
5. Neuman M, Edelhauser F, Tauschel D, et al. Empathy decline and its reasons: a systematic review of studies with medical students and residents. *Acad Med*. 2011;86:996–1009.
6. Ludmerer KM. The history of calls for reform in graduate medical education and why we are still waiting for the right kind of change. *Acad Med*. 2012;87:34–40.
7. Eden J, Berwick D, Wilensky G, eds. *Graduate Medical Education That Meets the Nation's Health Needs*. Washington, D.C.: National Academies Press; 2014.
8. Institute of Medicine. *Redesigning Continuing Education in the Health Professions*. Washington, D.C.: National Academies Press; 2010.
9. Cervero RM, Gaines JK. Effectiveness of continuing medical education: updated synthesis of systematic reviews [Internet]. Chicago. July 2014. Available at http://www.accme.org/sites /default/files/652_20141104_Effectiveness_of_Continuing_Medical_Education_Cervero _and_Gaines.pdf.
10. Cuff PA, Vanselow N, eds. *Improving Medical Education: Enhancing the Behavioral and Social Science Content of Medical School Curricula*. Washington, D.C.: National Academies Press; 2004.
11. Skochelak SE. A century of progress in medical education: what about the next 10 years? *Acad Med*. 2010;85:197–200.
12. Interprofessional Education Collaborative Expert Panel. *Core Competencies for Interprofessional Collaborative Practice: Report of an Expert Panel*. Washington, D.C.: Interprofessional Education Collaborative; 2011.
13. Cooke M, Irby DM, O'Brien BC. *Educating Physicians: A Call for Reform of Medical School and Residency*. Stanford, Calif.: Jossey-Bass; 2010.
14. Cooper RA, Tauber AI. Values and ethics: a collection of curricular reforms for a new generation of physicians. *Acad Med*. 2007;82:321–23.
15. Skochelak SE. A decade of reports calling for change in medical education: what do they say? *Acad Med*. 2010;85:S26–33.
16. Harden RM, Grant J, Buckley G, Hart IR. Best evidence medical education. *Adv Health Sci Educ Theory Pract*. 2000;5:71–90.
17. Best Evidence in Medical Education Collaboration.org [Internet]. Available at www.bemecol laboration.org.
18. Hafferty FW, O'Donnell JF, Baldwin DC, eds. *The Hidden Curriculum in Health Professional Education*. Hanover, N.H.: Dartmouth College Press; 2014.
19. Mann KE. Theoretical perspectives in medical education: past experience and future possibilities. *Med Educ*. 2011;45:60–68.
20. Englander R, Cameron T, Ballard AJ, et al. Toward a common taxonomy of competency domains for the health professions and competencies for physicians. *Acad Med*. 2013;88:1088–94.

CHAPTER ONE

Overview
A Six-Step Approach to Curriculum Development

David E. Kern, MD, MPH

ORIGINS, ASSUMPTIONS, AND RELATION TO ACCREDITATION

The six-step approach described in this monograph derives from the generic approaches to curriculum development set forth by Taba (1), Tyler (2), Yura and Torres (3), and others (4) and from the work of McGaghie et al. (5) and Golden (6), who advocated the linking of curricula to health care needs. It is similar to models for clinical, health promotions, and social services program development, with Step 4, Educational Strategies, replacing program intervention (7–9).

Underlying assumptions are fourfold. First, educational programs have aims or goals, whether or not they are clearly articulated. Second, medical educators have a professional and ethical obligation to meet the needs of their learners, patients, and society. Third, medical educators should be held accountable for the outcomes of their interventions. And fourth, a logical, systematic approach to curriculum development will help achieve these ends.

Accrediting bodies for undergraduate, graduate, and continuing medical education in the United States require formal curricula that include goals, objectives, and explicitly articulated educational and evaluation strategies (10–12). Undergraduate and postgraduate medical curricula must address core clinical competencies (10, 13). The achievement of milestones for each competency is required for residency training (13). Current trends in translating competencies into clinical practice, such as entrustable professional activities (EPAs) (14, 15) and observable practice activities (OPAs) (16), are likely to provide additional direction and requirements for Step 3 (Goals and Objectives), Step 4 (Educational Strategies), and Step 6 (Evaluation and Feedback), while grounding curricula in societal needs (Step 1, Problem Identification and General Needs Assessment).

A SIX-STEP APPROACH (FIGURE 1)

Step 1: Problem Identification and General Needs Assessment

This step begins with the *identification and critical analysis of a health care need or other problem*. The need may relate to a specific health problem, such as the provision of care to patients infected with human immunodeficiency virus (HIV), or to a group of problems, such as the provision of routine gynecologic care by primary care providers (PCPs). It may relate to qualities of the physician, such as the need for health care providers to develop as self-directed, lifelong learners who can provide effective care as medical knowledge and practice evolve. Or it may relate to the health care needs of society in general, such as whether the quantity and type of physicians being produced are appropriate. A complete problem identification requires an analysis of the *current approach* of patients, practitioners, the medical education system, and society, in general, to addressing the identified need. This is followed by identification of an *ideal approach* that describes how patients, practitioners, the medical education system, and society should be addressing the need. The difference between the ideal approach and the current approach represents a *general needs assessment*.

Step 2: Targeted Needs Assessment

This step involves assessing the needs of one's targeted group of learners and their medical institution/learning environment, which may be different from the needs of learners and medical institutions in general. It enables desired integration of a specific curriculum into an overall curriculum. It also develops communication with and support from stakeholders and aligns one's curriculum development strategy with potential resources.

EXAMPLE: *Problem Identification and General Needs and Targeted Needs Assessments*. The *problem identification and general needs assessment* for a curriculum designed to reduce adverse drug events (ADEs) in the elderly revealed that ADEs were a common cause of morbidity and mortality. Risk factors included age, number of diagnoses, number of medications, and high-risk medications. Most training for residents was inpatient-based. Primary care providers, who coordinated patients' overall care, seemed to be best situated to address the issue of polypharmacy. The *targeted needs assessment* revealed that residents scored very highly in geriatrics on the in-training examination, and faculty were satisfied with the residents' understanding of polypharmacy and ADEs. Most training was inpatient-based. Few residents identified or addressed polypharmacy during patients' hospitalization except when a drug was identified as a problem related to the cause for admission. There was reluctance to change a medication regimen already established by the patient and his or her PCP without an immediate medical rationale. Training related to medication regimens was primarily inpatient-based and focused on medication reconciliation. There was no outpatient curriculum related to reducing ADEs, and polypharmacy was seldom addressed as a problem or addressed in the outpatient record. Pharmacy support, available on the inpatient services, was not available in the outpatient practice. While the electronic medical record (EMR) could identify patients taking a large number of and high-risk medications, it would be too burdensome to develop the EMR to provide reminders or feedback to PCPs. Conversa-

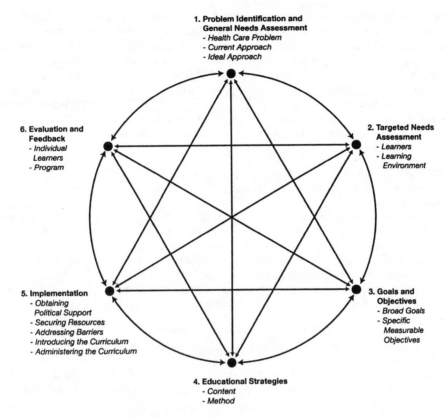

Figure 1.   A Six-Step Approach to Curriculum Development

tions with the residency program director, the outpatient practice director, and selected outpatient preceptors revealed strong support for the curriculum, but there was not time within the clinic schedule to house the proposed curriculum (17).

Step 3: Goals and Objectives

Once the needs of targeted learners have been identified, goals and objectives for the curriculum can be written, starting with *broad or general goals* and then moving to *specific, measurable objectives*. Objectives may include cognitive (knowledge), affective (attitudinal), or psychomotor (skill and behavioral) objectives for the learner; process objectives related to the conduct of the curriculum; or even health, health care, or patient outcome objectives. The development of goals and objectives is critical because they help to determine curricular content and learning methods and help to focus the learner. They enable communication of what the curriculum is about to others and provide a basis for its evaluation. When resources are limited, prioritization of objectives can facilitate the rational allocation of those resources.

Step 4: Educational Strategies

Once objectives have been clarified, *curriculum content is chosen and educational methods are selected that will most likely achieve the educational objectives.*

EXAMPLE: *Educational Strategies*. Based on the above example of a targeted needs assessment, objectives for the ADE curriculum focused on increasing awareness, skill development, and the reinforcement of desired behaviors. Two two-hour workshops were scheduled during protected educational time that engaged learners in applying an efficient, user-friendly worksheet to identify patients at risk, to identify high-risk medications, using Beers (18) and STOPP (19) criteria, that were candidates for removal or replacement, and to develop an action plan. The worksheet was applied to a sample case and two or three patients from the resident practice. Identifying and addressing ADE risk was reinforced through the distribution of pocket cards, placing the worksheets on the practice website for easy access, faculty development of clinic preceptors, and feedback of evaluation data from the electronic medical record (17).

EXAMPLES: *Congruent Educational Methods*.

Lower-level knowledge can be acquired from reading or lectures or, asynchronously, through online modules.

Case-based, problem-solving exercises that actively involve learners are methods that are more likely than attendance at lectures to improve clinical reasoning skills.

The development of physicians as effective team members is more likely to be promoted through their participation in and reflection on interprofessional cooperative learning and work experiences than through reading and discussing a book on the subject.

Interviewing, physical examination, and procedural skills will be best learned in simulation and practice environments that supplement practice with self-observation, observation by others, feedback, and reflection.

Step 5: Implementation

Implementation involves the implementation of both the educational intervention and its evaluation. It has *several components*: obtaining political support; identifying and procuring resources; identifying and addressing barriers to implementation; introducing the curriculum (e.g., piloting the curriculum on a friendly audience before presenting it to all targeted learners, phasing in the curriculum one part at a time); administering the curriculum; and refining the curriculum over successive cycles. Implementation is critical to the success of a curriculum. It is *the step that converts a mental exercise to reality*.

Step 6: Evaluation and Feedback

This step has several components. It usually is desirable to assess the performance of both *individuals* (individual assessment) and the *curriculum* (called "program evaluation"). The purpose of evaluation may be *formative* (to provide ongoing feedback so that the learners or curriculum can improve) or *summative* (to provide a final "grade" or evaluation of the performance of the learner or curriculum).

Evaluation can be used not only to drive the ongoing learning of participants and the improvement of a curriculum but also to gain support and resources for a curriculum and, in research situations, to answer questions about the effectiveness of a specific curriculum or the relative merits of different educational approaches.

THE INTERACTIVE AND CONTINUOUS NATURE OF THE SIX-STEP APPROACH

In practice, curriculum development does not usually proceed in sequence, one step at a time. Rather, it is a dynamic, interactive process. Progress is often made on two or more steps simultaneously. Progress on one step influences progress on another (as illustrated by the bidirectional arrows in Figure 1). As noted in the discussion and examples above, implementation (Step 5) actually began during the targeted needs assessment (Step 2). Limited resources (Step 5) may limit the number and nature of objectives (Step 3), as well as the extent of evaluation (Step 6) that is possible. Evaluation strategies (Step 6) may result in a refinement of objectives (Step 3). Evaluation (Step 6) may also provide information that serves as a needs assessment of targeted learners (Step 2). Time pressures, or the presence of an existing curriculum, may result in the development of goals, educational methods, and implementation strategies (Steps 3, 4, and 5) before a formal problem identification and needs assessment (Steps 1 and 2), so that Steps 1 and 2 are used to refine and improve an existing curriculum rather than develop a new one.

For a successful curriculum, curriculum development never really ends, as illustrated by the circle in Figure 1. Rather, the curriculum evolves, based on evaluation results, changes in resources, changes in targeted learners, and changes in the material requiring mastery.

REFERENCES

1. Taba H. *Curriculum Development: Theory and Practice*. New York: Harcourt, Brace, & World; 1962. Pp. 1–515.
2. Tyler RW. *Basic Principles of Curriculum and Instruction*. Chicago: University of Chicago Press; 1950. Pp. 1–83.
3. Yura H, Torres GJ, eds. *Faculty-Curriculum Development: Curriculum Design by Nursing Faculty*. New York: National League for Nursing; 1986. Publication No. 15-2164. Pp. 1–371.
4. Sheets KJ, Anderson WA, Alguire PC. Curriculum development and evaluation in medical education: annotated bibliography. *J Gen Intern Med*. 1992;7(5):538–43.
5. McGaghie WC, Miller GE, Sajid AW, Telder TV. *Competency Based Curriculum Development in Medical Education: An Introduction*. Geneva: World Health Organization; 1978. Pp. 1–99.
6. Golden AS. A model for curriculum development linking curriculum with health needs. In: Golden AS, Carlson DG, Hogan JL, eds. *The Art of Teaching Primary Care*. Springer Series on Medical Education, Vol. 3. New York: Springer Publishing Co.; 1982. Pp. 9–25.
7. Galley NG. *Program Development for the 21st Century: An Evidence-Based Approach to Design, Implementation, and Evaluation*. Thousand Oaks, Calif.: SAGE Publications; 2011.
8. McKenzie JF, Neiger BL, Thackeray R. *Planning, Implementing, and Evaluating Health Promotion Programs: A Primer*, 6th ed. San Francisco: Benjamin Cummings Publishing Co.; 2012.
9. Timmreck TC. *Planning, Program Development and Evaluation: A Handbook for Health Promotion, Aging and Health Services*, 2nd ed. Boston: Jones and Bartlett Publishers; 2003.
10. Liaison Committee on Medical Education.org [Internet]. Available at www.lcme.org.
11. Accreditation Council for Graduate Medical Education. Common Program Requirements [Internet]. Available at www.acgme.org.
12. Accreditation Council for Continuing Medical Education. Accreditation Requirements [Internet]. Available at www.accme.org.
13. Nasca TJ, Philibert I, Brigham T, Flynn TC. The next GME accreditation system—rationale and benefits. *N Engl J Med*. 2012;366:1051–55.
14. Ten Cate O. Nuts and bolts of entrustable professional activities. *J Grad Med Educ*. 2013;5:157–58.

15. Association of American Medical Colleges. Core Entrustable Professional Activities for Entering Residency (CEPAER) [Internet]. Washington, D.C. March 2014 Available at www .mededportal.org/icollaborative/resource/887.

16. Warm EJ, Mathis BR, Held JD, et al. Entrustment and mapping of observable practice activities for resident assessment. *J Gen Intern Med*. 2014;29 (8):1177–82.

17. Example adapted from the curricular project of Halima Amjad, MD, and Olivia Nirmalasari, MD, for the Johns Hopkins Longitudinal Program in Faculty Development, cohort 27, 2013–2014.

18. American Geriatrics Society 2012 Beers Criteria Update Expert Panel. American Geriatrics Society updated Beers Criteria for potentially inappropriate medication use in older adults. *J Am Geriatr Soc*. 2012;60(4):616–31.

19. Gallagher P, Ryan C, Byrne S, Kennedy J, O'Mahony D. STOPP (Screening Tool of Older Person's Prescriptions) and START (Screening Tool to Alert doctors to Right Treatment): consensus validation. *Int J Clin Pharmacol Ther*. 2008;46(2):72–83.

CHAPTER TWO

Step 1
Problem Identification and General Needs Assessment

. . . building the foundation for meaningful objectives

Eric B. Bass, MD, MPH, and Belinda Y. Chen, MD

Medical instruction does not exist to provide individuals with an
opportunity of learning how to make a living, but in order to make
possible the protection of the health of the public.
—Rudolf Virchow

Many reasons may prompt someone to begin work on a medical curriculum. Indeed, continuing developments in medical science and technology call for efforts to keep medical education up to date, whether it be new knowledge to be disseminated (e.g., effectiveness of a new therapy for hepatitis C infection) or a new technique to be taught (e.g., a robotic-assisted minimally invasive surgical technique). Sometimes, educational leaders issue a mandate to improve performance in selected areas, based on feedback from learners, suboptimal scores on standardized examinations, or recommendations from educational accrediting bodies. Other times, educators want to take advantage of new learning technology (e.g., a new simulation center) or need to respond to new national standards for competency-based training. Regardless of where one enters the curriculum development paradigm, it is critical to take a step back and consider the responsibilities of a medical educator. Why is a new or revised curriculum worth the time and effort needed to plan and implement it well? Since the ultimate purpose of medical education is to improve the health of the public, what is the health problem or outcome that needs to be addressed? What is the ideal role of a planned educational experience in improving such health outcomes? This chapter offers guidance on how to define the problem, determine the current and ideal approaches to the problem, and synthesize all of the information in a general needs assessment that clarifies the gap the curriculum will fill.

DEFINITIONS

The first step in designing a curriculum is to identify and characterize the health care problem that will be addressed by the curriculum, how the problem is currently being addressed, and how it ideally should be addressed. The difference between how the health care problem is currently being addressed, in general, and how it should be addressed is called a *general needs assessment*. Because the difference between the current and ideal approaches can be considered part of the problem that the curriculum will address, Step 1 can also simply be called *problem identification*.

IMPORTANCE

The better a problem is defined, the easier it will be to design an appropriate curriculum to address the problem. All of the other steps in the curriculum development process depend on having a clear understanding of the problem (see Figure 1). Problem identification (Step 1), along with targeted needs assessment (Step 2), is particularly helpful in focusing a curriculum's goals and objectives (Step 3), which in turn help to focus the curriculum's educational strategies and evaluation (Steps 4 and 6). Step 1 is especially important in justifying dissemination of a successful curriculum because it supports its generalizability. Steps 1 and 2 also provide a strong rationale that can help the curriculum developer obtain support for curriculum implementation (Step 5).

DEFINING THE HEALTH CARE PROBLEM

The ultimate purpose of a curriculum in medical education is to equip learners to address a problem that affects the health of the public or a given population. Frequently, the problem of interest is complex. However, even the simplest health care issue may be refractory to an educational intervention, if the problem has not been defined well. A comprehensive definition of the problem should consider the epidemiology of the problem, as well as the impact of the problem on patients, health care professionals, medical educators, and society (Table 2.1).

Table 2.1.   Identification and Characterization of the Health Care Problem

Whom does it affect?
    Patients
    Health care professionals
    Medical educators
    Society

What does it affect?
    Clinical outcomes
    Quality of life
    Quality of health care
    Use of health care and other resources
    Medical and nonmedical costs
    Patient and provider satisfaction
    Work and productivity
    Societal function

What is the *quantitative and qualitative importance* of the effects?

[handwritten note: ✓ this was done by previous research]

In defining the problem of interest, it is important to explicitly identify *whom* the problem affects. Does the problem affect people with a particular disease (e.g., frequent disease exacerbations requiring hospitalization for patients with asthma), or does the problem affect society at large (e.g., inadequate understanding of behaviors associated with acquiring an emerging infectious disease)? Does the problem directly or indirectly affect health professionals and their trainees (e.g., physicians inadequately prepared to participate effectively as part of interprofessional teams)? Does the problem affect health care organizations (e.g., a need to foster the practice of patient-centered care)? The problem of interest may involve many different groups. The degree of impact has implications for curriculum development because a problem that is perceived to affect many people may be granted more attention and resources than one that applies to only a small group. Educators will be able to choose the most appropriate target audience for a curriculum, formulate learning objectives, and develop curricular content when they know the characteristics and behaviors of those affected by the health care problem of interest.

Once those who are affected by the problem have been identified, it is important to elaborate on *how* they are affected. What is the effect of the problem on clinical outcomes, quality of life, quality of health care, use of health care services, medical and nonmedical costs, patient and provider satisfaction, work and productivity, and the functioning of society? How common and how serious are these effects?

EXAMPLE: *Partial Problem Identification for a Poverty in Health Care Curriculum.* "Thirty-seven million Americans live below the federal poverty threshold, representing 12.6% of the U.S. population. Even more—nearly 90 million Americans—live below 200% of the federal poverty threshold, an income at which many struggle to make ends meet. Given these realities, most physicians will work with low-income patients, regardless of their specialty or practice location. Countless studies have shown that lower socioeconomic status (SES) is associated with unique challenges to health, higher disease burden and poorer health outcomes" (1).

GENERAL NEEDS ASSESSMENT (TABLE 2.2)

Current Approach

Having defined the nature of the health care problem, the next task is to assess current efforts to address the problem. The process of determining the current approach to a problem is sometimes referred to as a "job analysis" because it is an assessment of the "job" that is currently being done to deal with a problem (2). To determine the current approach to a problem, the curriculum developer should ask what is being done by each of the following:

a. Patients (including their families, significant others, and caregivers)
b. Health care professionals
c. Medical educators
d. Society (including community networks, health care payers, and policymakers)

Knowing what *patients* are doing and not doing with regard to a problem may influence decisions about curricular content. For example, are patients using noneffective treatments or engaging in activities that exacerbate a problem, behaviors that need to be reversed? Or, are patients predisposed to engage in activities that could alleviate the problem, behaviors that need to be encouraged?

Knowing how *health care professionals* are currently addressing the problem is especially relevant because they are frequently the target audience for medical curricula. In the general needs assessment, one of the challenges is in determining how health care professionals vary in their approach to a problem. Many studies have demonstrated substantial variations in clinical practice within and between countries, in terms of both use of recommended practices and use of ineffective or harmful practices (3).

EXAMPLE: *Treatment of Diarrheal Illness among Private Practitioners in Nigeria.* Ninety-one doctors in Enugu, Nigeria, who had heard of oral rehydration therapy (ORT) and expressed belief in its efficacy were interviewed using a structured questionnaire to determine their knowledge of, attitude toward, and practice of treatment of diarrheal illness. Fifty percent said they would recommend salt-sugar solution (SSS) over standardized oral rehydration solutions due to availability and cost-effectiveness. However, only 55% knew how to prepare SSS correctly. Even though 76% of doctors believed that viral infections were a common cause of diarrhea, antibiotics were commonly used. The study revealed a high rate of inappropriate drug use and a deficiency in the knowledge and practice of ORT (4).

Most problems important enough to warrant a focused curriculum are encountered in many different places, so it is wise to explore what other *medical educators* are currently doing to help patients and health care professionals address the problem. Much can be learned from the previous work of educators who have tried to tackle the problem of interest. For example, curricular materials may exist already for medical trainees and may be of great value in developing a curriculum for one's own target audience. The existence of multiple curricula may highlight the need for evaluation tools to help educators determine which methods are most effective. This is particularly important in medical education, where the number of things that could be taught is constantly expanding while the time and resources available for education are finite. A dearth of relevant curricula will reinforce the need for innovative curricular work.

EXAMPLE: *Interprofessional Education.* Reports from the World Health Organization and the Institute of Medicine have called for greater interprofessional education (IPE) to improve health outcomes through fostering the development of coordinated interprofessional teams that work together to promote quality,

Table 2.2.   The General Needs Assessment

What is *currently* being done by the following?
    Patients
    Health care professionals
    Medical educators
    Society

What personal and environmental factors affect the problem?
    Predisposing
    Enabling
    Reinforcing

What *ideally* should be done by the following?
    Patients
    Health care professionals
    Medical educators
    Society

What are the key *differences* between the current and ideal approaches?

---

safety, and systems improvement. Those developing curricula in interprofessional education should be familiar with the guidelines and competencies established by various Interprofessional Health Collaboratives (5, 6). However, even within the guidelines, there is substantial room for variation. To assist other curriculum developers, a paper published in *Academic Medicine* describes the development, implementation, and assessment of IPE curricula in three different institutions, along with a discussion of lessons learned (7).

Curriculum developers should also consider what *society* is doing to address the problem. This will help to improve understanding of the societal context of current efforts to address the problem, taking into consideration potential barriers and facilitators that influence those efforts.

EXAMPLE: *Impact of Societal Approach on Curricular Planning.* In designing a curriculum to help health care professionals reduce the spread of HIV infection in a given society, it is necessary to know how the society handles the distribution of condoms and clean needles. As of 2010, 82 countries were reported to have some program for needle/syringe exchange. However, 76 countries/territories reported IV drug use activity but no needle/syringe exchange programs (8). If the distribution of clean needles is prohibited, an HIV infection prevention curriculum for health care professionals will need to address the most appropriate options acceptable in that society.

To understand fully the current approach to addressing a health care problem, curriculum developers need to be familiar with the ecological perspective on human behavior. This perspective emphasizes multiple influences on behavior, including at the individual, interpersonal, institutional, community, and public policy levels (9). Interventions are more likely to be successful if they address multiple levels of influence on behavior. Most educational interventions will focus primarily on individual and/or interpersonal factors, but some may be part of larger interventions that also target collective levels of influence.

When focusing on the individual and interpersonal levels of influence on behavior, curriculum developers should consider the fundamental principles of modern theories of human behavior change. While it is beyond the scope of this book to discuss specific theories in detail, three concepts are particularly important: 1) human behavior is mediated by what people know and think; 2) knowledge is necessary, but not sufficient, to cause a change in behavior; and 3) behavior is influenced by individual beliefs, motivations, and skills, as well as by the environment (9).

In the light of these key concepts, curriculum developers need to consider *multiple types of factors* that may aggravate or alleviate the problem of interest. Factors that can influence the problem can be classified as predisposing factors, enabling factors, or reinforcing factors (10). *Predisposing factors* refer to people's knowledge, attitudes, and beliefs that influence their motivation to change (or not to change) behaviors related to a problem. *Enabling factors* generally refer to personal skills and societal or environmental forces that make a behavioral or environmental change possible. *Reinforcing factors* refer to the rewards and punishments that encourage continuation or discontinuation of a behavior.

> **EXAMPLE:** *Predisposing, Enabling, and Reinforcing Factors.* In designing curricula for health professionals on the prevention of smoking-related illness, curriculum developers should be familiar with predisposing, enabling, and reinforcing factors that influence an individual's smoking behavior. The 2008 U.S. Public Health Service Clinical Practice Guideline *Treating Tobacco Use and Dependence* (11) summarizes available evidence to make recommendations for health professional interventions. One predisposing factor is an individual's self-defined readiness to quit—so the guidelines recommend strategies for assessing a patient's readiness to quit and describe different interventions based on whether a patient is willing or unwilling to make a quit attempt. An enabling factor would be the availability and cost of tobacco products and tobacco-cessation products. Reinforcing factors include the strength of physical and psychological addiction, personally defined benefits to smoking, personally defined motivators for stopping or not starting, and personally defined barriers to cessation.

By considering all aspects of how a health care problem is addressed, one can determine the most appropriate role for an educational intervention in addressing the problem, keeping in mind that an educational intervention by itself usually cannot solve all aspects of a complex health care problem.

Ideal Approach

After examination of the current approach to the problem, the next task is to determine the ideal approach to the problem. Determination of the ideal approach will require careful consideration of the multiple levels of influence on behavior, as well as the same fundamental concepts of human behavior change described in the preceding section. The process of determining the ideal approach to a problem is sometimes referred to as a "task analysis," which can be viewed as an assessment of the specific "tasks" that need to be performed to appropriately deal with the problem (2, 12). To determine the ideal approach to a problem, the curriculum developer should ask what each of the following groups should do to deal most effectively with the problem:

a. Patients
b. Health care professionals
c. Medical educators
d. Society

To what extent should *patients* be involved in handling the problem themselves? In many cases, the ideal approach will require education of patients and families affected by or at risk of having the problem.

EXAMPLE: *Role of Patients/Families.* Parents of children discharged from a neonatal intensive care unit (NICU) generally have not received any instruction about the developmental milestones that should be expected of their children. To foster timely and appropriate developmental assessment of children discharged from a NICU, neonatologists need to address the role that parents play in observing a child's development (13).

Which *health care professionals* should deal with the problem, and what should they be doing? Answering these questions can help the curriculum developer to target learners and define the content of a curriculum appropriately. If more than one type of health care professional typically encounters the problem, the curriculum developer must decide what is most appropriate for each type of provider and whether the curriculum will be modified to meet the needs of each type of provider or will target just one group of health care professionals.

EXAMPLE: *Role of Health Care Professionals.* A curriculum designed for physicians to practice developmental assessment of pediatric patients in a post-NICU follow-up clinic needed to accommodate general pediatric residents, neurology residents, and neonatal and neurodevelopmental fellows. The curriculum developers recognized that general pediatric physicians needed to know what to teach parents and which patients to refer for specialty evaluation. Neonatologists needed to learn the potential developmental complications of various NICU interventions. Neurodevelopmental specialists needed to learn not only how to formulate specific management plans but also how to teach key diagnostic assessment tools to referring pediatricians and neonatologists (13).

What role should *medical educators* have in addressing the problem? Determining the ideal approach for medical educators involves identifying the appropriate target audiences, the appropriate content, the best educational strategies, and the best evaluation methods to ensure effectiveness. Reviewing previously published curricula that address the health care problem often uncovers elements of best practices that can be used in new curricular efforts.

EXAMPLE: *Identifying Appropriate Audiences and Content.* Interns and residents have traditionally been trained to be on "code teams," but medical students can also be in clinical situations where improved competence in basic resuscitation can make a difference in patient outcomes. Basic life support (BLS) and advanced cardiovascular life support (ACLS) training can increase familiarity with cardiac protocols but have been shown to be inadequate in achieving competency as defined by adherence to protocols. Deliberative practice through simulation is an educational method that could potentially improve students' achievement of competency in these critical skills, so a curriculum was created, implemented, and evaluated with these outcomes in mind. (See Appendix A, Essential Resuscitation Skills for Medical Students.)

EXAMPLE: *Identifying Best Practices.* Since publication of the Institute of Medicine's report *Unequal Treatment* (14), there has been increasing attention to addressing health care disparities in undergraduate medical education. A curriculum developer searching PubMed might learn of a validated cultural assessment instrument, TACCT, that could be used in a needs assessment or post-curricular evaluation to assess cultural competency (15–17). A consortium of 18 U.S. medical schools funded by the National Heart, Lung, and Blood Institute to address health disparities through medical education has also collated and shared additional online curricular resources on this topic (18). Resources include tools for measuring implicit bias, case studies for use in workshops and local curricula, validated assessment tools, and sample curricular products. Curriculum developers tasked with developing approaches to health care disparities within their local environments should be familiar with such resources.

Keep in mind, however, that educators may not be able to solve the problem by themselves. When the objectives are to change the behavior of patients or health care professionals, educators should define their role relative to other interventions that may be needed to stimulate and sustain behavioral change.

What role should *society* have in addressing the problem? While curriculum developers usually are not in the position to effect *societal* change, some of their targeted learners may be, now or in the future. A curriculum, therefore, may choose to address current societal factors that contribute to or alleviate a problem (such as advertisements, political forces, organizational factors, and government policies). Sometimes, curriculum developers may want to target or collaborate with policymakers as part of a comprehensive strategy for addressing a public health problem.

> **EXAMPLE:** *Social Action Influenced by a Curriculum.* The Kellogg Health Scholars Program was a two-year postdoctoral fellowship program that trained academic leaders, not only in community-based participatory research related to the social determinants of health, but also in the application of research to effect policy changes (19).

> **EXAMPLE:** *Social Action Influenced by Curricula.* Medical school faculty published 12 tips for teaching social determinants of health in medical school, based on their review of the literature and their five-year experience in developing and teaching a longitudinal course at their institution. Their description includes a table of sample cases and action-oriented activities to engage students in the subject matter. These actions include looking at local data and discussing policy recommendations that could decrease health disparities (20).

The ideal approach should serve as an important, but not rigid, guide to developing a curriculum. One needs to be flexible in accommodating others' views and the many practical realities related to curriculum development. For this reason, it is useful to be transparent about the basis for one's "ideal" approach: individual opinion, consensus, the logical application of established theory, or scientific evidence. Obviously, one should be more flexible in espousing an "ideal" approach based on individual opinion than an "ideal" approach based on strong scientific evidence.

Differences between Current and Ideal Approaches

Having determined the current and ideal approaches to a problem, the curriculum developer should identify the differences between the two approaches. The differences identified by this *general needs assessment* should be the main target of any plans for addressing the health care problem. As mentioned above, the differences between the current and ideal approaches can be considered part of the problem that the curriculum will address, which is why Step 1 is sometimes referred to, simply, as *problem identification*.

OBTAINING INFORMATION ABOUT NEEDS

Each curriculum has unique needs for information about the problem of interest. In some cases, substantial information already exists and simply has to be identified. In other cases, much information is available, but it needs to be systematically reviewed and synthesized. Frequently, the information available is insufficient to guide a new curriculum, in which case new information must be collected. Depending on the availability of relevant information, different methods can be used to identify and characterize a health care problem and to determine the current and ideal approaches to that problem. The most commonly used methods are listed in Table 2.3.

Table 2.3.   Methods for Obtaining the Necessary Information

Review of Available Information
    Evidence-based reviews of educational and clinical topics
    Published original studies
    Clinical practice guidelines
    Published recommendations on expected competencies
    Reports by professional organizations or government agencies *ie CDC, HBB*
    Documents submitted to educational clearinghouses
    Curriculum documents from other institutions
    Patient education materials prepared by foundations or professional organizations
    Patient support organizations
    Public health statistics
    Clinical registry data
    Administrative claims data

Use of Consultants/Experts
    Informal consultation
    Formal consultation
    Meetings of experts

Collection of New Information
    Surveys of patients, practitioners, or experts
    Focus group(s)
    Nominal group technique
    Liberating structures
    Group judgment methods (Delphi method)
    Daily diaries by patients and practitioners
    Observation of tasks performed by practitioners
    Time and motion studies
    Critical incident reviews
    Study of ideal performance cases or role-model practitioners

By carefully obtaining information about the need for a curriculum, educators will demonstrate that they are using a scholarly approach to curriculum development. This is an important component of educational scholarship, as defined by a consensus conference on educational scholarship that was sponsored by the Association of American Medical Colleges (AAMC) (21). A scholarly approach is valuable because it will help to convince learners and other educators that the curriculum is based on up-to-date knowledge of the published literature and existing best practices.

Finding and Synthesizing Available Information

The curriculum developer should start with a *well-focused review of information that is already available.* A *review of the medical literature,* including journal articles and textbooks, is generally the most efficient method for gathering information about a health care problem, what is currently being done to deal with it, and what should be done to deal with it. A medical librarian can be extremely helpful in accessing the medical and relevant nonmedical (e.g., educational) literature, as well as in accessing databases that contain relevant but unpublished information. However, the curriculum developer should formulate specific questions to guide the search for relevant information. Without focused questions, the review will be inefficient and less useful.

The curriculum developer should look for published *reviews* as well as any *original studies* about the topic. If a systematic review has been performed recently, it may be possible to rely on that review, with just a quick look for new studies performed since the review was completed. The Best Evidence in Medical Education (BEME) Collaboration is a good source of high-quality evidence-based reviews of topics in medical education (22). Depending on the topic, other evidence-based medicine resources may also contain valuable information, especially the Cochrane Collaboration, which produces evidence-based reviews on a wide variety of clinical topics (23). If a systematic review of the topic has not yet been done, it will be necessary to search systematically for relevant original studies. In such cases, the curriculum developer has an opportunity to make a scholarly contribution to the field by performing a *systematic review* of the topic. A systematic review of a medical education topic should include a carefully documented and comprehensive search for relevant studies, with explicitly defined criteria for inclusion in the review, as well as a verifiable methodology for extracting and synthesizing information from eligible studies (24). By examining historical and social trends, the review may yield insights into future needs, in addition to current needs.

For many clinical topics, it is wise to look for pertinent *clinical practice guidelines* because the guidelines may clearly delineate the ideal approach to a problem. In some countries, practice guidelines can be accessed easily through a government health agency, such as the Agency for Healthcare Research and Quality (AHRQ) in the United States or the National Institute for Health and Care Excellence (NICE; formerly, the National Institute for Health and Clinical Excellence) in the United Kingdom, each of which sponsors a clearinghouse for practice guidelines (25, 26). With so many practice guidelines available, curriculum developers are likely to find one or more guidelines for a clinical problem of interest. Sometimes guidelines conflict in their recommendations. When that happens, the curriculum developer should critically appraise the methods used to develop the guidelines to determine which recommendations should be included in the ideal approach (27–29).

When designing a curriculum, educators need to be aware of any recommendations or statements by accreditation agencies or professional organizations about the *competencies* expected of practitioners. For example, any curriculum for internal medicine residents in the United States should take into consideration the core competencies set by the Accreditation Council for Graduate Medical Education (ACGME), requirements of the Internal Medicine Residency Review Committee, and the evaluation objectives of the American Board of Internal Medicine (ABIM) (30, 31). Similarly, any curriculum for medical students in the United States should take into consideration the accreditation standards of the Liaison Committee on Medical Education (LCME) and the core entrustable professional activities (EPAs) that medical school graduates should be able to perform when starting residency training, as defined by the AAMC (32, 33). Within any clinical discipline, a corresponding professional society may issue a consensus statement about core competencies that should guide training in that discipline. A good example is the Society of Hospital Medicine, a national professional organization of hospitalists, which commissioned a task force to prepare a framework for curriculum development based on the core competencies in hospital medicine (34). Often, the ideal approach to a problem will be based on this sort of authoritative statement about expected competencies.

EXAMPLE: *Use of Accreditation Body, Professional Organization, and Systematic Review.* In 2003 and 2007, respectively, the Institute of Medicine and the ACGME identified quality improvement as an important competency for physicians to acquire (35, 36). To guide the development of new curricula for medical trainees on the use of quality improvement methods in clinical practice, a group of educators performed a systematic review of the effectiveness of published quality improvement curricula for clinicians (37). The group found that most quality improvement curricula demonstrated improvement in knowledge or confidence to perform quality improvement, but additional studies were needed to determine whether such programs have meaningful clinical benefits.

Educational clearinghouses can be particularly helpful to the curriculum developer because they may provide specific examples of what is being done by other medical educators to address a problem. The most useful educational clearinghouses tend to be those that have sufficient support and infrastructure to have some level of peer review, as well as some process for keeping them up to date. One particularly noteworthy clearinghouse for medical education is the MedEdPORTAL launched in 2005 by the AAMC (38). This database includes a wide variety of educational documents and materials that have been prepared by educators from many institutions. Clearinghouses are also maintained by some specialty and topic-oriented professional organizations (see Appendix B).

Other sources of available information also should be considered, especially when the published literature is sparse (see Appendix B, Curricular Resources). Data sources such as government publications, preprint curricula, data collected for other organizations, patents, and informal symposia proceedings are termed the "grey literature." For example, the AAMC maintains a database of medical school curricular data collected from curriculum management systems in use at many U.S. and Canadian medical schools. The database includes information about the content, structure, delivery, and assessment of medical school curricula and aggregated reports. Data related to specific topics of interest may be accessible through its website (39). Other sources of information include *reports by professional societies or government agencies*, which can highlight deficiencies in the current approach to a problem or make recommendations for a new approach to a problem. In some cases, it may be worthwhile to contact *colleagues at other institutions* who are performing related work and who may be willing to share information that they have developed or collected. For some health care problems, foundations or professional organizations have prepared *patient education materials*, and these materials can provide information about the problem from the patient perspective, as well as material to use in one's curriculum. Consultation with a medical librarian or informationist can be very helpful in identifying relevant data sources from both the standard peer-reviewed journals and the educational and grey literature.

Public health statistics, *clinical registry data*, and *administrative claims data* can be used for obtaining information about the incidence or prevalence of a problem. Most medical libraries have reports on the vital statistics of the population that are published by the government. Clinical registry data may be difficult to access directly, but a search of the medical literature on a particular clinical topic can often identify reports from clinical registries. In the United States, the federal government and many states maintain administrative claims databases that provide data on the use of inpatient and outpatient medical services. Such data can help to define the magnitude of a clinical problem. Because of the enormous size of most claims databases, special expertise is needed to perform analyses of such data. Though these types of databases rarely have the depth of information that is needed to guide curriculum planning, they do have potential value in defining the extent of the health care problem.

Even though the curriculum developer may be expert in the area to be addressed by the curriculum, it frequently is necessary to ask other experts how they interpret the information about a problem, particularly when the literature gives conflicting information or when there is uncertainty about the future direction of work in that area. In such cases, *expert opinions* can be obtained by consultation or by organizing a meeting of experts to discuss the issues. For most curricula, this can be done on a relatively informal basis with local experts. Occasionally, the problem is so controversial or important that the curriculum developer may wish to spend the additional time and effort necessary to obtain formal input from outside experts.

Collecting New Information

When the available information about a problem is so inadequate that curriculum developers cannot draw reasonable conclusions, it is desirable to *collect new information* about the problem. Information gathering can take numerous forms involving both quantitative and qualitative methodologies. The key feature that differentiates Step 1 from Step 2 is that, in Step 1, the curriculum developer seeks information that is broadly generalizable, not targeted.

In-person interviews with a small sample of patients, students, practitioners, medical educators, or experts can yield information relatively quickly, but for a general needs assessment, the sample must be chosen carefully to be broadly representative. Such interviews may be conducted individually or in the format of a *focus group* of 8 to 12 people, where the purpose is to obtain in-depth views regarding the topic of concern (40–42). Obtaining consensus of the group is not the goal; rather, the goal is to elicit a range of perspectives. Another small group method occasionally used in needs assessment is the *nominal group technique*, which employs a structured, sometimes iterative approach to identifying issues, solutions, and priorities (43). The outcome of this technique is an extensive list of brainstormed and rank-ordered ideas. When the objective is not only to generate ideas or answers to a question but also to move a group toward agreement, an iterative process called the *Delphi method* can be used with participants who either meet repeatedly or respond to a series of questions over time. Participant responses are fed back to the group on each successive cycle to promote consensus (44–46). When seeking information from a diverse group of stakeholders, use of *liberating structures*, simple rules to guide interaction and innovative thinking about a shared issue, may help to organize and facilitate the experience (47, 48). When quantitative and representative data are desired, it is customary to perform a systematic *questionnaire or interview survey* (49–52) by mail, telephone, or Internet, or in person. For the general needs assessment, it is particularly important to ensure that questionnaires are distributed to an appropriate sample so that the results will be generalizable. (53). (See the General References at the end of this chapter and references in Chapter 3 for more information on survey methodology.)

Sometimes, more intensive methods of data collection are necessary. When little is known about the current approach to a clinical problem, educators may ask practitioners or patients to complete *daily diaries or records of activities*. Alternatively, they may use *observation* by work sampling (54), which involves direct observation of a sample of patients, practitioners, or medical educators in their work settings. Other options are *time and motion studies* (which involve observation and detailed analysis of how patients and/or practitioners spend their time) (2), *critical incident reviews* (in which cases having desired and undesired outcomes are reviewed to determine how the process of care relates to the outcomes) (55, 56), and *review of ideal performance cases* (using appreciative inquiry to discover what has enabled achievement in the past as a way to help to improve future performance) (57, 58). The latter methods require considerable time and resources but may be valuable when detailed information is needed about a particular aspect of clinical practice.

Regardless of what methods are used to obtain information about a problem, it is necessary to synthesize that information in an efficient manner. A logical, well-organized report with tables that summarize the collected information, is one of the most common methods for accomplishing the synthesis. A well-organized report has the advantages of efficiently communicating this information to others and being available for quick reference in the future. Collected reference materials and resources can be filed for future access.

TIME AND EFFORT

Those involved in the development of a curriculum must decide how much they are willing to spend, in terms of time, effort, and other resources, for problem identification and general needs assessment. A commitment of too little time and effort runs the risk of either having a curriculum that is poorly focused and unlikely to adequately address the problem of concern or "reinventing the wheel" when an effective curriculum already exists. A commitment of too much time and effort runs the risk of leaving insufficient resources for the other steps in the curriculum development process. Careful consideration of the nature of the problem is necessary to achieve an appropriate balance.

Some problems are complex enough to require a great deal of time to understand them adequately. It may also be the case that less complex problems that have been less well studied may require more time and effort than more complex problems that have been well studied because original data need to be collected.

One of the goals of this step is for the curriculum developer to become expert enough in the area to make decisions about curricular objectives and content. The curriculum developer's prior knowledge of the problem area, therefore, will also determine the amount of time and effort he or she needs to spend on this step.

The time and effort spent on defining the problem of interest in a scholarly manner may yield new information or new perspectives that warrant publication in the medical literature (see Chapter 9, Dissemination). However, the methods employed in the problem identification and general needs assessment must be rigorously applied and described if the results are to be published in a peer-reviewed journal. The curriculum developer must decide whether the academic value of a scholarly publication is worth the time and effort that would be diverted from the development of the curriculum itself. A sound, if less methodologically rigorous, problem identification and needs assessment that is used for planning the curriculum could also be used for the introduction and discussion of a scholarly publication about evaluation results or novel educational strategies.

Time pressures, or the inheritance of an existing curriculum, may result in a situation in which the curriculum is developed before an adequate problem identification and general needs assessment has been written. In such situations, a return to this step may be helpful in explaining or improving an existing curriculum.

CONCLUSION

To address a health care problem effectively and efficiently, a curriculum developer must define the problem carefully and determine the current and ideal approaches to the problem. A curriculum by itself may not solve all aspects of the problem, particularly if the problem is a complex one. However, the difference between the ideal and current approaches will often highlight deficiencies in the knowledge, attitudes, or skills of practitioners. Educational efforts can be directed toward closing those gaps. Thus, this step is essential in focusing a curriculum so that it can make a meaningful contribution to solving the problem.

The conclusions drawn from the general needs assessment may or may not apply to the particular group of learners or institution(s) targeted by a curriculum developer. For this reason, it is necessary to assess the specific needs of one's targeted learners and institution(s) (see Chapter 3) before proceeding with further development of a curriculum.

QUESTIONS

For the curriculum you are coordinating or planning, please answer the following questions:

1. What is the health care problem that will be addressed by this curriculum?

2. *Whom* does the problem affect?

3. *What* effects does the problem have on these people?

4. How important is the problem, *quantitatively and qualitatively*?

5. Based on your current knowledge, what are patients/families, health care professionals, educators, and policymakers doing *currently* to address the problem?

	Patients	Health Care Professionals	Medical Educators	Society
Current Approach				
Ideal Approach				

6. Based on your current knowledge, what should patients, health care professionals, educators, and policymakers *ideally* be doing to address the problem?

7. To complete a *general needs assessment*, what are the differences between the current and ideal approaches?

8. What are the key areas in which your knowledge has been deficient in answering these questions? Given your available resources, what *methods* would you use to correct these deficiencies? (See Table 2.3.)

GENERAL REFERENCES

Altschuld JA, ed. *The Needs Assessment Kit.* San Francisco: SAGE Publications; 2010.
This resource includes a set of five books that cover theory and tools for conducting needs assessments. Book 1: Needs Assessment, An Overview; Book 2: Phase 1, Pre-assessment (Getting the Process Started); Book 3: Phase 2, Assessment (Collecting Data); Book 4: Phase 2, Assessment (Analysis and Prioritization); Book 5: Phase 3, Post-assessment (Planning for Action and Evaluating the Needs Assessment). Each book is approximately 135 pages.

Altschuld JW, Witkin BR. *From Needs Assessment to Action: Transforming Needs into Solution Strategies.* Thousand Oaks, Calif. SAGE Publications; 2000.
Reviews earlier works referenced in this chapter, addresses the value of a multiple/mixed method approach to needs assessment, including both qualitative and quantitative methods, then focuses on the prioritization of needs and the transformation of needs assessments into action. Provides real-world examples. 282 pages.

Cooke M, Irby DM, O'Brien BC, Shulman LS. *Educating Physicians: A Call for Reform of Medical School and Residency.* San Francisco: Jossey-Bass; 2010.
A report based on the Carnegie Foundation–funded study of physician education that articulates the current and ideal approaches to general medical education. 320 pages.

Green LW, Kreuter MW. *Health Promotion Planning: An Educational and Environmental Approach*, 4th ed. New York: McGraw-Hill Publishing; 2005.
A dense but detailed text that provides a sound conceptual basis for developing plans to change health behaviors through the PRECEDE/PROCEED model. 600 pages.

Ludmerer KM. *Time to Heal: American Medical Education from the Turn of the Century to the Era of Managed Care.* Oxford: Oxford University Press; 1999.
The second in a trilogy of books written by Ken Ludmerer to chronicle the changes in medical education from World War I to the era of managed care. A good background to the Carnegie Foundation–funded report by Cooke et al. that illustrates the importance of considering overtly the connection between the training of medical professionals and the future of patient care. 544 pages.

SPECIFIC REFERENCES

1. Doran KM, Kirley K, Barnosky AR, Williams JC, Cheng JE. Developing a novel Poverty in Healthcare curriculum for medical students at the University of Michigan Medical School. *Acad Med.* 2008;83:5–13.
2. Golden AS. A model for curriculum development linking curriculum with health needs. In: Golden AS, Carlson DG, Hogan JL, eds. *The Art of Teaching Primary Care.* Springer Series on Medical Education, Vol. 3. New York: Springer Publishing Co.; 1982. Pp. 9–25.
3. Wennberg J. Practice variations and health care reform: connecting the dots. *Health Aff (Millwood).* 2004; Suppl Web Exclusives: VAR140–44.
4. Okeke TA, Okafor HU, Amah AC, Onwuasiqwe CN, Ndu AC. Knowledge, attitude, practice, and prescribing pattern of oral rehydration therapy among private practitioners in Nigeria. *J Diarrhoeal Dis Res.* 1996 Mar;14(1):33–36.
5. Canadian Interprofessional Health Collaborative. CIHC National Interprofessional Competency

Framework. Vancouver, BC, Canada, 2010. Available at www.cihc.ca/files/CIHC_IP Competencies_Feb1210.pdf.

6. Interprofessional Education Collaborative Expert Panel. *Core Competencies for Interprofessional Collaborative Practice: Report of an Expert Panel.* Washington, D.C.: Interprofessional Education Collaborative; 2011.

7. Aston SJ, Rheault W, Arenson C, et al. Interprofessional education: a review and analysis of programs from three academic health centers. *Acad Med.* 2012;87(7):949–55.

8. Global State of Harm Reduction 2010. Chap. 1.1, p. 10. Available at www.ihra.net/con tents/535.

9. Glanz K, Rimer BK. *Theory at a Glance: A Guide for Health Promotion Practice*, 2nd ed. Washington, D.C.: Department of Health and Human Services; 2005. Pp. 10–26.

10. Green LW, Kreuter MW. *Health Promotion Planning: An Educational and Environmental Approach.* New York: McGraw-Hill Publishing; 2005. Pp. 14–15.

11. Fiore MC, Jaén CR, Baker TB, et al. *Treating Tobacco Use and Dependence: 2008 Update.* Clinical Practice Guideline. Rockville, Md.: U.S. Department of Health and Human Services, Public Health Service; 2008.

12. Arsham GM, Colenbrander A, Spivey BE. A prototype for curriculum development in medical education. *J Med Educ.* 1973;48:78–84.

13. Example adapted with permission from the curricular project of Vera J. Burton, MD, PhD, and Mary L. Leppert, MBBCh, for the Johns Hopkins Longitudinal Program in Faculty Development, Cohort 26, 2012–2013.

14. Smedley BD, Stith AY, Nelson AR, eds, Committee on Understanding and Eliminating Racial and Ethnic Disparities in Health Care, Board on Health Sciences Policy, Institute of Medicine. *Unequal Treatment: Confronting Racial and Ethnic Disparities in Health Care.* Washington, D.C.: National Academies Press; 2003.

15. Carter MM, Lewis EL, Sbrocco T, et al. Cultural competency training for third-year clerkship students: effects of an interactive workshop on student attitudes. *J Natl Med Assoc.* 2006;98:1772–78.

16. Lie DA, Boker J, Crandall S, et al. Revising the Tool for Assessing Cultural Competence Training (TACCT) for curriculum evaluation: findings derived from seven US schools and expert consensus. *Med Educ Online.* 2008;13:11. doi:10.3885/meo.2008.Res00272.

17. Ko M, Heslin KC, Edelstein RA, Grumbach K. The role of medical education in reducing health care disparities: the first ten years of the UCLA/Drew Medical Education Program. *J Gen Intern Med.* 2007;22:625–31.

18. National Consortium for Multicultural Education for Health Professionals [Internet]. Available at http://culturalmeded.stanford.edu.

19. Kellogg Health Scholars.org [Internet]. Available at www.kellogghealthscholars.org.

20. Martinez IL, Artze-Vega I, Wells A, Mora J, Gillis M. Twelve tips for teaching social determinants of health in medicine. *Med Teach.* 2014;1–6. doi:10.3109/0142159X2014.975191.

21. Simpson D, Fincher RM, Hafler JP, et al. Advancing educators and education: defining the components and evidence of educational scholarship. *Med Educ.* 2007;41:1002–9.

22. Best Evidence in Medical Education Collaboration.org [Internet]. Available at www.bemecol laboration.org.

23. The Cochrane Collaboration.org [Internet]. Available at www.cochrane.org.

24. Reed D, Price EG, Windish DM, et al. Challenges in systematic reviews of educational intervention studies. *Ann Intern Med.* 2005;142:1080–89.

25. Agency for Healthcare Research and Quality. National Guideline Clearinghouse [Internet]. Available at www.guideline.gov.

26. National Institute for Health and Care Excellence.org [Internet]. Available at www.nice.org.uk.

27. Hayward RSA, Wilson MC, Tunis SR, Bass EB, Guyatt GH. Users' guides to the medical literature. VIII. How to use clinical practice guidelines. Part A. Are the results valid? Evidence-based Medicine Working Group. *JAMA.* 1995;274:570–74.

28. Wilson MC, Hayward RSA, Tunis SR, Bass EB, Guyatt GH. Users' guides to the medical literature. VIII. How to use clinical practice guidelines. Part B. What are the recommendations, and will they help you in caring for your patients? Evidence-based Medicine Working Group. *JAMA*. 1995;274:1630–32.
29. The AGREE Research Trust. AGREE, Appraisal of Guidelines for Research and Evaluation II [Internet]. Available at www.agreetrust.org.
30. Accreditation Council for Graduate Medical Education [Internet]. Available at www.acgme.org.
31. American Board of Internal Medicine. Certification Guide [Internet]. Available at www.abim .org/certification/policies/imss/im.aspx.
32. Liaison Committee on Medical Education. Functions and Structure of a Medical School Standards for Accreditation of Medical Education Programs Leading to the M.D. Degree [Internet]. Available at www.lcme.org.
33. Association of American Medical Colleges. Core Entrustable Professional Activities for Entering Residency [Internet]. 2014. Available at www.mededportal.org/icollaborative /resource/887.
34. McKean SCW, Budnitz TL, Dressler DD, Amin AN, Pistoria MJ. How to use the Core Competencies in Hospital Medicine: a framework for curriculum development. *J Hosp Med*. 2006;1(Suppl 1):57–67.
35. Greiner AC, Knebel E, eds, Institute of Medicine, Committee on Health Professions Education Summit. *Health Professions Education: A Bridge to Quality*. Washington, D.C.: National Academies Press; 2003. Pp. 45–96.
36. Swing, SR. The ACGME outcome project: retrospective and prospective. *Med Teach*. 2007;29(7):648–54.
37. Boonyasai RT, Windish DM, Chakraborti C, et al. Effectiveness of teaching quality improvement to clinicians: a systematic review. *JAMA*. 2007;298:1023–37.
38. Association of American Medical Colleges. MedEdPORTAL [Internet]. Available at www.med edportal.org.
39. Association of American Medical Colleges (AAMC). Curriculum Inventory and Reports (CIR)— part of the Medical Academic Performance Services (MedAPS). Available at www.aamc .org/initiatives/cir.
40. Krueger RA, Casey MA. *Focus Groups: A Practical Guide for Applied Research*, 5th ed. Thousand Oaks, Calif.: SAGE Publications; 2014.
41. Stewart DW, Shamdasani PN. *Focus Groups: Theory and Practice*, 3rd ed. Thousand Oaks, Calif.: SAGE Publications; 2014.
42. Morgan DL, Krueger RA, King JA. *The Focus Group Kit*. Thousand Oaks, Calif.: SAGE Publications; 1997.
43. Witkin BR, Altschuld JW. *Planning and Conducting Needs Assessments: A Practical Guide*. Thousand Oaks, Calif.: SAGE Publications; 1995. Pp. 167–71.
44. Witkin BR, Altschuld JW. *Planning and Conducting Needs Assessments: A Practical Guide*. Thousand Oaks, Calif.: SAGE Publications; 1995. Pp. 187–88, 193–203.
45. Keeney S, McKenna H, Hasson F. *The Delphi Technique in Nursing and Health Research*. Ames, Iowa: Wiley-Blackwell; 2011.
46. Fletcher AJ, Marchildon GP. Using the Delphi Method for qualitative, participatory action research in health leadership. *Int J Qual Methods*. 2014;13:1–18.
47. Lipmanowicz H, McCandless K. *The Surprising Power of Liberating Structures: Simple Rules to Unleash a Culture of Innovation*. Seattle: Liberating Structures Press; 2013.
48. Liberatingstructures.com [Internet]. Available at www.liberatingstructures.com.
49. Fink A. *How to Conduct Surveys: A Step-by-Step Guide*, 5th ed. Thousand Oaks, Calif.: SAGE Publications; 2012.
50. Fink A. *The Survey Kit*, 2nd ed. Thousand Oaks, Calif.: SAGE Publications; 2002.
51. Dillman DA, Smyth JD, Christian LM. *Internet, Phone, Mail, and Mixed-Mode Surveys: The Tailored Design Method*, 4th ed. Hoboken, N.J.: John Wiley & Sons; 2014.

52. Witkin BR, Altschuld JW. *Planning and Conducting Needs Assessments: A Practical Guide*. Thousand Oaks, Calif.: SAGE Publications, 1995. Pp. 150–51.
53. DiGaetano R. Sample frame and related sample design issues for surveys of physicians and physician practices. *Eval Health Prof.* 2013;36:296.
54. Sittig DF. Work-sampling: a statistical approach to evaluation of the effect of computers on work patterns in the healthcare industry. *Proc Annu Symp Comput Appl Med Care.* 1992:537–41.
55. Branch WT. Use of critical incident reports in medical education: a perspective. *J Gen Intern Med.* 2005;20(11):1063–67.
56. Flanagan JC. The critical incident technique. *Psycholl Bull.* 1954;51:327–58.
57. Whitney DD, Cooperrider DL, Stavros JM. *Appreciative Inquiry Handbook: For Leaders of Change*, 2nd ed. San Francisco: Berrett-Koehler Publishers, 2008.
58. Cockell J, McArthur-Blair J. *Appreciative Inquiry in Higher Education: A Transformative Force*. San Francisco: John Wiley & Sons; 2012.

CHAPTER THREE

Step 2
Targeted Needs Assessment

. . . refining the foundation

Mark T. Hughes, MD, MA

DEFINITION

A targeted needs assessment is a process by which curriculum developers apply the knowledge learned from the general needs assessment to their particular learners and learning environment. Curriculum developers must understand their learners and their learning environment to develop a curriculum that best suits their needs and addresses the health problem characterized in Step 1. In Step 2, curriculum developers identify specific needs by assessing *the differences between ideal and actual characteristics of the targeted learner group and the differences between ideal and actual characteristics of their learning environment.*

IMPORTANCE

The targeted needs assessment serves many functions. It allows the problem to be framed properly and allows stakeholders to be involved in the process of finding solutions. Those who are investing in the curriculum want to be confident that resources are being used effectively. Done appropriately, the targeted needs assessment prevents duplication of what is already being done, teaching what is already known, or teaching above the level of the targeted learners. The targeted needs assessment is one of the first steps in engaging and motivating learners in their own education. In addition, "a needs assessment can align resources with strategy, build relationships among those who have a stake in the situation, clarify problems or opportunities, set goals for future action, and provide data, insights, or justification for decision making" (1).

The targeted needs assessment should occur at two levels: 1) the targeted learners (their current and past experiences; their strengths and weaknesses in knowledge, attitudes, skills, and performance), and 2) the targeted learning environment (the existing curriculum; other characteristics of the learners' environment that influence whether/how learning occurs and is reinforced; the needs of key stakeholders).

The general needs assessment (GNA) from Step 1 can serve as a guide for developing the targeted needs assessment. The GNA can provide the rationale for a curricular approach, but that approach must still be considered in light of the characteristics of the targeted learners and their environment. A model curriculum from another institution, found in the literature search for Step 1, may require modification to fit one's own learners. Another caveat in adapting the general needs assessment involves the time lag between the gathering of GNA data from one or more institutions and the GNA's publication. The literature used to support the general needs assessment may be dated, and curriculum developers will need to update the targeted needs assessment based on current practice.

The needs of a curriculum's targeted learners are likely to be somewhat different from the needs of learners identified in the GNA (see Chapter 2). A curriculum's targeted learners may already be proficient in one area of general need but have particular learning needs in another area. Some objectives may already be taught in other parts of the overall teaching program but need to be further developed in the new curricular segment. Stakeholders, such as clerkship or program directors, may want specific learner objectives, competencies, or milestones to interact with and reinforce topics addressed in other curricula.

Curriculum developers must also assess their targeted learners' environment (or environments); otherwise, their curriculum may be inefficient because it devotes unnecessary resources to areas already addressed and mastered, or it may be suboptimally effective because it has devoted insufficient resources or attention to other areas of need or concern. Curriculum developers need to understand the culture of the targeted learning environment and how it may affect the attitudes and behaviors of the learners. In addition to developing the planned or formal curriculum, curriculum developers must be attentive to other learning experiences. These experiences that shape the values of learners during and after their training are known as the informal or collateral curriculum (2, 3). The unplanned sociopsychological interactions among student peers and between students and teachers create a learning environment that can have unintended consequences on learners' thought and behavior (4). The targeted learning environment can influence what is taught in the formal curriculum both positively, such as motivating learners and reinforcing knowledge or skills, and negatively, such as countering the attitudes educators wish to promote. As one example, not attending to the informal or hidden curriculum (5–7) can inhibit the translation of what has been learned in a specific curriculum on ethics into actual clinical practice and professional behavior. Priming students to attune themselves to the hidden curriculum within their environment can be one strategy within the formal curriculum to mitigate its influence (8).

IDENTIFICATION OF TARGETED LEARNERS

Before curriculum developers can proceed with the targeted needs assessment, they must first identify their targeted learners. Targeted learners can be patients, practitioners, practitioners-in-training, or students. Ideally, this choice of targeted learners would flow from the problem identification and general needs assessment. (See Chapter 2.) The targeted learners would be the group most likely, with further learning, to contribute to the solution of the problem. Frequently, however, curriculum developers have already been assigned their targeted learners, such as medical students or resident physicians-in-training. In this case, it is worth considering how an educational intervention directed at one's targeted learners could contribute to solving the health care problem of concern. Knowledge of the targeted learners can also help in determining the ideal timing for delivery of the curricular content, based on the learners' developmental stages.

CONTENT

Content about Targeted Learners

Once targeted learners have been identified, the next step in the targeted needs assessment is to decide on the information about the targeted learners that is most needed. Such information might include previous and already planned training and experiences; expectations regarding the scope of knowledge and skills needed (which will differ, for instance, between a medical student and a senior resident); existing proficiencies (cognitive, affective, psychomotor); perceived deficiencies and needs (from evaluators' and/or learners' perspectives); measured deficiencies in knowledge or skills; reasons for past poor performance; learners' capacities and motivations to improve performance; attitudes about the curricular topic; learning styles; preferred learning methods; and targeted learners' experiences with different learning strategies (Table 3.1).

> **EXAMPLE:** *Learners and Prior Experience.* Curriculum developers planning education programs for point-of-care ultrasound in resource-limited settings need to understand their trainees' prior experience with ultrasonography. For example: Have they referred a patient for ultrasonography at a health facility? Have they ever personally used an ultrasound machine before? Have they had formal instruction in ultrasonography? If so, was it lecture-based or hands-on skills training? Curriculum developers can include objective measures of the targeted learners' capabilities in diagnostic imaging to determine whether ultrasound training would aid the learners' diagnostic capacity. For learners with prior experience in the use of ultrasound, curriculum developers can design developmentally appropriate training to enhance their capacity. In addition, educators need to understand how the targeted learners anticipate applying ultrasound in their clinical practice and the barriers that can affect continuing education about and sustained use of ultrasonography (9).

Table 3.1.   Content Potentially Relevant to a Targeted Needs Assessment

Content about Targeted Learners
Expectations regarding scope of knowledge and skills needed
Previous training and experiences relevant to the curriculum
Already planned training and experiences relevant to the curriculum
Existing characteristics/proficiencies/practices
    Cognitive: knowledge, problem-solving abilities
    Affective: attitudes, values, beliefs, role expectations
    Psychomotor: skills/capabilities (e.g., history, physical examination, procedures,
        counseling), current behaviors/performance/practices
Perceived and measured deficiencies and learning needs
Attitudes and motivations of learners to improve performance
Preferences and experiences regarding different learning strategies
    Synchronous (educator sets time, such as with noon lecture)
    Asynchronous (learner decides on learning time, such as with e-learning)
    Duration (amount of time learner thinks is needed to learn or that he/she can devote to
        learning)
    Methods (e.g., readings, lectures, online learning resources, large and small group
        discussions, problem-based learning, team-based learning, peer teaching,
        demonstrations, role-plays/simulations, supervised experience)

Content about Targeted Learning Environment
Related existing curricula
Needs of stakeholders other than the learners (course directors, clerkship directors, program
directors, faculty, accrediting bodies, others)
Barriers, enablers, and reinforcing factors that affect learning by the targeted learners
    Barriers (e.g., time, unavailability, or competition for resources)
    Enablers (e.g., learning portfolios, electronic medical record reminders)
    Reinforcing factors (e.g., incentives such as grades, awards, recognition)
Resources (e.g., patients and clinical experiences, faculty, role models and mentors,
    information resources, access to hardware and software technology, audiovisual
    equipment, simulation center)
Informal and collateral curriculum

EXAMPLE: *Learners, Attitudes, and Barriers.* Curriculum developers designing a curriculum in spiritual care surveyed medical residents about their attitudes toward spirituality in the clinical context. They found that while the trainees thought that awareness of patients' faith, spirituality, or religious beliefs was important in their practice, the majority had difficulty identifying whether a patient desired a discussion about spiritual issues. Residents reported sometimes being unsure about how to respond to patients who brought up spiritual issues, such as asking the provider to pray. Time was also identified as a key barrier in engaging in spiritual discussions. The curricular objectives were then focused on these barriers. One of the objectives of the curriculum was to increase residents' comfort in raising and discussing issues of spirituality with patients. Another objective was to increase residents' knowledge and use of a brief spiritual assessment as a part of taking patients' medical histories (10).

For learners in a work environment, it may also be important to learn the scope of their work responsibilities, the competencies necessary to fulfill those responsibilities, and the training and nontraining requirements necessary for the learner to become competent (11).

Content about the Targeted Learning Environment

Concomitant with acquiring information about the learners, curriculum developers must also understand the environment in which their curriculum is to be delivered. For instance, does a curriculum addressing the problem already exist, and if so, what has been its track record (in terms of both learner satisfaction and achievement of learning objectives)? Curriculum developers may discover that the existing or planned curriculum is adequate to meet learners' knowledge and skill needs, but that programmatic or system changes are needed to facilitate subsequent application of the knowledge and skills in clinical settings.

> **EXAMPLE:** *Programmatic Change for Training on Clinical Record Keeping.* In designing a curriculum on the electronic medical record (EMR) for medical students about to embark on clinical rotations, curriculum developers planned online training to introduce students to the software program for the EMR used at the university hospital. However, the targeted needs assessment revealed that affiliated hospitals at which students also rotated either did not use the same software program or did not allow student access to the EMR. Programmatic changes needed to occur to ensure that students on clinical clerkships and elective rotations knew how to use the EMR at these other sites and had security clearance to do so in order to participate in patient care activities as part of their learning.

> **EXAMPLE:** *Programmatic Change for Interdisciplinary Clinical Experience.* In creating the curriculum on spiritual care, curriculum developers learned in focus groups with attending physicians and chaplain trainees that there could be mutual advantage in having chaplain trainees interact more directly with the medical team. It was recognized that chaplain trainees could role-model communication skills and act as a valuable liaison between the patient and the medical team, but that physicians were often limited in their knowledge about chaplains' roles and had difficulty finding time to include chaplain trainees' input. Chaplain trainees valued gaining a better understanding of the medical process. Both physician trainees and chaplain trainees could be taught how to do a spiritual assessment using the FICA (Faith and Belief; Importance; Community; Address in Care) tool (12, 13), but programmatic changes needed to be made to incorporate chaplain trainees into patient care rounds. The targeted needs assessment thus led to the curricular plan that chaplain trainees would join medical rounds at least once per week and, at the invitation of the attending physician, would share an "elevator speech" regarding the chaplain's role and offer a spiritual assessment of patients and their situations (10).

In assessing the learning environment, curriculum developers may find that the trainees' clinical training experiences do not match their learning needs, and this deficit will affect other stakeholders in the training environment.

> **EXAMPLE:** *Learners, Their Environment, and Other Stakeholders.* Curriculum developers designing a curriculum on minimally invasive gynecologic surgery found that learners rotated at four different hospitals and received little objective assessment of their surgical skills. In addition, the residency program had inadequate communication between training sites regarding the surgical proficiency of the trainees. Pilot studies with targeted learners showed that virtual reality robotic simulation training, with repetition, improved trainees' ability across a variety of performance metrics (14). Although case logs indicated involvement in about 50 minimally invasive hysterectomies by the time of graduation, upper-level residents reported less preparedness in performing laparoscopic and robotic hysterectomies relative to abdominal hysterectomies. Consequently, curriculum developers combined a multimodal training program that included simulation with linkage between case logs and procedural videos to allow faculty to electronically evaluate trainees across the four clinical sites. This approach led to better objective measurement of surgical performance and enhanced communication between stakeholders at the different hospitals (15).

Other information about the environment might include the needs of key stakeholders other than the learners (faculty, educational leaders, accrediting bodies). For instance, curriculum developers may find that faculty members are not prepared to teach what needs to be learned, and faculty development thus becomes an important factor in curricular planning.

> **EXAMPLE:** *Learners, the Existing Curriculum, and Need for Faculty Development.* Curriculum developers planning a quality improvement curriculum for residents in general preventive medicine sought to meet ACGME (Accreditation Council for Graduate Medical Education) requirements that preventive medicine residents incorporate a clinical component into their training and that primary care residencies implement quality improvement training. Although residents had been placed in community practices for three years and worked on projects that directly affected patient care, learning objectives were not well-defined for integrating clinical protocols with population-based health system improvement efforts. To assess the learning environment of the preventive medicine residents, preceptors at the clinical sites were surveyed. Preceptors expressed interest in working with the preventive medicine residents and thought their presence would improve care of preceptors' patient populations, but the preceptors lacked training in quality improvement and teamwork strategies. Thus, curriculum developers needed to modify their curricular approach by making the preceptors secondary targeted learners in order to enhance the educational experience of the primary targeted learners—the preventive medicine residents (16).

> **EXAMPLE:** *An Evolving Learning Environment and Need for Faculty Development.* A new Master of Education in the Health Professions (MEHP) degree program was developed to prepare health professionals to teach effectively, for schools and training programs related to medicine, public health, nursing, and other health professions. Curriculum developers planned to deliver the first year of the curriculum during in-person sessions, then, eventually, to transition to an exclusively online curriculum. In addition to recruiting faculty from various health professional schools and schools of education, curriculum developers learned in the targeted needs assessment that faculty members required training in how to deliver their content in an online format.

Curriculum developers must also assess whether faculty members are motivated and enthusiastic to teach and are sufficiently incentivized to deliver the curriculum.

> **EXAMPLE:** *Inadequate Team Skills Training, Need for Faculty Development.* Curriculum developers for a multifaceted interprofessional curriculum wanted to offer students various learning opportunities to learn and practice interprofessional teamwork competencies. A framework for creating opportunities for collaborative care was developed that included curricular and extracurricular learning experiences for students, as well as faculty development for team skills training. The targeted needs assessment revealed that successful implementation of the curriculum would require continuing education for faculty so that they would have the knowledge, skills, and values to work collaboratively in interprofessional teams and to role-model these behaviors for students. In addition to being taught basic team skills, faculty members were rewarded for work that involved interprofessional collaboration. Over time, demonstration of faculty interprofessional collaboration was acknowledged as a criterion for faculty promotion and existing university faculty awards (17).

It is also important to understand the barriers, enabling factors, and reinforcing factors (see Chapter 2) in the environment that affect learning by the targeted learners. For example, is there an ample supply of patients with whom learners can practice their clinical skills? Are technologies (e.g., computers, diagnostic equipment, simulation services) available? Is a resident too busy with clinical responsibilities to devote time to other educational pursuits? Are there established, designated time slots (e.g., noon conference) for delivering the formal curriculum? Are there aspects of the medical culture that promote or inhibit the application of learning? Are there incentives for learning or improving performance? Are there opportunities to collaborate with other departments or disciplines? Are sufficient resources available for learning and applying what is learned in practice? (See Table 3.1.)

METHODS

General Considerations

Curriculum developers may already have some of the information about their targeted learners and their environment; other information may have to be acquired. Data already in existence—such as the results of questionnaires (e.g., the Association of American Medical Colleges' matriculation and graduation questionnaires), standardized examinations (e.g., in-service training and specialty board examinations), procedure and experience logs, related curricula in which the targeted learners participate, and audit results—may provide information relevant to curriculum developers and obviate the need for independent data collection. Curriculum management software is another source of already collected data that can help curriculum developers determine what is happening in their institution with respect to a topic of interest. Such software is used to track information on a school's curricula, information that is increasingly being required by accreditation bodies. The Association of American Medical Colleges is attempting to collate information from U.S. and Canadian medical schools in a national data warehouse (18).

When the desired information about the targeted learners is not already available to or known by the curriculum developers, they must decide how to acquire it. As with problem identification and general needs assessment (see Chapter 2), curriculum developers must decide *how much time, effort, and resources should be devoted to this step*. A commitment of too little time and effort risks development of an inefficient or ineffective curriculum. A commitment of too much time and effort can diminish the resources available for other critical steps, such as the development of effective educational strategies, successful implementation of the curriculum, and evaluation. Because resources are almost always limited, curriculum developers will need to *prioritize* their information needs.

Once the information that is required has been decided on, curriculum developers should decide on the *best method to obtain this information, given available resources*. In making this decision, they should ask the following questions:

1. What standards of representativeness, validity, and accuracy will be required?
2. Will *subjective or objective* measures be used?
3. Will *quantitative or qualitative data* be preferable?

As with curriculum evaluation, a variety of measurement methods and analytic tools can be employed in the targeted needs assessment (see Chapter 7). The purpose and ultimate utility of the targeted needs assessment for aiding the curriculum development process can help in deciding which method to pursue. If there is strong disagreement within the group responsible for developing the curriculum about the knowledge, attitude, skill, or performance deficits of the targeted learners, a more rigorous, representative, objective, and quantitative assessment of learner needs may be required. If a curriculum developer is new to an institution or unfamiliar with the learners and the learning environment and needs to get a "big picture" sense of the targeted needs assessment, collection and analysis of in-depth qualitative data gathered from a sample of selected learners and faculty may be most useful. If the curriculum developers have limited or no experience in using a needs assessment method, it is wise to seek *advice or mentorship from those with expertise* in the method.

Before applying a method formally to the group of targeted learners, it is important to *pilot* the data collection instrument on a convenient, receptive audience. Piloting of a questionnaire on a few friendly learners and faculty can provide feedback on whether the questionnaire is too long or whether some of the questions are worded in a confusing manner. This kind of informal feedback can provide specific suggestions on improved wording and format, on what questions can be eliminated, and on whether any new questions need to be added before the questionnaire is sent to a larger pool of survey respondents. This ensures a better chance of acquiring valid information from the targeted learners or other stakeholders.

If publication or dissemination of the findings of one's targeted needs assessment is anticipated, the work is likely to be considered educational research. Issues related to the protection of human subjects may need to be contemplated, including whether study subjects perceive participation as voluntary or coercive. Before collecting data, curriculum developers should consider consultation with their institutional review board (see Chapters 6 and 9).

Specific Methods

Specific methods commonly used in the needs assessment of targeted learners include informal discussion or interviews with individual learners, their supervisors or observers, and other stakeholders; small group or focus group discussions with proposed participants in the curriculum; formal interviews and questionnaires; direct observation of targeted learners; pretests of knowledge, attitudes, or skills; audits of current performance; and strategic planning sessions for the curriculum (19). Strategic planning sessions with key stakeholders can promote successful implementation of the curriculum by engaging stakeholders (see Chapter 6). Strategic planning is an organizational process that assesses existing strengths and weaknesses, gauges readiness to change, and determines the steps needed to accomplish the change (20–22).

The advantages and disadvantages of each method of targeted needs assessment are shown in Table 3.2.

Surveys

Surveys are collections and/or reviews of data that are usually systematically performed. Three types of survey frequently used in curriculum development are interviews (questions asked and recorded by an interviewer), focus groups, and questionnaires (usually self-administered). Curriculum developers can decide which method best suits their needs. In designing a survey, curriculum developers must decide on the sample population to be surveyed, whether the sample is randomly or purposefully selected, and the design of the survey (cross-sectional vs. longitudinal). Regardless of the type of survey administered, each question should have clearly delineated objectives and justification for its inclusion in the survey. The length of a survey and/or the sensitivity of its questions will influence the response rate by the sample population. Because response rates are critical for acquisition of representative data, curriculum developers should generally include only questions that can be acted on (23). The sample population being surveyed should be notified about the survey, its purpose, what their responses will

Table 3.2.   Advantages and Disadvantages of Different Needs Assessment Methods

Method	Advantages	Disadvantages
Informal discussion (in-person, over phone, or by e-mail)	Convenient Inexpensive Rich in detail and qualitative information Method for identifying stakeholders	Lack of methodological rigor Variations in questions Interviewer biases
Formal interviews	Standardized approach to interviewee Methodological rigor possible Questions and answers can be clarified With good response rate, can obtain data representative of entire group of targeted learners Quantitative and/or qualitative information Means of gaining support from stakeholders	Methodological rigor requires trained interviewers and measures of reliability Costly in terms of time and effort, especially if methodological rigor is required Interviewer bias and influence on respondent
Focus group discussions	Efficient method of "interviewing" several at one time (especially those with common trait) Learn about group behavior that may affect job performance (especially helpful to understand team-based learning) Group interaction may enrich or deepen information obtained Qualitative information	Requires skilled facilitator to control group interaction and minimize facilitator influence on responses Need note taker or other means of recording information (e.g., audiotape) Views of quiet participants may not be expressed No quantitative information Information may not be representative of all targeted learners Time and financial costs involved in data collection and analysis
Questionnaires	Standardized questions Methodological rigor relatively easy With good response rate, can obtain representative data Quantitative and/or qualitative information Can assess affective traits (attitudes, beliefs, feelings) Respondents can be geographically dispersed (web-based questionnaires increase the ease of reaching geographically dispersed respondents)	Requires skill in writing clear, unambiguous questions Answers cannot be clarified without resurveying Requires time and effort to ensure methodological rigor in survey development, data collection, and data analysis Dependent on adequate response rate (and resources devoted to achieving this) Requires time, effort, and skill to construct valid measures of affective traits

Table 3.2.   *(continued)*

Method	Advantages	Disadvantages
Direct observation	Best method for assessing skills and performance Can be informal or methodologically rigorous Informal observations can sometimes be accomplished as part of one's teaching or supervisory role	Can be time-consuming, especially if methodological rigor is desired Guidelines must be developed for standardized observations Observer generally must be knowledgeable of behavior being observed Observer bias Impact of observer on observed Assesses ability, not real-life performance (unless observations are unobtrusive)
Tests	Efficient, objective means of assessing cognitive or psychomotor abilities Tests of key knowledge items relatively easy to construct	Requires time, effort, and skill to construct valid tests of skills and higher order cognitive abilities Test anxiety may affect performance Assesses ability, not real-life performance
Audits of current performance	Useful for medical record keeping and the provision of recorded care (e.g., tests ordered, provision of discrete preventive care measures, prescribed treatments) Potentially unobtrusive Assesses real-life performance Can be methodologically rigorous with standards, instructions, and assurance of inter- and intrarater reliability	Requires development of standards Requires resources to pay and train auditors, time and effort to perform audit oneself May require permission from learner and/or institution to audit records Difficult to avoid or account for recording omissions Addresses only indirect, incomplete measures of care
Strategic planning sessions for the curriculum	Can involve targeted learners as well as key faculty Can involve brainstorming of learner needs, as well as current program strengths and weaknesses Can involve prioritization as well as generation of needs Creates sense of involvement and responsibility in participants Part of a larger process that also identifies goals, objectives, and responsibilities	Requires skilled facilitator to ensure participation and lack of inhibition by all participants Requires considerable time and effort to plan and conduct successful strategic planning sessions and to develop the associated report

be used for, whether responses will be considered confidential, and the time needed to conduct the survey.

Interviews can be conducted in person, by phone, or electronically (e.g., instant messaging). Interviews can be structured, unstructured, or semi-structured. Structured interviews allow for consistency of questions across respondents so that responses can be compared/contrasted, whereas unstructured or semi-structured interviews allow spontaneity and on-the-spot follow-up of interesting responses. Several caveats should be kept in mind when developing, preparing for, and conducting an interview (Table 3.3) (24).

Focus groups bring together people with a common attribute to share their collective experience with the help of a skilled facilitator. Focus groups are well suited to explore perceptions and feelings about particular issues. The groups should be of a manageable size (7 ± 2 is a good rule) and should engender an atmosphere of openness and respectful sharing. The facilitator should be familiar with the topic area and use language understandable to the focus group participants (their typical jargon if a specialized group, layperson language if a mixed group). Questions asked in a focus group often come in three forms: 1) developing an understanding of a topic; 2) pilot-testing ideas, with attention to their advantages/disadvantages; and 3) evaluating a program based on the experiences of the focus group participants. The facilitator should encourage participation, acknowledge responses nonjudgmentally, manage those who are more willing or less willing to engage in the discussion, foster brainstorming in response to participants' answers, and keep track of time. After the focus group is completed, a report should be generated highlighting the key findings from the session (25, 26).

Questionnaires, as opposed to interviews and focus groups, are completed by the individual alone or with minimal assistance from another. They can be paper-based or

Table 3.3.   Tips for Developing, Preparing for, and Conducting an Interview

1. Decide how information will be collected (notes by interviewer vs. recorded and transcribed) and the time needed to document responses.

2. Develop an interview guide. This is especially important if multiple interviewers are used.

3. Structure interview questions to facilitate conversation, with more general, open-ended questions up front, important questions toward the beginning, and sensitive questions at the end.

4. Cluster questions with a common theme in a logical order.

5. Clarify responses when necessary (use prompts such as the following: "Describe for me . . . ," "Tell me more . . . ," "Can you say more about that . . .?" "Can you give me an example?").

6. Maintain a neutral attitude and avoid biasing interviewee responses (e.g., by discussing the responses of another interviewee).

7. At the end of the interview, express gratitude and offer the interviewee an opportunity to express any additional questions or comments.

8. Time permitting, summarize key points and ask permission to recontact interviewee for future follow-up questions.

Source: Sleezer et al., pp. 52–57 (24).

electronic. Electronic resources can be survey-focused (e.g., www.surveymonkey.com or www.qualtrics.com) or part of proprietary learning management systems (e.g., www.blackboard.com). Software programs offer design flexibility, and questionnaire design must attend to ease of survey navigation, choice of response formats, and typical interpretation of visual cues (27). Since online questionnaires can be accessed from a variety of platforms, including mobile devices, desktops, and laptops, curriculum developers need to be aware of the technological capabilities and preferences of the survey population (28). In addition, online surveys may need additional privacy protections (29). Often, websites for online questionnaires include software for data management and basic statistical analysis.

Curriculum developers need to be mindful of several issues with regard to questionnaires. A questionnaire must contain instructions on how to answer questions. It is also generally advisable to include a cover letter with the questionnaire, explaining the rationale of the questionnaire and what is expected of the respondent. The cover letter can be the first step to develop respondents' buy-in for questionnaire completion, if it provides sufficient justification for the survey and makes the respondent feel vested in the outcome. *Pilot-testing* to ensure clarity and understandability in both the format and the content of the questions is especially important, as no interviewer is present to explain the meaning of ambiguously worded questions.

Questions should relate to the questionnaire objectives, and the respondent should be aware of the rationale for each question. How questions are worded in a survey greatly affects the value of the information gleaned from them. Table 3.4 provides tips to keep in mind when writing questions (30–32). Curriculum developers must be cognizant of the potential for nonresponse to particular questions on the questionnaire and how this might affect the validity of the targeted needs assessment (33).

When representative data are desired, *response rate* is critical. Nonresponse can result from nondelivery of the survey request, a prospective respondent's refusal of the solicitation, or inability of the respondent to understand or complete the questionnaire (34). Overall questionnaire response rates will depend on the amount of burden (time, opportunity costs, etc.) placed on respondents in completing the questionnaire. Questionnaire designers have to decide on incentives for completion of the questionnaire. Where and when the questionnaire will be administered may also affect response rates (e.g., at the end of a mandatory training session when time can be allotted for completing the questionnaire, or asynchronously so that respondents can complete the questionnaire at their own pace). Methods for following up with questionnaire nonrespondents also have to be considered, as this may entail additional time and resources. For questionnaires targeting physicians, a general rule of thumb is to aim for response rates greater than 60% (35, 36). Tips for increasing response rates on health professional surveys are presented in Table 3.5 (37–42).

Sometimes, mixed methodologies for survey administration increase the yield of information (43). Learners may have preferred means of answering surveys, so offering options can enhance the chances of adequate response rates. The caveat for this, however, is that curriculum developers need to ensure that questions asked by different methodologies are being interpreted in the same way by survey respondents. Another strategy is to employ just-in-time techniques to engage learners in the needs assessment process. Appendix A provides an example of using an audience response system during a lecture to solicit attitudes about incorporating prognosis in the care of older patients with multimorbidity, and then following it up with audience discussion. Just-in-

Table 3.4.   Tips for Writing and Administering Questionnaire Questions

1. Ask for only one piece of information. The more precise and unambiguous the question is, the better.

2. Avoid biased, leading, or negatively phrased questions.

3. Avoid abbreviations, colloquialisms, and phrases not easily understood by respondents.

4. For paper-based questionnaires, make sure questions follow a logical order, key items are highlighted with textual elements (boldface, italics, or underline), the overall format is not visually complex or distracting, and the sequence of questions/pages is easy to follow.

5. For online questionnaires, develop a screen format that is appealing to respondents and displays easily across devices, highlight information that is essential to survey completion, provide error messages to help respondents troubleshoot issues, and use interactive and audiovisual capabilities sparingly to reduce respondent burden.

6. Decide whether an open-ended or closed question will elicit the most fitting response. Open-ended answers (e.g., fill in the blanks) will require more data analysis, so they should be used in a limited fashion when surveying a large sample. Closed questions are used when the surveyor wants an answer from a prespecified set of response choices.

7. Make categorical responses (e.g., race) mutually exclusive and exhaust all categories (if necessary, using "other") in the offered list of options.

8. When more than one response is possible, offer the option of "check all that apply."

9. In using ordinal questions (responses can be ordered on a scale by level of agreement, frequency, intensity, or comparison), make the scale meaningful to the topic area and easy to complete and understand based on the question thread and instructions. For potentially embarrassing or sensitive questions, it is generally best to put the negative end of the scale first.

10. For attitudinal questions, decide whether it is important to learn how respondents feel, how strongly they feel, or both.

11. If demographic questions are asked, know how this information will influence the data analysis, what the range of answers will be in the target population, how specific the information needs to be, and whether it will be compared with existing datasets (in which case common terms should be used). Sometimes asking respondents to answer in their own words or numbers (e.g., date of birth, zip code, income) allows the surveyor to avoid questions with a burdensome number of response categories.

time can also be used to determine the knowledge content of upcoming lectures in a curriculum.

> **EXAMPLE:** *Targeted Needs Assessment in Preparation for Teaching Sessions.* In a surgery residency training program, residents were sent short readings on an upcoming topic and required to complete online study questions before their weekly teaching sessions. In addition to five open-ended questions that addressed key concepts of the reading, a standard question was always added to the list of weekly questions: "Please tell us briefly what single point of the reading you found most difficult or confusing. If you did not find any part of it difficult or confusing, please tell us what parts you found most interesting." Faculty members reviewed the survey responses to tailor the session content to residents' learning needs (44).

Table 3.5.   Tips for Increasing Questionnaire Response Rates

1. Consider reasons that professionals refuse to participate.
   a. Lack of time
   b. Unclear or low salience of the study (i.e., need to establish relevance)
   c. Concerns about confidentiality of results
   d. Some questions seem biased or do not allow a full range of choices on the subject
   e. Volume and length of survey
   f. Office staff who pose barrier to accessing the professional (especially in private practice)
2. Offer incentives to increase participation and convey respect for professionals' time.
   a. Cash payment (even $1) > charitable inducement > donation to alma mater
   b. Not clear whether gift certificate has same motivating effect as cash
   c. Prepaid incentive > promised incentive (i.e., sent after survey returned)
   d. Small financial incentive > enrollment in lottery for higher amount
   e. For web survey, need to consider how liquid the monetary incentive is
   f. Token nonmonetary incentive has little to no impact on response rate
3. Design respondent-friendly questionnaire.
   a. Shorter survey (<1,000 words; <2 pages)
   b. Attractive business format helps, but paper quality does not make a difference
   c. Standard-size paper (8.5 x 11 inches) works better than booklet
   d. Single-sided vs. double-sided print format does not make a difference
   e. Closed questions get higher response rate than open-ended questions
   f. Mixed-methods reply approach helps (e.g., postal and/or electronic options)
4. Use several contacts (e.g., by first class mail) and one additional special contact (e.g., certified mail or telephone call).
   a. Prenotification about survey works best when mode of prenotification is different from survey mode (e.g., postal prenotification for web survey)
   b. Direct contact by professional peer helps
   c. Vary the type of appeal (i.e., value, utility, personal) made to motivate sample members in each contact
   d. Inclusion of replacement questionnaire with follow-up contact helps
   e. Recorded delivery or registered mail may prioritize survey into important mail
   f. For web surveys, send e-mail reminders and postal mail for final reminder
   g. For e-mail follow-up to web surveys, provide inviting subject line, avoid terms used by spammers, include URL to the survey, and ensure confidentiality
5. Make it easy for sample member to respond (e.g., include return envelope with first class stamp)
   a. Envelope size does not matter, but stamp is better than metered envelope
   b. For web surveys, provide estimate of survey length and have easy navigability
6. Personalize contact (cover letter, hand-written note, personalized envelope, phone)
   a. Sample members with a close relationship to surveyor are more likely to respond
   b. Endorsement by opinion leader or professional association has mixed results

Sources: Adapted from Kellerman and Herold (36), Field et al. (37), VanGeest et al. (38), Thorpe et al. (39), Martins et al. (40), Dykema et al. (41), and Cho et al. (42).
Note: Most evidence comes from mailed surveys. Data on response rates for web surveys are limited.

Whatever survey method is used, the data need to be systematically collected and analyzed (see Chapter 7 for more detail on data analysis). In performing the targeted needs assessment, curriculum developers should ask whether useful information was collected and what was learned in the process (45). Regardless of whether curriculum developers are analyzing quantitative data (46, 47) or qualitative data (48–50), they must always keep in mind that the targeted needs assessment is intended to focus the problem in the context of the targeted learners and their learning environment and to help shape the subsequent steps in curriculum development.

RELATION TO OTHER STEPS

The information one chooses to collect as part of the targeted needs assessment may be influenced by what one expects will be a *goal or objective* of the curriculum or by the *educational* and *implementation strategies* being considered for the curriculum. Subsequent steps—*Goals and Objectives, Educational Strategies, Implementation*, and *Evaluation and Feedback*—are likely to be affected by what is learned in the targeted needs assessment. The process of conducting a needs assessment can serve as advance publicity for a curriculum, engage stakeholders, and ease a curriculum's *implementation*. Information gathered as part of the targeted needs assessment can serve as *"pre-" or "before" data for evaluation* of the impact of a curriculum. For all of these reasons, it is wise to think through other steps, at least in a preliminary manner, before investing time and resources in the targeted needs assessment.

> **EXAMPLE:** *Interaction with Implementation.* A targeted needs assessment of internal medicine residents revealed performance barriers in terms of equipment and support staff, as well as skill deficits, that prevented residents from including cervical cancer screening in the care of their ambulatory continuity patients. The curriculum developers were able to convince the clinic administrator to purchase the necessary equipment and to redefine nursing staff roles with respect to availability for pelvic examinations (51).

> **EXAMPLE:** *Interaction with Evaluation and Feedback.* As part of a targeted needs assessment for a new curriculum on transitions in care for medical students, third- and fourth-year students were surveyed about how often they performed discharge-related tasks, such as reconciling medication lists, writing discharge summaries, and communicating with outpatient providers. After the curriculum was implemented, part of the evaluation included asking students similar questions about the frequency of performing discharge-related tasks before the training session and at the end of the clerkship (52).

It is also worth realizing that one can learn a lot about a curriculum's targeted learners in the course of conducting the curriculum. This information can then be used as a targeted needs assessment for the next cycle of the curriculum (see Chapter 10).

> **EXAMPLE:** *Evaluation That Serves as Targeted Needs Assessment.* As part of their ambulatory medicine clinic experience, residents were evaluated by their preceptors through EMR review of their patient panels. The evaluation found that, for the most part, residents were unskilled in incorporating preventive care into office visits and in motivating patients to follow through with cancer screening recommendations. Focused training in these areas was developed for the next cycle of the ambulatory medicine clinic experience, and preceptors were prompted to ask about these issues during case presentations.

SCHOLARSHIP

A well-done targeted needs assessment allows curriculum developers to provide specific information about learners and the learning environment that facilitates adaptation of the curriculum by other institutions or training programs. This is a critical step in dissemination of the curriculum beyond one's own institution. (See Chapter 9.)

CONCLUSION

By clarifying the characteristics of one's targeted learners and their environment, the curriculum developer can help ensure that the curriculum being planned not only addresses important general needs but also is relevant and applicable to the specific needs of its learners and their learning institution. Steps 1 and 2 provide a sound basis for the next step, choosing the goals and objectives for the curriculum.

QUESTIONS

For the curriculum you are coordinating, planning, or would like to be planning, please answer or think about the following questions:

1. *Identify your targeted learners.* From the point of view of your problem identification and general needs assessment, will training this group as opposed to other groups of learners make the greatest contribution to solving the health care problem? If not, who would be a better group of targeted learners? Are these learners an option for you? Notwithstanding these considerations, is it nevertheless important to train your original group of targeted learners? Why?

2. To the extent of your current knowledge, *describe your targeted learners and their environment.* What are your targeted learners' previous training experiences, existing proficiencies, past and current performance, attitudes about the topic area and/or curriculum, learning style and needs, and familiarity with and preferences for different learning methods? What key characteristics do the learners share? What areas of heterogeneity should be highlighted? In the targeted learning environment, what other curricula exist or are being planned, what are the enabling and reinforcing factors and barriers to development and implementation of your curriculum, and what are the resources for learning? Who are the stakeholders (course directors, faculty, school administrators, clerkship and residency program directors, and accrediting bodies), and what are their needs with respect to your curriculum?

3. *What information* about your learners and their environment *is unknown* to you? *Prioritize* your information needs.

4. *Identify one or more methods* (e.g., informal and formal interviews, focus groups, questionnaires) by which you could obtain the most important information. For each method, *identify the resources* (time, personnel, supplies, space) required to develop the necessary data collection instruments and to collect and analyze the needed data. To what degree do you feel that each method is feasible?

5. Identify individuals on whom you could *pilot* your needs assessment instrument(s).

6. After conducting the targeted needs assessment, systematically ask whether useful information was collected and *what was learned in the process*.

7. Define how the targeted needs assessment *focuses the problem* in the context of your learners and their learning environment and *prepares you for the next steps*.

GENERAL REFERENCES

Learning Environment

Hafferty FW, O'Donnell JF, eds. *The Hidden Curriculum in Health Professional Education.* Lebanon, N.H.: Dartmouth College Press / University Press of New England; 2014.
Published 20 years after a landmark article in *Academic Medicine*, this book is a compilation of essays exploring the informal or hidden curriculum. It discusses the theoretical underpinnings of the concept and methodical approaches for assessing and addressing it. The curriculum developer in medical education will gain a better understanding of the social, cultural, and organizational contexts within which professional development occurs. 320 pages.

Needs Assessment

Altschuld JW, ed. *The Needs Assessment KIT*. Thousand Oaks, Calif.: SAGE Publications; 2010.
This resource includes a set of five books that cover theory and tools for conducting needs assessments. Book 1: Needs Assessment, An Overview; Book 2: Phase 1, Pre-assessment (Getting the Process Started); Book 3: Phase 2, Assessment (Collecting Data); Book 4: Phase 2, Assessment (Analysis and Prioritization); Book 5: Phase 3, Post-assessment (Planning for Action and Evaluating the Needs Assessment). Each book approximately 135 pages.

Altschuld JW, Witkin BR. *From Needs Assessment to Action: Transforming Needs into Solution Strategies.* Thousand Oaks, Calif.: SAGE Publications; 2000.
Reviews earlier work (Witkin and Altschuld, see below), addresses the value of the multiple/mixed method approach to needs assessment, including both qualitative and quantitative methods, and then focuses on the prioritization of needs and the transformation of needs assessments into action. Provides real-world examples. 282 pages.

Morrison GR, Ross SM, Kalman HK, Kemp JE. *Designing Effective Instruction*, 7th ed. Hoboken, N.J.: John Wiley & Sons; 2013.
A general book on instructional design, including needs assessment, instructional objectives, instructional strategies, and evaluation. Chapters 2–4 (pp. 26–98) deal with needs assessment. 453 pages.

Sleezer CM, Russ-Eft DF, Gupta K. *A Practical Guide to Needs Assessment*, 3rd ed. San Francisco: John Wiley & Sons (published by Wiley); 2014.
Practical how-to handbook on conducting a needs assessment, with case examples and toolkit. 402 pages.

Survey Design

Books

Dillman DA, Smyth JD, Christian LM. *Internet, Phone, Mail, and Mixed-Mode Surveys: The Tailored Design Method*, 4th ed. Hoboken, N.J.: John Wiley & Sons; 2014.
Topics include writing questions, constructing questionnaires, survey implementation and delivery, mixed mode surveys, and Internet surveys. Presents a stepwise approach to survey implementa-

tion that incorporates strategies to improve rigor and response rates. Clearly written, with many examples. 509 pages.

Fink A. *How to Conduct Surveys: A Step-by-Step Guide*, 5th ed. Thousand Oaks, Calif.: SAGE Publications; 2013.
Short, basic text that covers question writing, questionnaire format, sampling, survey administration design, data analysis, creating code books, and presenting results. 173 pages.

Fink A. *The Survey Kit*, 2nd ed. Thousand Oaks, Calif.: SAGE Publications; 2003.
Practical 10-volume set: 1. Fink A. *The Survey Handbook.* 2. Fink A. *How to Ask Survey Questions.* 3. Bourque LB, Fielder EP. *How to Conduct Self-Administered and Mail Surveys.* 4. Bourque LB, Fielder EP. *How to Conduct Telephone Surveys.* 5. Oishi SM. *How to Conduct In-Person Interviews for Surveys.* 6. Fink A. *How to Design Survey Studies.* 7. Fink A. *How to Sample in Surveys.* 8. Litwin MS. *How to Assess and Interpret Survey Psychometrics.* 9. Fink A. *How to Manage, Analyze, and Interpret Survey Data.* 10. Fink A. *How to Report on Surveys.*

Fowler FJ. *Survey Research Methods (Applied Social Research Methods)*, 5th ed. Thousand Oaks, Calif.: SAGE Publications; 2014.
Short text on survey research methods, including chapters on sampling, nonresponse, data collection, designing questions, evaluating survey questions and instruments, interviewing, data analysis, and ethical issues. Focuses on reducing sources of error. 171 pages.

Krueger RA, Casey MA. *Focus Groups: A Practical Guide for Applied Research*, 5th ed. Thousand Oaks, Calif.: SAGE Publications; 2015.
Practical how-to book that covers uses of focus groups, planning, developing questions, determining focus group composition, moderating skills, data analysis, and reporting results. 252 pages.

Journal

VanGeest JB, Johnson TP, eds. Special issue: Surveying clinicians. *Eval Health Prof.* 2013;36: 275–407.
A theme issue reviewing methodologies for collecting information from physicians and other members of the interdisciplinary health care team. 1) Facilitators and Barriers to Survey Participation by Physicians: A Call to Action for Researchers. 2) Sample Frame and Related Sample Design Issues for Surveys of Physicians and Physician Practices. 3) Estimating the Effect of Nonresponse Bias in a Survey of Hospital Organizations. 4) Surveying Clinicians by Web: Current Issues in Design and Administration. 5) Enhancing Surveys of Health Care Professionals: A Meta-Analysis of Techniques to Improve Response.

Internet Resources

American Association for Public Opinion Research.
The American Association for Public Opinion Research (AAPOR) is a U.S. professional organization of public opinion and survey research professionals, with members from academia, media, government, the nonprofit sector, and private industry. It provides educational opportunities in survey research, provides resources for researchers on a range of survey and polling issues, and publishes the print journal *Public Opinion Quarterly* and the e-journal *Survey Practice*. Available at www.aapor.org.

Survey Research Methods Section, American Statistical Association.
Provides a downloadable "What Is a Survey" booklet on survey methodology and links to other resources. Available at www.amstat.org/sections/SRMS/index.html.

SPECIFIC REFERENCES

1. Sleezer CM, Russ-Eft DF, Gupta K. *A Practical Guide to Needs Assessment*, 3rd ed. San Francisco: John Wiley & Sons (published by Wiley); 2014. P. 24.
2. Tanner D, Tanner L. *Curriculum Development: Theory into Practice*, 4th ed. Upper Saddle River, N.J.: Pearson; 2007. Pp. 116–23, 186–87.
3. Tyler RW. *Basic Principles of Curriculum and Instruction*. Chicago: University of Chicago Press; 2013. Pp. 63–82.
4. Ornstein AC, Hunkins FP. *Curriculum: Foundations, Principles, and Issues*, 6th ed. Harlow, Essex, U.K.: Pearson; 2014. Pp. 9–14.
5. Hafferty FW, Franks R. The hidden curriculum, ethics teaching, and the structure of medical education. *Acad Med*. 1994;69:861–71.
6. Hundert EM, Hafferty F, Christakis D. Characteristics of the informal curriculum and trainees' ethical choices. *Acad Med*. 1996;71:624–42.
7. Hafferty FW. Beyond curriculum reform: confronting medicine's hidden curriculum. *Acad Med*. 1998;73:403–7.
8. Holmes CL, Harris IB, Schwartz AJ, Regehr G. Harnessing the hidden curriculum: a four-step approach to developing and reinforcing reflective competencies in medical clinical clerkship. *Adv Health Sci Educ Theory Pract*. 2014; Oct 16. doi:10.1007/s10459-014-9558-9.
9. Henwood PC, Mackenzie DC, Rempell JS, et al. A practical guide to self-sustaining point-of-care ultrasound education programs in resource-limited settings. *Ann Emerg Med*. 2014; 64(3):277–85.e2.
10. Example adapted with permission from the curricular project of Tahara Akmal, MA, Ty Crowe, MDiv, Patrick Hemming, MD, MPH, Tommy Rogers, MDiv, Emmanuel Saidi, PhD, Monica Sandoval, MD, and Paula Teague, DMin, MBA, for the Johns Hopkins Longitudinal Program in Faculty Development, cohort 26, 2012–2013.
11. Sleezer CM, Russ-Eft DF, Gupta K. *A Practical Guide to Needs Assessment*, 4th ed. San Francisco: John Wiley & Sons (published by Wiley); 2014. Pp. 117–71.
12. Puchalski C, Romer AL. Taking a spiritual history allows clinicians to understand patients more fully. *J Palliat Med*. 2000;3(1):129–37.
13. Borneman T, Ferrell B, Puchalski CM. Evaluation of the FICA tool for spiritual assessment. *J Pain Symptom Manage*. 2010;40(2):163–73.
14. Sheth SS, Fader AN, Tergas AI, Kushnir CL, Green IC. Virtual reality robotic surgical simulation: an analysis of gynecology trainees. *J Surg Educ*. 2014 Jan–Feb;71(1):125–32.
15. Example adapted with permission from the curricular project of Amanda Nickles Fader, MD, for the Johns Hopkins Longitudinal Program in Faculty Development, cohort 25, 2011–2012.
16. Example adapted with permission from the curricular project of Sajida Chaudry, MD, MPH, Clarence Lam, MD, MPH, Elizabeth Salisbury-Afshar, MD, MPH, and Miriam Alexander, MD, MPH, for the Johns Hopkins Longitudinal Program in Faculty Development, cohort 26, 2012–2013.
17. Blue AV, Mitcham M, Smith T, Raymond J, Greenberg R. Changing the future of health professions: embedding interprofessional education within an academic health center. *Acad Med*. 2010;85(8):1290–95.
18. Association of American Medical Colleges. Medical Academic Performance Services (MedAPS) [Internet]. Available at www.aamc.org/initiatives/medaps.
19. Altschuld JW, ed. *The Needs Assessment KIT*. Thousand Oaks, Calif.: SAGE Publications; 2010.
20. Altschuld JW. *Bridging the Gap between Asset/Capacity Building and Needs Assessment: Concepts and Practical Applications*. Thousand Oaks, Calif.: SAGE Publications; 2015. Pp. 25–49.

21. Bryson JM. *Strategic Planning for Public and Nonprofit Organizations*, 4th ed. San Francisco: Jossey-Bass, John Wiley & Sons; 2011.
22. Bryson JM, Alston FK. *Creating Your Strategic Plan: A Workbook for Public and Nonprofit Organizations*, 3rd ed. San Francisco: Jossey-Bass, John Wiley & Sons; 2011.
23. Fink A. *How to Conduct Surveys: A Step-by-Step Guide*, 5th ed. Thousand Oaks, Calif.: SAGE Publications; 2013. Pp. 29–56.
24. Sleezer CM, Russ-Eft DF, Gupta K. *A Practical Guide to Needs Assessment*, 3rd ed. San Francisco: John Wiley & Sons; 2014. Pp. 52–57.
25. Krueger RA, Casey MA. *Focus Groups: A Practical Guide for Applied Research*, 5th ed. Thousand Oaks, Calif.: SAGE Publications; 2015.
26. Sleezer CM, Russ-Eft DF, Gupta K. *A Practical Guide to Needs Assessment*, 3rd ed. San Francisco: John Wiley & Sons; 2014. Pp. 57–59.
27. Tourangeau R, Conrad FG, Couper MP. *The Science of Web Surveys.* Oxford: Oxford University Press; 2013. Pp. 57–98.
28. Dillman DA, Smyth JD, Christian LM. *Internet, Phone, Mail, and Mixed-Mode Surveys: The Tailored Design Method*, 4th ed. Hoboken, N.J.: John Wiley & Sons; 2014. Pp. 303–10.
29. Fink A. *How to Conduct Surveys: A Step-by-Step Guide*, 5th ed. Thousand Oaks, Calif.: SAGE Publications; 2013. Pp. 11–25.
30. Fink A. *The Survey Kit*, 2nd ed. *Volume 2: How to Ask Survey Questions.* Thousand Oaks, Calif.: SAGE Publications; 2003. Pp. 1–91.
31. Sleezer CM, Russ-Eft DF, Gupta K. *A Practical Guide to Needs Assessment*, 3rd ed. San Francisco: John Wiley & Sons; 2014. Pp. 59–71.
32. Dillman DA, Smyth JD, Christian LM. *Internet, Phone, Mail, and Mixed-Mode Surveys: The Tailored Design Method*, 4th ed. Hoboken, N.J.: John Wiley & Sons; 2014. Pp. 301–18.
33. Fink A. *The Survey Kit*, 2nd ed. *Volume 9: How to Manage, Analyze, and Interpret Survey Data.* Thousand Oaks, Calif.: SAGE Publications; 2003. Pp. 1–24.
34. Groves RM, Dillman DA, Eltinge JL, Little RJA. *Survey Nonresponse* (Wiley Series in Survey Methodology). Hoboken, N.J.: John Wiley & Sons; 2001. Pp. 3–26.
35. Asch DA, Jedrziewski MK, Christakis NA. Response rates to mail surveys published in medical journals. *J Clin Epidemiol*. 1997;50(10):1129–36.
36. Kellerman SE, Herold J. Physician response to surveys: a review of the literature. *Am J Prev Med*. 2001;20(1):61–67.
37. Field TS, Cadoret CA, Brown ML, et al. Surveying physicians: do components of the "Total Design Approach" to optimizing survey response rates apply to physicians? *Med Care*. 2002;40(7):596–605.
38. VanGeest JB, Johnson TP, Welch VL. Methodologies for improving response rates in surveys of physicians: a systematic review. *Eval Health Prof*. 2007;30(4):303–21.
39. Thorpe C, Ryan B, McLean SL, et al. How to obtain excellent response rates when surveying physicians. *Fam Pract*. 2009;26(1):65–68.
40. Martins Y, Lederman RI, Lowenstein CL, et al. Increasing response rates from physicians in oncology research: a structured literature review and data from a recent physician survey. *Br J Cancer*. 2012;106(6):1021–26.
41. Dykema J, Jones NR, Piché T, Stevenson J. Surveying clinicians by web: current issues in design and administration. *Eval Health Prof*. 2013;36:352–81.
42. Cho YI, Johnson TP, VanGeest JB. Enhancing surveys of health care professionals: a meta-analysis of techniques to improve response. *Eval Health Prof*. 2013;36:382–407.
43. Dillman DA, Smyth JD, Christian LM. *Internet, Phone, Mail, and Mixed-Mode Surveys: The Tailored Design Method*, 4th ed. Hoboken, N.J.: John Wiley & Sons; 2014. Pp. 398–449.
44. Schuller MC, DaRosa DA, Crandall ML. Using just-in-time teaching and peer instruction in a residency program's core curriculum: enhancing satisfaction, engagement, and retention. *Acad Med*. 2015;90(3):384–91.

45. Stevahn L, King JA. *Needs Assessment Phase III: Taking Action for Change* (Needs Assessment KIT Book 5). Thousand Oaks, Calif.: SAGE Publications; 2010. Pp. 133–49.

46. Fink A. *The Survey Kit*, 2nd ed. *Volume 9: How to Manage, Analyze, and Interpret Survey Data.* Thousand Oaks, Calif.: SAGE Publications; 2003. Pp. 25–121.

47. Altschuld JW, White JL. *Needs Assessment: Analysis and Prioritization* (Needs Assessment KIT Book 4). Thousand Oaks, Calif.: SAGE Publications; 2010.

48. Miles MB, Huberman AM. *Qualitative Data Analysis: A Methods Sourcebook*, 3rd ed. Thousand Oaks, Calif.: SAGE Publications; 2014.

49. Richards MG, Morse JM. *README FIRST for a User's Guide to Qualitative Methods*, 3rd ed. Thousand Oaks, Calif.: SAGE Publications; 2013.

50. Lichtman M. *Understanding and Evaluating Qualitative Educational Research.* Thousand Oaks, Calif.: SAGE Publications; 2011.

51. Wolfe L, Ryden J. Primary care gynecology for internal medicine residents. Appendix A in: Kern DE, Thomas PA, Hughes MT. *Curriculum Development for Medical Education: A Six-Step Approach*, 2nd ed. Baltimore: Johns Hopkins University Press; 2009. Pp. 201–16.

52. Example adapted with permission from the curricular project of Lauren Block, MD, MPH, Melissa Morgan-Gouveia, MD, Samuel Williams, MD, and Danelle Cayea, MD, MS, for the Johns Hopkins Longitudinal Program in Faculty Development, cohort 25, 2011–2012.

Step 3
Goals and Objectives

. . . focusing the curriculum

Patricia A. Thomas, MD

DEFINITIONS

Once the needs of the learners have been clarified, it is desirable to target the curriculum to address these needs by setting goals and objectives. *A goal or objective is defined as an end toward which an effort is directed. In this book, the term "goal" will be used when broad educational objectives are being discussed. The term "objective" will be used when specific measurable objectives are being discussed.*

EXAMPLE: *Goal versus Specific Measurable Objective.* A *goal* (or broad educational objective) of a transitions of care curriculum for internal medicine residents is that the residents develop the knowledge, attitudes, and skills necessary to effect safe transitions of care in both inpatient and outpatient settings. A *specific measurable objective* of the curriculum might be that, by the end of the orientation curriculum week, each resident will have demonstrated, at least once, the appropriate technique, as defined on a check sheet, for a verbal and a written handoff of patient care to a colleague.

IMPORTANCE

Goals and objectives are important because they do the following:

- help direct the choice of curricular content and the assignment of relative priorities to various components of the curriculum;
- suggest what learning methods will be most effective;
- enable evaluation of learners and the curriculum, thus permitting demonstration of the effectiveness of a curriculum;
- suggest what evaluation methods are appropriate;
- clearly communicate to others, such as learners, faculty, program directors, department chairs, and individuals from other institutions, what the curriculum addresses and hopes to achieve.

Broad educational goals communicate the overall purposes of a curriculum and serve as criteria against which the selection of various curricular components can be judged. The development and the prioritization of *specific measurable objectives* permit further refinement of the curricular content and guide the selection of appropriate educational and evaluation methods.

WRITING OBJECTIVES

Writing educational objectives is an underappreciated skill. Despite the importance of objectives, learners, teachers, and curriculum planners frequently have difficulty in formulating or explaining the objectives of a curriculum. Poorly written objectives can result in a poorly focused and inefficient curriculum, prone to "drift" over time from its original goals.

A key to writing useful educational objectives is to make them *specific and measurable*. *Five basic elements* should be included in such objectives (1):

<u>Who</u> <u>will do</u> <u>how much (how well)</u> <u>of what</u> <u>by when</u>?

1)   2)   3)   4)   5)

EXAMPLE: *Specific Measurable Objective.* The example provided at the beginning of the chapter contains these elements: Who (each resident) will do (demonstrate) how much/how well (once/the appropriate protocol per checklist) of what (communicating both written and verbal handoff of patient care) by when (by the end of resident orientation)? That objective could be measured by observation using a checklist.

In other words, the specific measurable objective should include 2) a verb and 4) a noun that describe a *performance*, as well as 3) a *criterion* and 3) and 5) *conditions* of the performance. In writing specific measurable objectives (as opposed to goals), one should *use verbs that are open to fewer interpretations* (e.g., to list or to demonstrate) rather than words that are open to many interpretations (e.g., to know or to be able). Table 4.1 lists more precise and less precise words to use in writing objectives. It is normal for objectives to go through several revisions. Before finalizing, it is important to *have people such as content experts and potential learners review the objectives*, to ensure that others understand what the objectives are intended to convey. Table 4.2 provides some examples of poorly written and better written objectives.

Table 4.1.   Verbs Open to More and Fewer Interpretations

Verbs Open to More Interpretations	Verbs Open to Fewer Interpretations	
Verbs that frequently apply to cognitive objectives:		
	Taxonomy of cognitive objectives (2, 3)	Verb
know	*Remember* (recall of facts)	identify list recite define recognize retrieve
understand	*Understand*	define contrast interpret classify describe sort explain illustrate
be able know how appreciate	*Apply*	implement execute use (a model, method) complete
	Analyze	differentiate distinguish organize deconstruct discriminate
	Evaluate	detect judge critique test
know how	*Create*	design hypothesize construct produce
Verbs that frequently apply to affective objectives:		
appreciate grasp the significance of	rate as valuable, rank as important	
believe	identify, rate, or rank as a belief or opinion	
enjoy	rate or rank as enjoyable	
internalize	use one of above terms	

Verbs that frequently apply to psychomotor objectives:

Skill/Competence:
be able	demonstrate
know how	show

Behavior/Performance
Internalize	use or incorporate into performance (as measured by)

Other Verbs:
learn	(use one of the above terms)
teach	(use one of the above terms; do not confuse the teacher and the learner in writing learner objectives)

TYPES OF OBJECTIVE

In constructing a curriculum, one should be aware of the different types and levels of objective. *Types of objective* include objectives related to the learning of *learners*, to the educational *process* itself, and to health care and other *outcomes* of the curriculum. These types of objective can be written at the level of the *individual learner* or at the level of the *program* or of all learners in *aggregate*. Table 4.3 provides examples of the different types of objective for a curriculum on smoking cessation.

Learner Objectives

Learner objectives include objectives that relate to learning in the cognitive, affective, and psychomotor domains. The identification of the learning needs in these domains occurred in Step 1, Problem Identification and General Needs Assessment. Learner objectives that pertain to the *cognitive* domain of learning are often referred to as "knowledge" objectives. The latter terminology, however, may lead to an overemphasis on factual knowledge. Objectives related to the cognitive domain of learning should take into consideration a spectrum of mental skills relevant to the goals of a curriculum, from simple factual knowledge to higher levels of cognitive functioning, such as problem solving and clinical decision making.

> **EXAMPLE:** *Cognitive Objective.* By the end of the neurology curriculum, the learner will describe in writing a cost-effective approach to the initial evaluation and management of a patient presenting with dementia (an approach that includes at least six of the eight elements listed on the handout).

Bloom's taxonomy was the first attempt to describe this potential hierarchy of mental skills (2). At the time of its development in the mid-twentieth century, Bloom's taxonomy of cognitive learning objectives conceptualized a process of learning that occurred through a series of steps, which were referred to as six levels in the cognitive domain: knowledge (i.e., recall of facts), comprehension, application, analysis, synthesis, and evaluation (2). By the turn of the century, these categories were revised by Anderson and Krathwohl to incorporate modern cognitive psychology and understanding of learning (3). This version describes the second level, "understand," as constructing meaning from information, interpreting, explaining or summarizing, and the highest level, "create," as "to put elements together, generate hypotheses, plan a project" (3).

Table 4.2.   Examples of Less-Well-Written and Better-Written Objectives

Less-Well-Written Objectives	Better-Written Objectives
▪ Residents will learn the techniques of joint injections. [*The types of injection to be learned are not specified. The types of resident are not specified. It is unclear whether cognitive understanding of the technique is sufficient, or whether skills must be acquired. It is unclear by when the learning must have occurred and how proficiency could be assessed. The objective on the right addresses each of these concerns.*]	▪ By the end of the residency, each family practice resident will have demonstrated at least once (according to the attached protocol) the proper techniques for the following: - subacromial, bicipital, and intra-articular shoulder injection; - intra-articular knee aspiration and/or injection; - injections for lateral and medial epicondylitis; - injections for de Quervain's tenosynovitis; - aspiration and/or injection of at least one new bursa, joint, or tendinous area, using appropriate references and supervision.
▪ By the end of the internal medicine clerkship, each third-year medical student will be able to diagnose and manage common ambulatory medical disorders. [*This objective specifies "who" and "by when" but is vague about what it is the medical students are to achieve. The two objectives on the right add specificity to the latter.*]	▪ By the end of the internal medicine ambulatory medicine clerkship, each third-year medical student will have achieved cognitive proficiency in the diagnosis and management of hypertension, diabetes, angina, chronic obstructive pulmonary disease, hyperlipidemia, alcohol and drug abuse, smoking, and asymptomatic HIV infection, as measured by acceptable scores on interim tests and the final examination. ▪ By the end of the internal medicine clerkship, each third-year medical student will have seen and discussed with the preceptor, or discussed in a case conference with colleagues, at least one patient with each of the above disorders.
▪ Physician practices whose staff complete the three-session communication skills workshops will have more satisfied patients. [*This objective does not specify the comparison group or what is meant by "satisfied." The objective on the right specifies more precisely which practices will have more satisfied patients, what the comparison group will be, and how satisfaction will be measured. It specifies one aspect of performance as well as satisfaction. One could look at the satisfaction questionnaire and telephone management monitoring instrument for a more precise description of the outcomes being measured.*]	▪ Physician practices that have ≥50% of their staff complete the three-session communication skills workshops will have lower complaint rates, higher patient satisfaction scores on the yearly questionnaire, and better telephone management, as measured by random simulated calls, than practices that have lower completion rates.

Table 4.3.   Types of Objective: Examples from a Smoking Cessation Curriculum for Residents

	Individual Learner	Aggregate or Program
Learner		
Cognitive (knowledge)	By the end of the curriculum, each resident will be able to list the five-step approach to effective smoking cessation counseling.	By the end of the curriculum, ≥80% of residents will be able to list the five-step approach to effective smoking cessation counseling, and ≥90% will be able to list the four critical (asterisked) steps.
Affective (attitudinal)	By the end of the curriculum, each primary care resident will rank smoking cessation counseling as an important and effective intervention by primary care physicians (≥3 on a 4-point scale).	By the end of the curriculum, there will have been a statistically significant increase in how primary care residents rate the importance and effectiveness of smoking cessation counseling by primary care physicians.
Psychomotor (skill or competence)	During the curriculum, each primary care resident will demonstrate in role-play a smoking cessation counseling technique that incorporates the attached five steps.	During the curriculum, ≥80% of residents will have demonstrated in role-play a smoking cessation counseling technique that incorporates the attached five steps.
Psychomotor (behavioral or performance)	By 6 months after completion of the curriculum, each primary care resident will have negotiated a plan for smoking cessation with ≥60% of his/her smoking patients or have increased the percentage of such patients by ≥20% from baseline.	By 6 months after completion of the curriculum, there will have been a statistically significant increase in the percentage of GIM residents who have negotiated a plan for smoking cessation with their patients.
Process	Each primary care resident will have attended both sessions of the smoking cessation workshop.	≥80% of primary care residents will have attended both sessions of the smoking cessation workshop.
Patient outcome	By 12 months after completion of the curriculum, the smoking cessation rate (for ≥6 months) for the patients of each primary care resident will have increased twofold or more from baseline or be ≥10%.	By 12 months after completion of the curriculum, there will have been a statistically significant increase in the percentage of primary care residents' patients who have quit smoking (for ≥6 months).

Marzano and Kendall further refined the taxonomy based on their review of the literature (4). They identify four levels: retrieval of knowledge, comprehension, analysis, and use of knowledge. They also emphasize the importance of *learner motivation*, beliefs and emotions (self-system), and goal setting and self-monitoring (metacognition) in learning.

To some extent, these taxonomies are hierarchical, although cognitive expertise is no longer assumed to develop linearly through these levels. Curriculum planners usually specify the highest-level objective expected of the learner. The level of objectives is implied by the choice of verbs (see Table 4.1). The ability to *explain* and *illustrate*, for example, is a higher-level objective than the ability to *list* or *recite*. Planners should also recognize that there are *enabling objectives* necessary to attain a certain level. In the example above, learners will need to know the differential diagnosis of dementia and the operating characteristics of diagnostic tests before they can implement a cost-effective approach. Understanding the need for these enabling objectives will help curriculum developers to plan educational strategies.

Learner objectives that pertain to the *affective* domain are frequently referred to as "attitudinal" objectives. They may refer to specific attitudes, values, beliefs, biases, emotions, or role expectations that can affect a learner's learning or performance. Affective objectives are usually more difficult to express and to measure than cognitive objectives (5). Indeed, some instructional design experts maintain that, because attitudes cannot be accurately assessed by learner performance, attitudinal objectives should not be written (6). Affective objectives, however, are implicit in most health professions' educational programs. Nearly every curriculum, for instance, holds as an affective objective that learners will value the importance of learning the content, which is critical to attaining other learner objectives. This objective relates to Marzano and Kendall's "self-system" (see above), which includes motivation, emotional response, perceived importance, and efficacy, and which they argue is an important underpinning of learning. Actual experiences within and outside medical institutions (termed the "informal" and "hidden" curricula) may run counter to what is formally taught (7, 8). Therefore, it behooves curriculum developers to recognize and address such attitudes and practices.

To the extent that a curriculum involves learning in the affective domain, having a written objective will help to alert learners to the importance of such learning. Such objectives can help direct educational strategies, even when there are insufficient resources to objectively assess their achievement.

> **EXAMPLE:** *Affective Objective.* By the end of the Health Care Disparities course week, first-year medical students will have demonstrated a deeper awareness of their own biases, as demonstrated in a reflective writing assignment.

Learner objectives that relate to the *psychomotor* domain of learning are often referred to as "skill" or "behavioral" objectives. These objectives refer to specific psychomotor tasks or actions that may involve hand or body movements, vision, hearing, speech, or the sense of touch. Medical interviewing, patient education and counseling, interpersonal communication, physical examination, record keeping, and procedural skills fall into this domain. In writing objectives for relevant psychomotor skills, it is helpful to indicate whether learners are expected only to achieve the ability to perform a skill (a "skill" objective) or are also expected to incorporate the skill into their actual behavior *in the workplace* (a "behavioral" or "performance" objective). This book will use the term *behavioral objective* to mean an observable skill in the workplace environment that is done repeatedly or habitually, such as routinely using a surgery checklist before starting an operating room procedure. The term *performance objective* will be used to indicate a skill that has been observed at least once in the workplace setting, such as adherence to Advanced Cardiovascular Life Support (ACLS) protocol for a cardiac arrest. Whether a psychomotor skill is written as a skill or as a behavioral objective has important implications for the choice of evaluation strategies and may influence the choice of educational strategies (see Chapter 5).

> **EXAMPLE:** *Skill Objective.* By the end of the curriculum, all medical students will have demonstrated proficiency in assessing alcohol use, using all four of the CAGE questions with one simulated and one real patient. (This skill objective can be assessed by direct or video-recorded observation by an instructor.)

> **EXAMPLE:** *Behavioral Objective.* All students who have completed the curriculum will routinely (>80% of time) use the CAGE questions to assess their patients' alcohol use. (This behavioral objective might be indirectly assessed by reviewing a random sample of student write-ups of the new patients they evaluate during their core medicine clerkship.)

Another way to envision the learner objectives related to clinical competence is in the hierarchy implied by Miller's assessment pyramid (9). The pyramid implies that clinical competence begins with building a knowledge base (knows) and proceeds to learning a related skill (knows how), demonstrating the skill (shows how), and finally performing in actual clinical practice (does). While the learning objective may be stated as the highest objective of the pyramid, it is important, again, to recognize that there are *enabling objectives* necessary to achieve this objective that may require the attention of the curriculum developer. Attainment of a skill objective usually implies attainment of prerequisite knowledge. Attainment of a performance objective implies attainment of prerequisite knowledge, attitudes, and skills. Because some objectives encompass more than one domain, efficiency may be achieved by clearly articulating the highest-order objective, without separately articulating the underlying cognitive, affective, and skill objectives. This approach is the hallmark of competency-based frameworks (see below), which state the outcomes of educational programs as integrated competencies. From the evaluation perspective, achievement of a performance objective implies achievement of the prerequisite underlying objectives. However, educational strategies must still address the knowledge, attitudes, and skills that the learner requires to perform well.

> **EXAMPLE:** *Multidomain Objective.* At the completion of a continuing medical education course, "Update in Cardiology," participants will uniformly implement the ACC/AHA clinical practice guidelines for care of adults with ST-elevation myocardial infarction. (This objective implies knowledge of guidelines, valuing the importance of the guidelines in improving patient outcomes, and skill in patient care.)

Process Objectives

Process objectives relate to the implementation of the curriculum. They may indicate the degree of participation that is expected from the learners (see Table 4.3). They may indicate the expected learner or faculty response to or satisfaction with a curriculum. *Program process objectives* address the success of the implementation at the program level and are often aggregated learner process objectives.

> **EXAMPLE:** *Individual Process Objective.* Each resident during the PGY-2 year will participate in a critical incident root cause analysis as part of a multidisciplinary team.

> **EXAMPLE:** *Program Process Objectives.* By the end of this academic year, 90% of PGY-2 residents will have participated in a critical incident root cause analysis and in a hospital patient safety initiative.

Outcome Objectives

In this book, we use the term *outcome objectives* to refer to *health, health care, and patient outcomes* (i.e., the impact of the curriculum beyond that delineated in its learner and process objectives). Outcomes might include health outcomes of patients or career choices of physicians. More proximal outcomes might include changes in the behaviors of patients, such as smoking cessation (10). Outcome objectives relate to the health care problem that the curriculum addresses. Unfortunately, the term "outcome objectives" is not consistently used, and learner cognitive, affective, and psychomotor objectives are sometimes referred to as outcomes, such as knowledge, attitudinal, or skill outcomes. To avoid confusion, it is best to describe the objective by using precise language that includes the specific type of outcome that will be measured.

> **EXAMPLE:** *Career Outcome Objective.* Eighty percent or more of the graduates of our primary care residency programs will be pursuing careers in primary care five years after graduation.

> **EXAMPLE:** *Behavioral and Health Outcome Objectives.* Physicians who have completed the two-session continuing education course on basic interviewing skills will demonstrate, during audio-recorded doctor-patient encounters 1 to 2 months later, a significantly greater use of taught skills in their practice setting than control group physicians (*learner psychomotor behavioral objective*). Their emotionally disturbed patients, as determined by General Health Questionnaire (GHQ) scores of 5 or more, will show significantly greater improvement in GHQ scores at 2 weeks, 3 months, and 6 months following the course (*health outcome objective*) (11).

It is often unrealistic to expect medical curricula to have easily measurable effects on quality of care and patient outcomes. (Medical students, for example, may not have responsibility for patients until years after completion of a curriculum.) However, most medical curricula should be designed to have positive effects on quality of care and patient outcomes. Even if outcomes will be difficult or impossible to measure, the inclusion of some health outcome objectives in a curriculum plan will emphasize the ultimate aims of the curriculum and may influence the choice of curricular content and educational methods.

At this point, it may be useful to review Table 4.3 for examples of each type and level of objective.

COMPETENCY AND COMPETENCY-BASED EDUCATION

Competency-based education (CBE) is a new paradigm of medical education that is driven by systems needs rather than by learner needs and is outcomes-defined, time-variable rather than time-defined, outcomes-variable (12, 13). The goals of a CBE program are the attainment of health system or patient outcomes. (Notice the relationship to Step 1, Problem Identification). Learner outcomes in CBE are articulated as achievement of *competencies*, which are observable behaviors that result from the integration of knowledge, attitudes, and psychomotor skills. Competencies are often grouped into *domains of competence*, with more specific professional behaviors subsumed in the domain. For example, the competency domains for residency education in North America were first published as part of the Accreditation Council for Graduate Medical Education (ACGME) Outcome Project in 1999, as follows: Patient Care, Medical Knowledge, Interpersonal and Communication Skills, Practice-Based Learning and Improvement, Professionalism, and Systems-Based Care (14). These six core competencies continue to be refined and enhanced as training programs acquire more experience with them, and seek a connection with patient and systems outcomes (14, 15).

Learner progression in CBE is described as progression from novice to competent to master level. The progression is tracked by achievement of *milestones* rather than by documentation of time in the program. Recent publications have argued that competence is a trait of the learner and that the behaviors that are being assessed should be termed *activities*. The point at which the learner has demonstrated an activity at the level that no longer requires direct supervision is termed an *entrustable professional activity* (EPA) (15).

> **EXAMPLE:** *Patient Care.* One domain of General Physician Competencies is: "Patient Care: Provide patient-centered care that is compassionate, appropriate, and effective for the treatment of health problems and the promotion of health." Within this domain, one of several more specific behaviors is: "Interpret laboratory data, imaging studies and other tests required for the area of practice" (16).

Note that while attainment of competency is clearly a learner objective, the written descriptor is far more general than a specific learning objective as defined in this book and better fits the definition of a "goal" than an "objective" in the six-step approach.

> **EXAMPLE:** *Practice-Based Learning and Improvement Competency and Milestone.* Competencies specified by the American Board of Pediatrics include: "Practice-based Learning and Improvement: Use information technology to optimize learning and care delivery." The second-level *developmental milestone* for this competency is described as: "Demonstrates a willingness to try new technology for patient care assignments or learning. Able to identify and use several available databases, search engines, or other appropriate tools, resulting in a manageable volume of information, most of which is relevant to the clinical question. Basic use of an EHR [electronic health record] is improving, as evidenced by greater efficacy and efficiency in performing needed tasks. Beginning to identify shortcuts to getting the right information quickly, such as use of filters" (17).

Note that the developmental milestone is more specific but also implies that *habitual and ongoing development of attitudes and skills* has been directly observed by a faculty member and, as written, is not clearly measurable.

A 2013 review of multiple international health professions competency frameworks found surprising consistency in these domains, adding only two to the six ACGME competencies (16). The additional domains are *Interprofessionalism* and *Personal and Professional Identity Formation*. The competencies related to interprofessionalism were published as a consensus statement from the Interprofessional Education Collaborative in 2011 (18). *Professional Formation* was defined in the 2010 Carnegie Report as "habits of thought, feeling and action that allow learners to *demonstrate compassionate, communicative, and socially responsible physicianhood*" (19). Competence in this domain is envisioned as a professional with "a deep sense of commitment and responsibility to patients, colleagues, institutions, society and self and an unfailing aspiration to perform better and achieve more" (19). Behaviors in this domain include resilience, searching for improvements in care, wellness, and effective work-life balance.

Medical education is clearly moving to standardize the competency language used across the continuum from medical student to practicing physician. In 2013, the

Association of American Medical Colleges (AAMC) published its *Reference List of General Physician Competencies* (16) and requested that all medical schools map their educational program objectives to this taxonomy. The discipline descriptors of these competencies will, in all likelihood, continue to be refined and codified by the specialties. EPAs for medical students, the *Core Entrustable Professional Activities for Entering Residency*, were also published by the Association for American Medical Colleges in 2013 and are in pilot implementation as of this writing (20). For curriculum developers, it is most important to be aware of these overarching goals and to consider how specific learning objectives for the planned curriculum could support and map to competency development.

ADDITIONAL CONSIDERATIONS

While educational objectives are a crucial part of any curriculum, it is important to remember that *most educational experiences encompass much more than a list of preconceived objectives* (21, 22). For example, on clinical rotations, much learning derives from unanticipated experiences with individual patients. In many situations, the most useful learning derives from learning needs identified and pursued by individual learners and their mentors. An exhaustive list of objectives in such settings can be overwhelming for learners and teachers alike, stifle creativity, and limit learning related to individual needs and experiences. On the other hand, if no goals or objectives are articulated, learning experiences will be unfocused, and important cognitive, affective, or psychomotor objectives may not be achieved.

Goals provide desired overall direction for a curriculum. An important and difficult task in curriculum development is to develop a *manageable number of specific measurable objectives* that:

- interpret the goals;
- focus and prioritize curricular components that are critical to realization of the goals; and
- encourage (or at least do not limit) creativity, flexibility, and nonprescribed learning relevant to the curriculum's goals.

> **EXAMPLE:** *Use of Goals and Objectives to Encourage Learning from Experience.* A broad goal for a residency in general internal medicine might be for learners to become proficient in the cost-effective diagnosis and management of common clinical problems. Once these clinical problems have been identified, patient case-mix can be assessed to determine whether or not the settings used for training provide the learners with adequate clinical experience.
>
> Broad goals for clinical rotations in the same residency program might be that residents develop as self-directed learners, develop sound clinical reasoning skills, and use evidence-based and patient-centered approaches in the care they provide. Specific measurable *process objectives* could promote the achievement of these goals without being unnecessarily restrictive. One such objective might be that each resident, during the course of a one-month clinical rotation, will present a 15-minute report on a patient management question encountered during that month that incorporates principles of clinical epidemiology, evidence-based medicine, clinical decision making, cost-effectiveness, and an assessment of patient or family preferences. A second objective might be that, each week during the rotation, each resident identifies a question relevant to the care of one of his or her patients and briefly reports, during morning rounds, the sources used, the search time required, and the answer to the question.

Usually, several cycles of writing objectives are required to achieve a manageable number of specific measurable objectives that truly match the needs of one's targeted learners.

EXAMPLE: *Refining and Prioritizing Objectives.* Faculty developing a curriculum on diabetes for the residency in the above example might begin with the following objectives:

1. By the end of the curriculum, each resident will be able to list each complication of diabetes mellitus.
2. By the end of the curriculum, each resident will be able to list atherosclerotic cardiovascular disease, retinopathy/blindness, nephropathy, neuropathy, and foot problems/amputation as complications of diabetes and will be able to list specific medical interventions that prevent each of these complications or their sequelae.
3. By the end of the curriculum, each resident will be able to list all of the medical and sensory findings seen in each of the neuropathies that can occur as a complication of diabetes mellitus. (Similar objectives might have been written for other complications of diabetes.)
4. Residents will know how to use insulin.

After reflection and input from others, objective 1 might be eliminated because remembering every complication of diabetes, regardless of prevalence or management implications, is felt to be of little value. Objective 3 might be eliminated as consisting of too many components and containing detail unnecessary for management by the generalist. Objective 4 might be rejected as being too general and could be rewritten in specific measurable terms. Objective 2 might be retained because it is felt that it is sufficiently detailed and relevant to the goal of training residents to be proficient in the cost-effective diagnosis and management of clinical problems commonly encountered in medical practice. In the above process, the curriculum team would have reduced the number of objectives while ensuring that the remaining objectives are sufficiently specific and relevant to direct and focus teaching and evaluation.

CONCLUSION

Writing goals and objectives is a critically important skill in curriculum development. Well-written goals and objectives define and focus a curriculum. They provide direction to curriculum developers in selecting educational strategies and evaluation methods.

QUESTIONS

For the curriculum you are coordinating, planning, or would like to be planning, please answer or think about the following questions:

1. Write one to three broad educational goals.

2. Do these goals relate to a defined competency set for the profession?

3. Write one specific measurable educational objective of each type, using the template provided.

Level of Objective

	Individual Learner	Aggregate or Program
Learner (cognitive, affective, or psychomotor)		
Process		
Health, health care, or patient outcome		

Check each objective to make sure that it includes all five elements of a specific measurable objective (Who will do how much of what by when?). Check to see that the words you used are precise and unambiguous (see Table 4.1). Have someone else read your objectives and see whether they can explain them to you accurately.

4. Do your specific measurable objectives support and further define your broad educational goals? If not, you need to reflect further on your goals and objectives and change one or the other.

5. Can you map these objectives to the defined competency set identified in Question 2?

6. Reflect on how your objectives, as worded, will focus the content, educational methods, and evaluation strategies of your curriculum. Is this what you want? If not, you may want to rewrite, add, or delete some objectives.

GENERAL REFERENCES

Anderson LW, Krathwhol DR, eds. *A Taxonomy for Learning, Teaching, and Assessing: A Revision of Bloom's Taxonomy of Educational Objectives.* New York: Longman; 2001.
A revision of Bloom's taxonomy of cognitive objectives that presents a two-dimensional framework for cognitive learning objectives. Written by cognitive psychologists and educators, with many useful examples to illustrate the function of the taxonomy. 302 pages.

Bloom BS. *Taxonomy of Educational Objectives: A Classification of Educational Objectives. Handbook 1: Cognitive Domain.* New York: Longman; 1984.
Classic text that presents a detailed classification of cognitive educational objectives. A condensed version of the taxonomy is included in an appendix for quick reference. 207 pages.

Cooke M, Irby DM, O'Brien BC. *Educating Physicians: A Call for Reform of Medical School and Residency.* San Francisco: Jossey-Boss; 2010.
This report, commissioned by the Carnegie Foundation for the Advancement of Teaching on the hundredth anniversary of the Flexner Report, takes a comprehensive look at current medical education, its strengths and limitations, and calls for four new goals of medical education: 1) standardization of learning outcomes and individualization of the learning process; 2) integration of

formal knowledge and clinical experience; 3) development of habits of inquiry and innovation; and 4) focus on professional identity formation.

Green L, Kreuter M, Deeds S, Partridge K. *Health Education Planning: A Diagnostic Approach*. Palo Alto, Calif.: Mayfield Publishing; 1980.
Basic text of health education program planning that includes the role of objectives in program planning. 306 pages.

Gronlund NE. *Writing Instructional Objectives for Teaching and Assessment*, 7th ed. Upper Saddle River, N.J.: Pearson/Merrill/Prentice Hall; 2004.
Comprehensive and well-written reference that encompasses the cognitive, affective, and psychomotor domains of educational objectives. It provides a useful updating of Bloom's and Krathwohl et al.'s texts, with many examples and tables. 136 pages.

Krathwohl DR, Bloom BS, Masia BB. *Taxonomy of Educational Objectives: Affective Domain*. New York: Longman; 1964.
Classic text that presents a detailed classification of affective educational objectives. A condensed version of the taxonomy is included in an appendix for quick reference. 196 pages.

Mager RF. *Preparing Instructional Objectives: A Critical Tool in the Development of Effective Instruction*, 3rd ed. Atlanta: CEP Press; 1997.
Readable, practical guidebook for writing objectives. Includes examples. Popular reference for professional educators, as well as health professionals who develop learning programs for their students. 185 pages.

Marzano RJ, Kendall JS. *The New Taxonomy of Educational Objectives*, 2nd ed. Thousand Oaks, Calif.: Corwin Press; 2007.
Yet another revision of Bloom's taxonomy. Based on three domains of knowledge: information, mental procedures, and psychomotor procedures. Well-written and thoughtful, this work argues for well-researched models of knowledge and learning. 167 pages.

SPECIFIC REFERENCES

1. Green L, Kreuter M, Deeds S, Partridge K. *Health Education Planning: A Diagnostic Approach*. Palo Alto, Calif.: Mayfield Publishing; 1980. Pp. 48, 50, 64–65.
2. Bloom BS. *Taxonomy of Educational Objectives: Cognitive Domain*. New York: Longman; 1984.
3. Anderson LW, Krathwohl DR, eds. *A Taxonomy for Learning, Teaching, and Assessing: A Revision of Bloom's Taxonomy of Educational Objectives*. New York: Addison Wesley Longman; 2001.
4. Marzano RJ, Kendall JS. *The New Taxonomy of Educational Objectives*, 2nd ed. Thousand Oaks, Calif.: Corwin Press; 2007.
5. Henerson ME, Morris LL, Fitz-Gibbon CT. *How to Measure Attitudes.* Book 6 in: Herman JL, ed. *Program Evaluation Kit*. Newbury Park, Calif.: SAGE Publications; 1987. Pp. 9–13.
6. Mager RF. *Preparing Instructional Objectives: A Critical Tool in the Development of Effective Instruction*, 3rd. ed. Atlanta: CEP Press; 1997. Pp. 151–54.
7. Hafferty FW. Beyond curriculum reform: confronting medicine's hidden curriculum. *Acad Med.* 1998;73:403–7.
8. Martinez W, Lehmann LS. The "hidden curriculum" and residents' attitudes about medical error disclosure: comparison of surgical and nonsurgical residents. *J Am Coll Surg.* 2013;217: 1145–50.
9. Miller G. The assessment of clinical skills/competence/performance. *Acad Med.* 1990; 65(Suppl):S63–67.
10. Cornuz J, Humair JP, Seematter L, et al. Efficacy of resident training in smoking cessation: a

randomized control trial of a program based on application of behavioral theory and practice with standardized patients. *Ann Intern Med.* 2002;136:429–37.

11. Roter DL, Hall JA, Kern DE, et al. Improving physicians' interviewing skills and reducing patients' emotional distress: a randomized clinical trial. *Arch Intern Med.* 1995;155: 1877–84.

12. Frank JR, Mungrood R, Ahmad Y, et al. Toward a definition of competency-based education in medicine: a systematic review of published definitions. *Med Teach.* 2010;32:631–37.

13. Fernandez N, Dory V, Louis-Georges S, et al. Varying conceptions of competence: an analysis of how health sciences educators define competence. *Med Educ.* 2012;46:357–65.

14. Swing SR. The ACGME outcome project: retrospective and prospective. *Med Teach.* 2007;29:648–54.

15. ten Cate O, Snell L, Carraccio C. Medical competence: the interplay between individual ability and the health care environment. *Med Teach.* 2010;32:669–75.

16. Englander R, Cameron T, Ballard AJ, et al. Toward a common taxonomy of competency domains for the health professions and competencies for physicians. *Acad Med.* 2013;88:1088–94.

17. The Pediatrics Milestone Project: A Joint Initiative of the Accreditation Council for Graduate Medical Education and the American Board of Pediatrics [Internet]. 2015. Available at https://www.acgme.org/acgmeweb/Portals/0/PDFs/Milestones/PediatricsMilestones .pdf.

18. Interprofessional Education Collaborative Expert Panel. *Core Competencies for Interprofessional Collaborative Practice: Report of an Expert Panel.* Washington, D.C.: Interprofessional Education Collaborative; 2011.

19. Cooke M, Irby DM, O'Brien BC. *Educating Physicians: A Call for Reform of Medical School and Residency.* San Francisco: Jossey-Bass; 2010. P. 41.

20. Association of American Medical Colleges. Core Entrustable Professional Activities for Entering Residency (CEPEAR) [Internet]. Washington, D.C. March 2014. Available at www .mededportal.org/icollaborative/resource/887.

21. Ende J, Atkins E. Conceptualizing curriculum for graduate medical education. *Acad Med.* 1992;67:528–34.

22. Ende J, Davidoff F. What is curriculum? *Ann Intern Med.* 1992;116:1055–57.

Step 4
Educational Strategies

. . . accomplishing educational objectives

Patricia A. Thomas, MD, and Chadia N. Abras, PhD

*True teaching is not an accumulation of knowledge; it is an awakening
of consciousness which goes through successive stages.*
—From a temple wall inside an Egyptian pyramid

*Education is what survives when what has been learned has
been forgotten.*
—B. F. Skinner

DEFINITIONS

Once the goals and specific measurable objectives for a curriculum have been determined, the next step is to *develop the educational strategies* by which the curricular objectives will be achieved. Educational strategies involve both content and methods. *Content* refers to the specific material to be included in the curriculum. *Methods* are the ways in which the content is presented.

IMPORTANCE

Educational strategies provide the means by which a curriculum's objectives are achieved. They are the heart of the curriculum, the educational intervention itself. There is a natural tendency to think of the curriculum in terms of this step alone. As we shall see, the groundwork of Steps 1 through 3 guides the selection of educational strategies.

LEARNING THEORY AND LEARNING SCIENCE

As curriculum developers think through the educational strategies that will be employed, they should be aware of some of the principles and cognitive science related to learning, and to learning by adults in particular. (See Bransford et al. and Brookfield in General References.) *Teaching* is what educators do, but *learning* is what happens within the learner. The job of curriculum developers, therefore, is largely to *facilitate* learning in curriculum participants.

In the past century, the understanding of learning was initially based on studies of children. In 1973, Malcolm Knowles published his observations that learning in adulthood was a far more complex process, influenced by differences in adult self-concept and motivation; prior experience; readiness to learn—that is, when needed rather than in advance; and orientation to learning. (See Knowles et al. in General References.) Knowles reasoned that effective curricula would engage these unique characteristics of adult approaches to learning. Knowles's learning theory was termed *andragogy*, to distinguish it from the previous child-centered theories of pedagogy. Much of the innovation in health professions education in the twentieth century, such as problem-based learning and independent study, reflected attempts to adopt an *andragogical* approach.

More recently, a body of research from cognitive science and neuroscience has built on this approach, identifying three core elements in effective learning, regardless of age: addressing preconceptions, building expertise, and developing a metacognitive approach to learning (1). Adult learners bring a wealth of different *experiences and cultures* to the learning situation that shape their interpretation of reality and their approach to learning and that should be recognized and engaged to facilitate learning. Surveying learners about prior knowledge and experience before a learning event and tailoring the event to the learners, as in *just-in-time teaching* (JiTT) pedagogy, is an approach that addresses this need (2). The *JiTT* method relies on completion of a preclass assignment (often web-based) designed to evaluate students' prior knowledge in order to tailor class instruction accordingly. This method is student-centered and promotes interactive learning. More importantly, it gives the faculty member the opportunity to correct students' prior knowledge before building new knowledge. The method creates an effective feedback loop that may lead to more effective personalized instruction.

Constructivist learning theory reasons that learners actively build knowledge by imparting meaning to new information that builds on prior knowledge and creates a conceptual framework (3). When learners repeatedly access this conceptual framework to solve problems, they develop a fluency of retrieval termed "automatism" that frees working memory for more complex thinking tasks. With experience and practice, learners can elaborate that framework to include multiple examples of its use. This elaborated framework and fluency of retrieval forms the basis of *expertise*. Educational methods should facilitate the acquisition of that conceptual framework, emphasizing a core set of principles and "big ideas," as well as practice in retrieval through application of knowledge (1).

The third element of effective learning is termed "metacognition." *Metacognition* implies assessing what one knows or needs to know in a problem-solving situation. Metacognitive thinking is embedded in the *problem-based learning* and *inquiry-based learning* approaches discussed below and is closely linked to habits of *reflection*. The skill of metacognition, or the awareness or analysis of one's own learning or thinking processes, also supports maintenance of expertise in the rapidly evolving context of health professions education, often referred to as *lifelong learning*.

Transformative learning occurs when learners change in meaningful ways—the core of *professional identity formation* in health professions education. It usually involves experiences that promote the questioning of assumptions, beliefs, and values, as well as the consideration of multiple points of view, followed by *reflection* on these experiences, a key component of *experiential learning*. Such change tends to be resisted. Transformative learning is promoted by skillful facilitation and a safe and supportive *learning environment*. The quotations at the beginning of this chapter remind us that a goal of combining educational objectives with congruent and resourceful educational strategies should be to stimulate learning that is meaningful, profound, and enduring.

DETERMINATION OF CONTENT

The content of the curriculum flows from its learning objectives. Listing the nouns used in these objectives (see Chapter 4) should outline the content of the curriculum. The amount of material presented to learners should not be too little (lacking key substance) or too much (cluttering rather than clarifying). Curriculum developers should aim to have just the right amount of detail to achieve the desired objectives and outcomes. For some curricula, it is helpful to group or sequence objectives and their associated content in a manner that is logical and promotes understanding. It is usually helpful to construct a *syllabus* for the curriculum that includes: 1) an explicit statement of learning objectives and methods, to help focus learners; 2) a schedule of the curriculum events and other practical information, such as locations and directions; 3) curricular resources (e.g., readings, cases, questions); and 4) plans for assessment. The use of learning management software allows course directors to easily provide and update these resources. When using software to deliver online content, however, it is important to attend to the issues of interface design and "cognitive load" (4). Developers should partner with an expert in instructional design to plan for efficient use of electronic resources.

CHOICE OF EDUCATIONAL METHODS

General Guidelines (Table 5.1)

Recognizing that the educational method should be consistent with principles of learning discussed above, it is helpful to keep the following additional principles in mind when considering educational methods for a curriculum.

- **Maintain Congruence between Objectives and Methods.** Choose educational methods that are most likely to achieve a curriculum's goals and objectives. One way to approach the selection of educational methods is to group the specific measurable objectives of the curriculum as cognitive, affective, or psychomotor objectives (see Chapter 4) and select educational methods most likely to be effective for the type of objective (see Table 5.2).

- **Use Multiple Educational Methods.** Individuals have different preferences for approaches to learning, sometimes referred to as *learning styles* or *learning preferences* (5). These preferences are probably dictated by both hereditary and environmental factors, but there is also a developmental aspect, since preferences can change over time (3). There has been much research on learning styles over the past decade, and many conceptual models of learning styles have been published. While the validity of designing curricula to meet learning styles has been questioned, it is clear that certain approaches work for some students and not for others (3, 6). Using an educational method that meets the learner's preference for learning promotes a learner-centered curriculum (see below) and avoids a mismatch between the educational method and the learner, which would impair successful learning. Ideally, the curriculum would use those methods that work best for individual learners. However, few curricula can be that malleable; often, a large number of learners need to be accommodated in a short period of time. The use of *different* educational methods helps to overcome the problem of presenting the information in different formats to accommodate learning preferences.

  The use of different educational methods also helps to maintain *learner interest* and provides opportunities for retrieval and *reinforcement of learning*. Such reinforcement can deepen learning, promote retention, and enhance the application of what has been learned. It is particularly relevant for curricula extending over longer time periods.

  Finally, for *curricula attempting to achieve higher-order or complex objectives that span several domains* (see Chapter 4), as is often the case with competency-based frameworks, the use of multiple educational methods facilitates the integration of several lower-level objectives.

- **Choose Educational Methods That Are Feasible in Terms of Resources.** Resource constraints may limit implementation of the ideal approach in this step, as

Table 5.1.   Guidelines for Choosing Educational Methods

- Maintain congruence between objectives and educational methods
- Use multiple educational methods
- Choose educational methods that are feasible in terms of resources

Table 5.2.   Matching Educational Methods to Objectives

Educational Method*	Cognitive: Knowledge	Cognitive: Problem Solving	Affective: Attitudinal	Psychomotor: Skills or Competence	Psychomotor: Behavioral or Performance
	Type of Objective				
Readings	+++	+	+	+	
Lectures	+++	+	+	+	
Online learning resources	+++	++	+	+	
Discussion (large or small groups)	++	++	+++	+	+
Problem-based learning/Inquiry-based learning	++	+++	+	+	+
Team-based learning	+++	+++	++	+	+
Peer teaching	+++	+++	++	+	+
Real-life and supervised clinical experiences	+	++	++	+++	++
Reflection on experience, e.g., writing	+	+	+++	+	++
Role models	+	+	+++	+	++
Demonstration	+	+	+	++	+
Simulation and artificial models†	+	++	++	+++	++
Role-plays	+	+	+++	+++	++
Standardized patients†	+	++	++	+++	++
Audio or video review of learner†			++	+++	+++
Behavioral/environmental interventions‡			+	+	+++

Note: Blank = not recommended; + = appropriate in some cases, usually as an adjunct to other methods; ++ = good match; +++ = excellent match (consensus ratings by author and editors).
*For the purposes of this table, the methods refer to chapter text descriptions.
†Assumes feedback on performance is integrated into the method.
‡Removal of barriers to performance; provision of resources that promote performance; reinforcements that promote performance.

well as in other steps. Curriculum developers will need to consider faculty time, space, availability of clinical material and experiences, and costs, as well as the availability of learner time. Faculty are often a critical resource; faculty development may be an additional consideration, especially if an innovative instructional method is chosen. Use of technology may involve initial cost but save faculty resources over the time course of the curriculum. When resource limitations threaten the achievement of curricular outcomes, objectives and/or educational strategies (content and methods) will need to be further prioritized and selectively limited. The question then becomes: What is the most that can be accomplished, given the resource limitation?

When the curriculum developer selects educational methods for a curriculum, it is helpful to weigh the advantages and disadvantages of each method under consideration. Advantages and disadvantages of commonly used educational methods are summarized for the reader in Table 5.3. Specific methods are discussed below, in relation to their function.

Methods for Achieving Cognitive Objectives

Methods that are commonly used to achieve cognitive objectives include the following:

- Readings
- Lecture
- Online learning resources or learning objects
- Discussion
- Problem-based learning
- Inquiry-based learning
- Team-based learning
- Peer teaching

For learners early in the introduction to a topic or discipline, new information can be presented as readings or lectures or through the use of online learning resources. The use of targeted *readings* can be an efficient method of presenting information. The completion of readings, however, depends on protected time for the learner to read and on the motivation of individual learners. Before they are assigned, existing publications should be assessed to ensure that they efficiently target a curriculum's objectives. Learners can be directed to use readings more effectively if the syllabus gives explicit objectives and content for individual readings.

> **EXAMPLE:** *Syllabus Materials.* To teach medical students how to critically appraise the literature, a curriculum was designed that introduced problem-based educational materials into the weekly clerkship tutorial, including 1) a set of objectives and guidelines for how to use the package, 2) a patient scenario presenting a clinical dilemma, 3) a relevant journal article, and 4) an essay defining and discussing quality standards that should be met by the article. A worksheet was provided for each journal article (7).

Perhaps the most universally applied method for addressing cognitive objectives is the *lecture*, which has the advantages of structure, low technology, and the ability to teach many learners in a short period of time. Faculty generally approach a lecture with an accompanying visual "slide" presentation program; few understand, however, that there are critical design elements in such a presentation that result in better learning (4).

> **EXAMPLE:** *Incorporating Design Principles into Lecture Presentation.* A traditional lecture on shock in a surgery clerkship was modified using multimedia design principles. Surgery clerkship students in one

Table 5.3.   Summary of Advantages and Limitations of Different Educational Methods

Educational Method	Advantages	Disadvantages
Readings	Low cost Covers fund of knowledge Transportable	Passive learning Learners must be motivated to complete Readings need updating
Lectures	Low cost Accommodates large numbers of learners Can be transmitted to multiple locations Can be recorded	Passive learning Teacher-centered Quality depends on speaker and media
Online learning resources	Does not need clinical material at hand Accessible for learners across time and space Can be interactive and provide immediate feedback	Developmental costs if not commercially available Learners need device and Internet access to use
Discussion, large group	Active learning Permits assessment of learner needs; can address misconceptions Allows learner to apply newly acquired knowledge; constructivist Suitable for higher-order cognitive objectives Exposes learners to different perspectives Technology can support	More faculty-intensive than readings or lectures Cognitive/experience base required of learners Learners need motivation to participate Group-dependent Usually facilitator-dependent Teaching space needs to facilitate with use of microphones, etc.
Discussion, small group	Active learning Reinforces other learning methods Addresses misconceptions Suitable for higher-order cognitive objectives More suitable for discussion of sensitive topics; opportunity to create a "safe environment" for students	Requires more faculty than lecture or large group discussion Faculty development in small group teaching and in session objectives Cognitive/experience base required of learners Learners need motivation to participate Teaching space should facilitate, e.g., room configuration

Table 5.3.   *(continued)*

Educational Method	Advantages	Disadvantages
Problem-based learning (PBL)/Inquiry-based learning	Active learning Facilitates higher cognitive objectives: problem solving and clinical decision making Can incorporate objectives that cross domains, such as ethics, humanism, cost-efficiency Case-based learning provides relevance and facilitates transfer of knowledge to clinical setting	Case development costs Requires faculty facilitators Faculty time to prepare exercises Learners need preparation in method and expectation of accountability for learning
Team-based learning (TBL)	Active learning Facilitates higher cognitive objectives Application exercises are relevant and facilitate transfer of problem-solving skills Collaborative Students are accountable for learning Uses less faculty than PBL and other small group learning methods	Developmental costs (Readiness Assurance Tests, application exercises) Learners need preparation in method and expectation of accountability for learning Learners may be uncomfortable with ambiguity of application exercises Requires orientation to the process of teamwork and peer evaluation
Peer teaching	Increases teacher-to-student ratio Safe environment for novice learners (more comfortable asking questions) Student/peer teachers are motivated to learn content and practice retrieval Student/peer teachers acquire teaching skills	Student/peer teachers' availability Student/peer teachers need additional development in teaching skills as well as orientation to the curriculum Need to ensure student/peer teachers receive feedback on teaching skills
Real-life and supervised clinical experiences	Relevant to learner Learners may draw on previous experiences Promotes learner motivation and responsibility Promotes higher-level cognitive, attitudinal, skill, and performance learning	May require coordination to arrange opportunities with patients, community, etc. May require clinical material when learner is ready Clinical experiences require faculty supervision and feedback Learner needs basic knowledge or skill Clinical experience needs to be monitored for case mix, appropriateness Requires reflection, follow-up

Educational Method	Advantages	Disadvantages
Reflection on experience	Promotes learning from experience Promotes self-awareness/mindfulness Can be built into discussion/group learning activities Can be done individually through assigned writings/portfolios Can be used with simulation, standardized patients, role-play, and clinical experience	Requires protected time Usually requires scheduled interaction time with another/others Often facilitator-dependent Learners may need orientation and/or motivation to complete the activity
Role models	Faculty are often available Impact often seems profound Can address the hidden curriculum	Requires valid evaluation process to identify effective role models Specific interventions usually unclear Impact depends on interaction between specific faculty member and learner Outcomes multifactorial and difficult to assess
Demonstration	Efficient method for demonstrating skills/procedures Effective in combination with experience-based learning (e.g., before practicing skill in simulated or real environment)	Passive learning Teacher-oriented Quality depends on teacher/audiovisual material
Simulation and artificial models	Excellent environment to demonstrate and practice skills Can approximate clinical situations and facilitate transfer of learning Learners can use at own pace Facilitates kinesthetic approach in visuospatial learning Facilitates deliberate practice Facilitates mastery learning approach Can be used for team skills and team communications	Requires dedicated space and models/simulators, which can be expensive; may not be available Faculty facilitators need training in teaching with simulation Multiple sessions often required to reach all learners

Table 5.3. *(continued)*

Educational Method	Advantages	Disadvantages
Role-play	Suitable for objectives that cross domains of knowledge, attitudes, and skill Efficient Low cost Can be structured to be learner-centered Can be done "on the fly"	Requires trained faculty facilitators Learners need some basic knowledge or skills Can be resource-intensive if there are large numbers of learners Artificiality, learner discomfort
Standardized patients	Ensures appropriate clinical material Approximates "real life" more closely than role-play and facilitates transfer of learning Safe environment for practice of sensitive, difficult situations with patients, families, etc. Can give feedback to learners on performance and repeat; deliberate practice model Can reuse for ongoing curricula	Cost of patients, trainers, and in some cases, dedicated space Requires an infrastructure to find and train standardized patients and coordinate them with curriculum Faculty facilitators
Audio or video review of learner	Provides accurate feedback on performance Provides opportunity for self-observation Can be used with simulation, standardized patients, role-play, and clinical experience	Requires reflection, follow-up Requires trained faculty facilitators Requires patients' permission to record, when recording interactions with real patients
Behavioral/ environmental interventions*	Influences performance	Assumes competence has been achieved Requires control over learners' real-life environment

*Removal of barriers to performance; provision of resources that promote performance; reinforcements that promote performance.

medical school were divided into three groups; two of the groups received the modified design lecture, and one group received the traditional design lecture. All students showed improved knowledge in pretest and posttest assessments, but students in the modified design group had significantly greater improvements in retention and total knowledge scores (8).

Successful lecturers develop skills that promote the learners' interest and acquisition of knowledge, such as control of the physical environment, assessing and engaging their audience, organizing their material, making transitional and summary statements, presenting examples, using emphasis and selected repetition, effectively using audiovisual aids, and facilitating an effective question-and-answer period (8–10). Medical lectures are often topic-based, with the learners serving as passive recipients of information. The inclusion of problem-solving exercises or case discussions can engage the learners in a more active process that helps them to recognize what they may not know (i.e., set learning objectives) and to apply new knowledge as it is learned.

> **EXAMPLE:** *Lecture Combined with Cases and Testing.* Endocrinology lectures in a year 1 physiology course begin with a brief overview of one to three simplified cases, followed by the didactic lecture. At the end of the lecture, the cases are reviewed in detail, and the whole class is invited to respond to a series of questions (11).

The use of *audience response systems* has also increased the interactivity of the lecture, allowing faculty to pose questions and solicit commitments (answers) from the learners. Technology employed in *classroom communication systems* has helped to engage individual learners attending large, lecture-based classes in higher education. Faculty using these systems can send tasks or problems to individual students or groups of students, who respond via mobile devices; the faculty can display results in real time and address learning needs immediately. (Note the similarity to the JiTT approach discussed earlier in this chapter.)

Video files can be used to present a lecture when a lecturer is unavailable or to provide an online resource for review by learners at an unscheduled time. Video can also be used to demonstrate standardized techniques such as taking a sexual history, appropriate surgical gowning and gloving, or performing a bedside procedure, providing the basis for actual practice (see the section on psychomotor objectives, below). Videos also have the potential to put students into clinical scenarios and improve the authenticity of case-based learning. The effective use of videos requires some redesign from the previous face-to-face lecture, such as attention to the length of the video, inclusion of interactive elements, and avoidance of cognitive overloading (4, 12).

Online resources, which have been carefully constructed to convey conceptual understanding with a combination of visual, animation, and auditory media, are proliferating in health professions education. These files, referred to as "learning objects" or, more specifically, as *reusable learning objects* (RLOs), are increasingly available for use on mobile devices and facilitate repetition and access across a longitudinal program. RLOs have proven effective in e-learning, especially since they target the needs and learning preferences of the millennial generation (13). RLOs are interactive, visual, and small in size, and they can be used and repurposed for different activities and situations to address the needs of students, which makes them learner-centered and highly effective (13). An attraction of these learning objects is that they are self-contained and give the flexibility of studying anytime, anywhere, at the student's own pace. Moreover, these objects can be very effective in training medical personnel at a distance and on the fly. Existing RLOs can be restructured with specific activities for targeted training of personnel around the world, as long as Internet access is available (14).

The use of the *flipped classroom* has been popularized in health professions education (15, 16). In this model, learners are assigned the task of mastering factual content with readings, learning objects (as noted above), or other resources before arriving at formal curricular events, which are designed as active "application exercises" such as problem solving or discussions. The faculty facilitator monitors and models critical thinking skills rather than serving as an information resource. This design emphasizes to learners the importance of problem solving and critical thinking over memorizing factual content.

> **EXAMPLE:** *Use of RLOs and the Flipped Classroom.* The Kahn Academy hosts a series of seven video files, each 8 to 12 minutes in length, that present the concepts of respiratory gas exchange (17). Students in a respiratory physiology course are directed to view these files before small group case-based discussions.

Online resources also facilitate self-paced learning, which refers to the use of programmed textbooks or software that present material organized in a sequential fashion. Learners using these systems can proceed at their own pace, identify their own knowledge deficiencies, and receive immediate feedback.

> **EXAMPLE:** *Internet-Based Curriculum, Programmed Learning.* An ambulatory curriculum for internal medicine residents was developed and delivered online. The curriculum covered 16 topics with programmed pretest-didactics-posttest. The didactics included immediate feedback to answers and links to abstracts or full-text articles. Comparison of pre- and posttests of knowledge showed improved knowledge of curricular content (18).

As noted earlier, learning and retention are enhanced when learners practice or repeatedly retrieve information from memory, and they are further enhanced when that retrieval is spaced over time (19). There is active research on the optimal timing of that spacing. Online software can facilitate the spacing and practice to improve learning. *Spaced retrieval* refers to the use of online software to trigger repeated retrieval, based on the learner's prior performance.

> **EXAMPLE:** *Online Spaced Education.* Participants attending a face-to-face continuing medical education course were randomized to receive a spaced education (SE) intervention of 40 validated questions and explanations covering four clinical topics. Repetition intervals (8-day and 16-day) were adapted to the participants based on performance; questions were retired after being correctly answered 2 weeks in a row. At week 18, a behavior survey demonstrated that participants who received the SE reported significantly greater change in their clinical behaviors than the controls (20).

Discussion moves the learner further from a passive to an active role and also facilitates retrieval of previously learned information or opportunity to add meaning to new information. Much of the learning that occurs in a discussion format depends on the skills of the instructor to create a supportive learning climate, to assess learners' needs, and to effectively use a variety of interventions. such as maintaining focus, questioning, generalizing, and summarizing for the learner (21). *Group discussion* of cases, as in attending rounds or morning report, is a popular method that allows learners to process new knowledge with faculty and peers and to identify specific knowledge deficiencies. Group discussions are most successful when facilitated by teachers trained in the techniques of small group teaching (21–24) and when participants have some background knowledge or experience. Preparatory readings can help. The *combination of lecture and small group discussion* can be extremely effective in imparting knowledge, as well as in learners' practicing the higher-order cognitive skills of assessment and integration of medical facts.

Educators can also use *asynchronous* group discussions to engage a community of learners in problem solving and discussion through the use of blogs or discussion group sites within learning management software. In health professions education, the use of online discussions has facilitated the interaction of learners across disciplines and geographic boundaries.

> **EXAMPLE:** *Online Discussion and Problem Solving.* The NYU3T curriculum is a longitudinal program for medical students and nursing students, which begins with completion of web-based modules on teamwork, conflict resolution, and communication (25). Interprofessional teams of students work together on solving problems using an instant messaging platform. In the second half of the curriculum, pairs of medical and nursing students are assigned a virtual ambulatory patient and manage that patient through acute and chronic illness (26).

Problem-based learning (PBL) is a particular use of small groups that was designed to promote learning principles of being constructivist, collaborative, self-directed, and contextual (27). In PBL, learner groups are presented with a case and set their own learning objectives, often dividing the work and teaching each other, guided by a tutor-facilitator. In a case of renal failure in a child, for instance, the learning objectives may include genitourinary anatomy, renal physiology, calcium metabolism in renal failure, and genetic disorders of renal function. Students bring new knowledge back to the PBL group, and the group problem-solves the case together. PBL is highly dependent on the tutor-facilitators and requires intensive faculty and case development. After decades of use in medical education, the efficacy of PBL compared with conventional approaches in achieving cognitive objectives is still debated, although learners report higher levels of satisfaction with this method (28, 29).

Inquiry-based learning is an extension of PBL, with the objective of acquisition of knowledge through students' independent investigation of questions for which there is often no single answer (30). Inquiry-based learning presupposes that such active engagement results in deeper understanding and internalization of knowledge than do traditional didactic approaches (31). Inquiry-based learning involves the following process: 1) taking responsibility for learning; 2) engaging with and exploring an issue; 3) developing a good question; 4) determining the information needed; 5) accessing information effectively and efficiently; 6) critically evaluating information and its sources; 7) synthesizing a coherent whole; and 8) communicating the product and process of inquiry effectively.

> **EXAMPLE:** *Inquiry-Based Learning.* A four-year medical school curriculum is revised using student-centered inquiry-based learning groups (32). For the population health objectives, the first block in year 1 introduces students to public health and to the care of individual patients, including the context of society, culture, economics, and behavioral factors. After week 1, the students explore in depth, through a series of cases, issues relevant to population health (33).

Team-based learning (TBL) is another application of small groups that requires fewer faculty than PBL. (See Michaelsen et al. in General References.) It combines reading, testing, discussion, and collaboration to achieve both knowledge and higher-order cognitive learning objectives. The process of TBL is as follows:

Phase I:
1.   Students are assigned readings or self-directed learning before class.

Phase II:
2.   On arrival to class, students take a brief knowledge test, the *Readiness Assurance Test* (RAT), and are individually scored.
3.   Students work in teams of six to seven to retake the RAT and turn in consensus answers for immediate scoring and feedback (Group or GRAT).

Phase III (may last several class periods):
4.   Groups work on problem-solving or application exercises that require use of knowledge objectives.
5.   Groups eventually share responses to exercise with entire class, and discussion is facilitated by instructor.

Regardless of the intent to emphasize critical thinking over memorization, there are some content areas in health professions education, such as gross anatomy (see Example below) and pharmacology, that require significant use of memory to become facile with concepts. The use of multimodal methods that enhance achievement of deep factual knowledge is an ideal strategy in these situations.

> **EXAMPLE**: *Integrated Multimodal Multidisciplinary Teaching of Anatomy.* A medical school gross anatomy course consisted of lectures and hours of cadaveric dissection. To enhance and contextualize learning, traditional teaching with lectures and dissection was supplemented with 3D models, imaging, computer-assisted learning, problem-based learning, surface anatomy, clinical correlation lectures, peer teaching, and team-based learning (34).

Peer teaching or near-peer (one or two levels above the learner) teaching is frequently used in medical education, although there are few published reports of its outcomes (35). Although often initiated to relieve teaching pressures for faculty, there may be solid learning benefits for a peer teaching approach. For learners, the peer facilitator may be more effective because she or he is closer to the learner's fund of knowledge and better able to understand the conceptual challenges. Learners often find the learning environment to be more comfortable with peers and are more likely to seek clarification with peers than with faculty. For the peer teachers, there is additional effort to learn the material as preparation for teaching, as well as practice with retrieval, which should reinforce retention. Students who have learned teaching and learning principles may be better learners themselves and may further develop their metacognitive skills.

Methods for Achieving Affective Objectives

Methods that are commonly used to achieve affective objectives include the following:

-    Exposure (readings, discussions, experiences), such as narrative medicine, experiential learning
-    Reflective writing
-    Facilitation of openness, introspection, and reflection
-    Role models

Attitudes can be difficult to measure, let alone change (36). Some undesirable attitudes are based on insufficient knowledge and will change as knowledge is expanded in a particular area. Others may be related to insufficient skill or lack of confidence.

Attitudinal change requires exposure to knowledge, experiences, or the views of respected others that contradict undesired and confirm desired attitudes (37). A number of educational methods have attempted to deliver this exposure. Debriefing of experiences, in the form of role-play, simulation, or clinical practice, may reveal feelings, biases, or psychological defenses that have affected performance and can be discussed. Positive experiences can reinforce desired and contradict undesired attitudes. Charon (38) has promulgated the use of *narrative medicine*, defined as the competence to recognize, interpret, and be moved by stories of illness, and linked this competence to improved clinical effectiveness. *Reflective writing*, in which students are encouraged to write about their experiences and reactions and then share them in open discussions with a trained facilitator, builds on the use of narrative (39). Targeted readings may be helpful adjuncts to other methods for developing desirable attitudes. Probably more than any other learning objective, attitudinal change is helped by the use of *facilitation techniques that promote openness, introspection, reflection, and a safe and supportive learning environment* (40–42). These facilitation methods can be incorporated into skill-building methods, such as role-plays or simulated patient exercises, where the learner may be encouraged by the group process to explore barriers to performance. Properly facilitated *small group discussions* can also promote changes in attitudes, by bringing into awareness the interests, attitudes, values, and feelings of learners and making them available for discussion. Finally, *role-model* health professionals can help change attitudes by demonstrating successful approaches to a particular problem. Interestingly, the professional attitudes that educators often aim to instill in students, such as competency, excellence, sensitivity, enthusiasm, and genuineness, are those attributes most valued by students in their teachers (43, 44).

EXAMPLE: *Attitude toward Role, Role Modeling Combined with Reflection and Discussion.* A geriatrics curriculum has as an objective that primary care residents will believe that it is their role to document the advance directive wishes of their elderly outpatients. A needs assessment instrument discovered that most residents believed that their patients did not want these discussions or had no biases about advance directives. A video interview of a respected geriatrician with several of his patients was used to model the technique of the advance directive interview, as well as the reaction of patients to the discussion. The video was used as a trigger in residents' small group discussions to talk about patient reactions to advance directives and residents' barriers to initiating these discussions.

EXAMPLE: *Attitude toward Socioeconomic Class, Experience Combined with Reflection and Discussion.* Senior nursing students participated in a one-day *poverty simulation*. In this simulation, participants assume the roles of different families living in poverty. Volunteers serve the roles of resources. The families are tasked to provide for basic necessities of food and shelter for one month, consisting of four 15-minute weeks. Exercises included applying for a job, negotiating a delayed utility bill, and applying for welfare assistance. The simulation concluded with facilitated reflection and discussion. Following the simulation, scores on a validated Attitudes about Poverty and Poor Populations Scale showed significant changes on the factor of stigma of poverty (45).

EXAMPLE: *Awareness and Management of Negative Feelings, Trigger Tape Combined with Reflection and Discussion, Role-Modeling Success.* In a substance abuse and HIV curriculum, residents watch a trigger tape of a difficult interaction between a substance-abusing HIV-infected patient and a physician. They identify and discuss the emotions and attitudes evoked by the tape and reflect on how these might influence their management of such patients. Subsequently, residents work with a highly respected role-model physician in a practice that successfully manages such cases.

Methods for Achieving Psychomotor Objectives

Skill Objectives. Methods commonly used to achieve skill objectives include the following:

- Supervised clinical experience
- Demonstration
- Simulations and artificial models
- Role-plays
- Standardized patients
- Audio or visual review of skills

Rarely is knowledge the sole prerequisite to a learner's achievement of competence in a health-related area. Health professional learners need to develop a variety of skills, such as conducting a physical examination, performing procedures, and communicating with patients and team members. The learning of skills can be facilitated when learners 1) are *introduced* to the skills by didactic presentations, demonstration, and discussion; 2) are given the opportunity to *practice* the skill; 3) are given the opportunity to *reflect* on their performance; 4) receive *feedback* on their performance; and then 5) *repeat the cycle* of discussion, practice, reflection, and feedback until mastery is achieved. This structured practice, termed *deliberate practice*, is critical to the development of expertise (46).

The development of *experiential learning* methods that promote the achievement of psychomotor objectives can be a creative process for curriculum developers. Experiential learning can be challenging for the learner and teacher alike. Experiential learning requires learners to expose their strengths and weaknesses to themselves and others. As discussed above, interpersonal skills, feelings, biases, and psychological defenses, as well as previous experiences, may affect performance and need to be discussed. Creation of a *safe and supportive learning environment* is, therefore, helpful. Methods include the development of faculty-learner rapport, disclosure by faculty of their own experiences and difficulties with the material, explicit recognition and reinforcement of the learner's strengths, and provision of feedback about deficiencies in a factual, non-judgmental, helpful, and positive manner (47).

With appropriate supervision, this cycle of learning can occur in clinical settings, such as the classic *"see one–do one–teach one"* approach. Inherent in the success of this method is modeling of the ideal behavior or skill by an experienced clinician, the availability of clinical opportunities for the learner to practice the skill under observation, time to reflect and receive feedback on performance (47), and, last, the opportunity to teach the skill to another generation of learners. Effective clinical teachers can facilitate this type of experience (see General References, below).

A number of difficulties have been noted with this approach to skills training, however, especially in an era of patient safety and patient-centeredness. In medicine, the shortened length of stay in inpatient settings and the reduced work hours for resident and student trainees have decreased the opportunities to acquire sufficient practice in real-life settings to achieve competence. When expert clinicians are not readily available for demonstration or the appropriate clinical situations are not available for practice, supplementary methods should be considered. *Videos* can be used to demonstrate a skill before the learner practices in another situation. *Simulations* of clinical situations provide the opportunity for learners to practice skills in a "safe" learning environment in which risks can be taken and mistakes made without harm (48).

Simulation has been defined as "a person, device, or set of conditions which attempts to present . . . problems authentically. The student . . . is required to respond to the problems as he or she would under natural circumstances" (49). Simulations include the use of standardized patients, partial task trainers (e.g., pelvic models), manikins with computer technology to reproduce physiology (e.g., anesthesia simulators), and virtual reality high-fidelity simulators (e.g., laparoscopic surgery simulators). In situ simulations involve the use of simulations, models and practice in the actual clinical site, such as team practice before a complicated procedure.

> **EXAMPLE:** *Simulation with Manikin: Cardiac Patient Simulator.* Medical students enrolled in a cardiology elective were randomized to a two-week multimedia educational intervention including the "Harvey" patient simulator plus 2 weeks of ward work versus 4 weeks of ward work. In posttest analysis, intervention students acquired nearly twice the core bedside cardiology skills in half the time compared with the control group (50).

> **EXAMPLE:** *In Situ Simulation: Mock Codes.* To improve the performance of pediatric cardiopulmonary resuscitation interprofessional teams, monthly "mock" cardiac arrests were staged with a human simulator on hospital floor units, without prior notice to the teams. Video recordings of the mock codes were debriefed with a trained facilitator. After 48 months of random mock codes, resuscitation survival increased from 30% to 50% and remained stable for 3 years of follow-up (51).

A critical review of simulation in medical education research focused on 12 features and best practices in simulation-based educational interventions (52). Curriculum developers should keep these features in mind when making the decision to incorporate this methodology. They are:

1. Feedback
2. Deliberate practice
3. Curriculum integration
4. Outcome measurement
5. Simulation fidelity
6. Skill acquisition maintenance
7. Mastery learning
8. Transfer to practice
9. Team training
10. High-stakes testing
11. Instructor training
12. Educational and professional context

The importance of debriefing the simulation as a team to provide a structured reflection on the experience cannot be overemphasized (53).

Role-playing, during which the learner plays one role (e.g., clinician) and another learner or faculty member plays another role (e.g., patient), provides the opportunity for learners to experience different roles (54). It is most useful for teaching communication skills, physical examination techniques, and the recognition of normal physical examination findings. It permits the learner to try, observe, and discuss alternative techniques until a satisfactory performance has been achieved. It is efficient, inexpensive, and portable and can be used spontaneously in any setting. It may be as effective as the use of simulated patients (55). Role-plays can be constructed on the spot to address individual learner needs as they are identified. Limitations include variable degrees of artificiality and learner and faculty discomfort with the technique. Facilitators can alleviate students' initial discomfort by discussing it at the outset, by establishing ground rules for the role-play, and by attending to the creation of a safe and supportive learning environment (see above).

EXAMPLE: *Role-Play, Video Review.* A group of medical school faculty sought additional training in the skills of the medical interview, as part of a faculty development program. Participants were videotaped in a role-play of giving bad news to a patient. The participants reflected on their performance, received feedback from the other participants in the role-play and from the group at large, and defined areas for continued improvement. (Note the use of deliberate practice in this example.)

Role-playing works best when *ground rules for role-play* are used to prepare learners and to structure the activity. These are:

Phase of Role-play	Facilitator Task
Preparation	Choose a situation that is relevant and readily conceptualized by the learners.
	Describe the situation and critical issues for each role-player.
	Choose/assign roles and give learners time to assimilate and add details.
	Identify observers and clarify their functions.
	Establish expectations for time-outs by the learner and interruptions by others (e.g., time limits).
Execution	Ensure compliance with agreed-upon ground rules.
	Ensure that learners emerge comfortably from their roles.
Debriefing	First give the principal learners the opportunity to self-assess what they did well, what they would want to do differently, and what they would like help with.
	Assess the feelings and experiences of other participants in the role-play.
	Elicit feedback from all observers on what seemed to go well.
	Elicit suggestions regarding alternative approaches that might have been more effective.
Replay	Give the principal learners the opportunity to repeat the role-play using alternative approaches.

Standardized (simulated) patients are actors or real patients trained to play the roles of patients with specific problems. As with role-play, the use of standardized patients ensures that important content areas will be covered and allows learners to try new techniques, make mistakes, and repeat their performance until a skill is achieved. In addition to basic communication and physical diagnosis skills, professionalism and ethics teaching cases have been developed using standardized patients (56). Standardized patients can be trained to provide feedback and instruction, even in the absence of a faculty member. The method has proven efficacy, both for teaching and for evaluating learners (57). The major limitation is the need to recruit, train, schedule, and pay standardized patients. Following the introduction of USMLE Step 2 Clinical Skills in 2004–5, most medical schools in the United States now have active standardized patient programs or access to partner institutions with standardized patient programs.

Reviews of recorded (audio or video) performances of role-play, standardized patient, or real patient encounters can serve as helpful adjuncts to experiential learning (58, 59). The files can provide information on learner and patient behaviors that the participants may not have noticed or remembered. They provide learners with the rare opportunity to observe their own performance from outside themselves. Properly facilitated audio or video reviews promote helpful reflection on and discussion of a learner's performance.

EXAMPLE: *Review of Observed Performance.* Surgical residents were videotaped performing a laparoscopic cholecystectomy. Residents who performed elements of the surgery below a predetermined level of performance were required to complete practice on a virtual reality simulator for each task performed below a predetermined cutoff level (deliberative practice). The deliberative practice group performed better than the control group on a subsequent videotaped laparoscopic cholecystectomy (60). (This is also an example of mastery level strategy, discussed below.)

- *Behavioral or Performance Objectives.* Methods commonly used to achieve behavioral or performance objectives include the following:

- Removal of barriers to performance
- Provision of resources that facilitate performance
- Provision of reinforcements for performance

Changing learners' behaviors can be one of the more challenging aspects of a curriculum. There is no guarantee that helping learners develop new skills and/or improved attitudes will result in the desired performance when the learners are in actual clinical situations. Skills training is necessary but not sufficient to ensure performance in real settings. To promote desired performance, curriculum developers may need to address *barriers to performance* in the learners' environment, provide *resources that promote performance*, and design *reinforcements* that will encourage the continued use of the newly acquired skills. Attention to the learner's subsequent environment can reduce or eliminate the decay of performance that often occurs after an educational intervention.

> **EXAMPLE:** *Systems Improvements and Feedback.* One of the pediatric residency competencies is the provision of safe transfer of patient care. A milestone for this competency states that the trainee adapts and applies a standardized template, relevant to individual contexts, reliably and reproducibly, with minimal errors of omission or commission (61). To address this milestone, trainees in one program are introduced to a standardized template with an interactive workshop that includes presentation of relevant communication theory, case-based examples emphasizing the importance of handoffs, and video demonstration of appropriate handoffs. A pocket card reminder of the standardized template is provided. Trainees are then evaluated by residents also trained in the template with an Objective Structured Hand-Off Exercise. Finally, trainees receive feedback in the workplace on the efficacy of observed written and verbal handoffs (62).

Methods for Promoting Learner-Centeredness

Methods for promoting learner-centeredness include the following:

- Formal or informal assessment of learners' needs
- Tailoring of educational content and methods to meet learners' needs

A curriculum is learner-centered to the extent that it is tailored to meet the specific needs of its individual learners and its targeted group of learners. This could mean 1) adapting methods to specific learning styles or preferences; 2) addressing specific learner needs in the cognitive, affective, or psychomotor areas related to established curricular objectives; 3) allowing flexibility in both the timing of the method and the time required to achieve objectives; or 4) accommodating specific learner objectives not included in the curriculum.

The *needs assessment of targeted learners* discussed in Step 2 and at the start of this chapter is the first step in tailoring a curriculum to a specific group of learners. *Formal evaluations of individual learners*, such as pretests, and *informal observations of individual learners*, which can occur during small group and one-on-one teaching sessions, can help the faculty identify the needs of individual learners, as can *discussion with individual learners*, during which learners are asked about their learning style preferences and perceived needs. This discovery process is more likely to occur when the faculty use observational, listening, and question-asking skills. As noted in the opening paragraphs of this chapter, identifying learners' needs and addressing preconceptions and prior experiences is the foundation of effective learning. Once the faculty are aware of these specific needs, they may be able to modify or add to the curriculum's educational strategies to address the specific needs. Such accommodation is more likely to be possible in *one-on-one and small group teaching* than in lecture situations, although online lectures allow flexibility in timing for learners.

This approach to learner-centered instruction is not new. Bloom proposed the *mastery learning instructional strategy* more than four decades ago as a method to narrow achievement gaps in education (63, 64). The mastery learning instructional process begins with identification of core concepts and organization into a unit of study; this is followed by a formative assessment (see Chapter 7) of learners. Learners who have mastered the concepts then go on to enrichment activities, and those who have not done so receive corrective instruction, often utilizing a *different educational method*. When all learners have mastered the concept, the next unit begins. Bloom showed that the application of mastery learning strategy narrowed the usual spread of student achievement in group instruction. Mastery learning, while difficult in a time-based curriculum, is eminently achievable with online learning software and resources, fits well with the outcomes-based, competency-based frameworks discussed in Chapter 4, and is being applied increasingly in medical education.

Generally speaking, learner-centered approaches to education require more time and effort on the part of educators than teacher-centered approaches. They are more likely, however, to engage the learner and succeed in helping the learner achieve agreed-upon objectives. The curriculum developer will need to decide to what extent learner-centered approaches are critical for the achievement of curricular objectives, are desirable but not critical, and are feasible within resource constraints.

> **EXAMPLE:** *Curriculum with Built-in Flexibility in Terms of Depth and Pace, and Remedial Instruction for Those Who Do Not Achieve Competency.* Students studying biochemistry receive a set of objectives that outlines both the minimum requirement of the course and those areas that they can study in more depth. Students study the subject individually from printed material or programmed tape/slide presentations at their own pace. They may also choose those materials that best suit their learning preferences. When the students feel that they have mastered a phase of the course, they arrange for an assessment. If they have not achieved an acceptable level of competency, a remedial program of instruction is developed by the staff and student (65).

Methods for Promoting Achievement of Selected Competencies

As noted in Chapter 4, six core competencies were introduced into graduate medical education in 1999 by the U.S. Accreditation Council for Graduate Medical Education (ACGME) and have influenced the approach to learning outcomes in all phases of medical training. In 2012, the Association of American Medical Colleges (AAMC) added two additional competencies: *Interprofessionalism* and *Personal and Professional Development* (66). While some of these competencies relate more directly to previous types of objectives, such as medical knowledge as a cognitive objective and patient care and interpersonal/communication skills as psychomotor objectives, others require integrative approaches. This section discusses five of the competencies: Practice-Based Learning and Improvement, Systems-Based Practice, Interprofessionalism, Professionalism, and Personal and Professional Formation.

- *Practice-Based Learning and Improvement (PBLI).* The Practice-Based Learning and Improvement competency requires that trainees examine, evaluate, and improve the care they provide, appraising and assimilating scientific evidence in the process (66). The habits of *lifelong learning* and *self-directed learning* are included in this competency.

Methods for promoting PBLI and self-directed learning (67, 68) include the following:

- Training in skills relevant to self-directed learning, such as inquiry-based learning including self-assessment, audits of one's own patient care / clinical practice, information searching, critical appraisal, clinical decision making
- Independent learning projects
- Personal learning plans or contracts
- Use of learning portfolios (69, 70)
- Role-modeling
- Training in teaching skills

In an era of burgeoning information and ever-evolving advances in medical care, it is important for curriculum developers to consider how learners will continue to develop in relevant cognitive, affective, and psychomotor areas after completion of the curriculum. Most overall educational programs have as a stated or unstated goal that their learners, by the end of the program, will be effective self-directed learners. *Effective self-directed learners* take primary responsibility for their own learning, accurately identify their own learning needs, clarify their learning goals and objectives, successfully identify and use resources and educational strategies that can help them achieve their goals and objectives, accurately assess their achievements, and repeat the learning cycle if necessary. By its very nature, self-directed learning is learner-centered. An advantage of self-directed learning is that active learners are said to learn more things more efficiently, to retain that knowledge better, and to use it more effectively than passive learners (68).

A self-directed learning approach is most applicable when the learner already has some relevant knowledge and experience. It is easiest when the learner already possesses *skills that facilitate self-directed learning*, such as self-assessment skills, library and informatics skills for searching the health care literature and other databases, skills in reading and critically appraising the medical literature, and clinical decision-making skills.

Curriculum developers must decide how their curriculum will fit into an educational program's overall approach to promoting the development of self-directed learners. If a focused curriculum is toward the beginning of a multifaceted educational program, it may need to take responsibility for teaching learners skills relevant to a self-directed learning approach (see above). If learners have already developed these fundamental skills but are relatively inexperienced in self-directed learning, they may benefit from a special orientation to self-directed learning and from an intensive mentoring process. If an effective self-directed learning approach has already been established in the overall program, a curriculum can simply include methods with which the learners are already familiar.

Required *independent learning projects and reports* are the method that is most commonly used to promote self-directed learning. Curricula can also require that learners develop a *personal learning plan or contract* (71), usually in combination with a preceptor or mentor, which specifies learning objectives, learning methods, resources, and evaluation methods. Faculty can promote self-directed learning by encouraging *targeted independent reading or consultation* related to clinical or other problems that are encountered, by *encouraging and helping learners to answer some of their own questions*, and by *modeling* self-directed learning themselves.

A curriculum is most likely to be successful in promoting self-directed learning if it schedules sufficient protected time for the activity, clearly communicates expectations to the learner, requires products (e.g., formal or informal presentations or reports), provides ongoing mentoring and supervision throughout the process, and provides training for learners in skills that facilitate self-directed learning, if they are lacking.

> **EXAMPLE:** *Training in Skills Relevant to Self-directed Learning.* Medical students in a PBL curriculum work in small groups throughout the basic science curriculum. The curriculum opens with training in effective search and appraisal of information. In a given session, students are presented with a case, discuss potential explanations for the presentation, and then identify learning objectives for the case. Between the group meetings, students independently identify information resources and synthesize the information needed to meet the learning objectives. In a follow-up meeting, students share and synthesize the information they have acquired; structured summaries encourage critical analysis of the source and information (33).

> **EXAMPLE:** *Self-audit, Patient and Systems Surveys, Reflection and Study.* For maintenance of certification, the American Board of Internal Medicine has developed Practice Improvement Modules (PIMs) to help physicians self-assess and apply quality improvement principles to their practices. The web-based module requires completion of four steps: 1) collect practice data (chart audit, patient survey, practice survey); 2) review and reflect on performance; 3) develop and implement an improvement plan; and 4) report on the plan and its outcomes. A review of the preventive cardiology PIM completed by 179 physicians found significant gaps in physician knowledge and skills in quality improvement. Targets for improvement included achieving goal LDL-cholesterol levels and systolic blood pressure measurement. Systems improvements included implementing chart forms, patient education, and care management processes (72).

▪ *Systems-Based Practice and Teamwork.* The Systems-Based Practice competency is demonstrated by "an awareness of and responsiveness to the larger context and system of health care and the ability to effectively call on system resources to provide care that is of optimal value." Competence in this area includes knowledge of health care delivery systems and costs of care, as well as the skills to work with other health care team members within a system to improve care outcomes. In this respect, this competency overlaps with the *Interprofessionalism* and *Interpersonal and Communications Skill* competencies, which include effective teamwork with other health care professionals.

Methods that can be used to help develop knowledge of health care systems include the following:

- Simulation exercises that include interprofessional teams
- Inclusion of other health professionals on health care teams
- Providing feedback on costs of care
- Case conferences focused on cost-effectiveness and quality of care
- Opportunities to work in disease management programs
- Appreciative inquiry to promote organizational change
- Participation in quality improvement and safety teams

EXAMPLE: *Quality Improvement Project.* A quality improvement project was designed to reduce drug-prescribing errors in a teaching hospital intensive care unit. Inclusion of a senior pharmacist on daily rounds who was available for consultation significantly decreased adverse drug events when compared with a control unit (73).

EXAMPLE: *Revised Morbidity and Mortality Conference, Use of a Health Care Matrix.* A residency program revised its morbidity and mortality conference to include the use of a health care matrix, which linked the Institute of Medicine aims for quality improvement and the ACGME core competencies. The discussant was charged with completing the matrix as it related to the case under discussion, identifying which quality improvement goals and which competencies were unfulfilled in the case (74).

EXAMPLE: *Appreciative Inquiry to Identify Best Practices.* A residency program surveyed its residents to identify the top five exemplar residents for effective patient sign-out. Appreciative inquiry interviews of these residents were used to develop a model of "best practices" for patient handoffs. Residents then worked together with a larger group of residents to develop a template for improved patient sign-out (75).

▪ *Interprofessionalism and Teamwork.* As medical knowledge has increased, and as societal expectations for customer-friendly, high-quality, cost-effective care have risen, the mechanisms for providing the best health care have become more complex. Health care professionals will have to work effectively in teams to accomplish desired goals of access, quality, and cost-effectiveness. Traditional medical curricula that have fostered a competitive approach to learning and an autocratic approach to providing care now need to foster collaborative approaches to learning and to prepare learners to be effective team members. Health care professionals need to become knowledgeable about and skilled in facilitating group process, in running and participating in meetings, in being appropriately assertive, in managing conflict, in facilitating organizational change, in motivating others, in delegating to and supervising others, and in feedback and general communication skills. Baker et al. (76) elucidated a framework of principles that characterize effective teamwork, including leadership skills, elucidation of shared goals and objectives, effective communication, trust, task sharing and backup behavior, adaptability, and performance monitoring/feedback. TeamSTEPPS is an evidence-based teamwork system that emphasizes team leadership, situational monitoring, mutual support, and communication behaviors and is increasingly being used as the model for medical education training in team skills (77, 78).
Methods for promoting and reinforcing team skills include the following:

▪ Focused curricula on team functioning and related skills
▪ Involvement of trainees in collaborative versus competitive approaches to learning, such as team-based learning (TBL)
▪ Learner participation in multidisciplinary teams and in work environments that model effective teamwork
▪ Having learners assess and discuss the functioning of the teams in which they are involved

EXAMPLE: *Focused Curricula on Team Skills: TeamSTEPPS Training.* A half-day workshop with first-year nursing students and third-year medical students used TeamSTEPPS as an educational intervention. Following a didactic introduction and simulation training exercise, students were better able to identify the presence and quality of team skills in video vignettes (79).

As noted in Chapter 4, the competencies for the domain of Interprofessionalism describe a breadth of knowledge, attitude, and skills to achieve collaborative practice with other health professionals (80). The World Health Organization (WHO) has emphasized that the development of interprofessional competencies is best done when interprofessional students learn together. Successful models include introduction to the competencies in didactic formats and discussions, followed by actual practice (81). Finding the optimal timing to do this is difficult in the crowded curricula of modern health education programs. Ideally, clinical rotations would occur in model collaborative practice sites, but that may also be challenging for some programs to identify.

> **EXAMPLE**: *Interprofessionalism.* First- and second-year medical students (MS), undergraduate nursing students (NS), and social work students partnered to design and implement a weekend urban Student Run Free Clinic. The students designed a process that included intake by a case manager (NS), evaluation by a junior (MS or NS) and a senior (MS or NS) clinician, presentation to a faculty preceptor, and then sign-out by a social work student. In both the design and the implementation of the clinic, students expressed respect for the other professions, comfort with interprofessional teams, and increased understanding of roles and responsibilities of the other professions (82).

- *Professionalism.* While not new, professionalism has been given increased emphasis by the ACGME and others (83–85). Professionalism includes respect for others; compassion; cross-cultural sensitivity; effective communication; shared decision making; honesty and integrity; self-awareness; responsiveness to the needs of patients and society that supersedes self-interest; accountability; sense of duty; a commitment to ethical principles; confidentiality; appropriate management of conflicts of interest; and a commitment to excellence, scientific knowledge, and ongoing professional development.

- *Personal and Professional Formation.* This has been used to describe the continuous development of these personal characteristics during training, as identity evolves from layperson to physician. Professional formation is a more complicated construct than professionalism because of its developmental nature, and it includes elements of social learning and identity formation (86). Cook et al. (85) have noted three aspects of professional formation that facilitate this development: 1) self-awareness and reflective practice, 2) interpersonal relationships, and 3) acculturation. Linking attention to these aspects to the methods listed below may be critical to their effectiveness. Unfortunately, there is evidence that some elements of professionalism deteriorate with training and that lapses of professionalism are common in medical settings (87, 88).

Methods for promoting professionalism and professional identity formation include the following:

- Faculty role-modeling (87, 89)
- Facilitated reflection on and discussion of experiences embodying professionalism (87)
- Participation in writing professionalism goals (90)
- Symbolic events such as White Coat Ceremony
- Appreciative inquiry, reflection, and narrative medicine (38, 91)
- Ethics consultation rounds
- Peer evaluations
- Participation in patient advocacy groups

- Service learning and volunteerism
- Attention of institutional and program leaders to the policies and culture of the training institution, as well as to the hidden and informal curricula that influence trainees (90, 92–94)

EXAMPLE: *Summer Internship with Seminars and Community Experience.* A summer internship for medical students included seminars related to professionalism and clinical experience in community-based organizations with community mentors. Students reported that the internship taught them about influences on professionalism, especially that of pharmaceutical companies; the role of physician advocacy for patients; and the experience of vulnerable populations with the health care system (95).

EDUCATIONAL TECHNOLOGY

Educational technology is growing at an exponential rate and is quickly being adopted in health professions education. Learners, especially the millennial generation, are adept at using technology and are expecting it to be implemented in their daily environment and education. Educators need to be facile at using evolving technologies if their instructional designs are to be learner-centered and presented in a way that is familiar to students. In addition, evolving technologies create new opportunities to increase access to learners, regardless of location and time, and to use data to drive learning. Technology also presents learning challenges (4, 8). Simulation, online learning, mobile technology, social networking, gaming, and learning analytics are examples of the use of educational technology in medical education.

- *Simulation.* The use of high-fidelity simulation to train professionals and health care teams has shown dramatically improved outcomes in performance and patient safety indicators. As discussed in this chapter's section on psychomotor objectives, simulation frees learning, to some extent, from constraints in clinical experience. The most common form of simulation is the use of life-size mannequins to mimic various functions of the human body. According to the AAMC, as of 2011, 95% of medical schools are using this technology. A meta-analysis of 609 studies of the effect of technology-enhanced simulation on students' learning outcomes determined that these simulations were associated with improved learning outcomes when coupled with traditional practice (96). Evidence of a positive impact on patient outcomes through simulation-based training is increasingly reported (48).

Another form of simulation is *virtual reality*, a computer-generated simulation of a three-dimensional environment, which provides a sense of physical presence for the learner. Sometimes termed "immersive multimedia," virtual reality can task the learner to respond to problems or manipulate the environment. To expand the reach of health care education beyond traditional academic medical centers, some centers are adopting mobile simulation units that include mannequin and virtual reality units and can be used by rural practitioners (97).

- *Online Education.* Online learning resources can transcend location and time constraints by permitting learners to access the resources in different places and at different times (asynchronous learning). Online education can be administered in several forms (98):

- *Web-enhanced learning*, in which the instructor and students still meet face to face, but technology is used to enhance learning. In this instance, technology could be in the form of media presentations, virtual reality simulation, social media, and/or gaming, among other technologies.
- *Blended learning* or *hybrid learning*, a combination of face-to-face and online instruction. The blend could be between 30% and 80% online and involves very careful instructional design to ensure that the two blended environments are seamless (99). Blended learning offers the best of online and face-to-face learning. The *flipped classroom* (16) could be a form of blended or web-enhanced learning. In a hybrid environment, the instructor is able to utilize the Internet to present the lectures, readings, and examples, while leaving class time for applications and discussions of the material.
- *Online learning, per se*, a method that is almost all online and uses web technology to deliver instruction. The instructor and students are separated by time and space. Online learning has a global reach and affords students in remote locations access to an education that might otherwise be unattainable. Because online learning can be isolating, curriculum developers need strategies to create online learning communities. Instruction in online learning can be synchronous or asynchronous or a combination of both methods, depending on the content, the audience, and the desired outcome (100).
- *Massive open online courses (MOOCs)*, open-source, web-based courses that are also growing in popularity because of their global reach. A review of 225 MOOCs in health- and medicine-related fields found that the duration varied from 3 to 20 weeks, with an average length of 7 weeks. On average, the MOOCs expected participants to work on material for four hours a week. Several offered certificates or other professional recognition of passing the course (101).

EXAMPLE: *Online Learning Transcending Location and Time.* A school of public health needs to train personnel on the ground in remote locations. Bringing personnel to one location for training could be prohibitive. The school decides to deliver the training via the Internet, using e-learning technologies. The lessons and training are designed using an inquiry-based instructional model, in which the learners are introduced to the concepts via media lectures and readings. They are asked to interact with the content and with each other. Then they are asked to apply the knowledge through carefully designed activities (102).

- *Mobile Technology and Social Networking.* Social networking can facilitate the use of collaborative learning approaches and lends itself well to the millennial generation. Mobile technology is widely available globally and even allows access to learners without computers. Mobile devices can be used to customize educational content to fit individual students' needs and interests, thereby enabling a personalized approach to instruction. In a study conducted by the Brookings Institution, 52% of teachers reported that their students were *more motivated* to learn when mobile digital technology was employed in education (103). A 2013 systematic review found that the most commonly reported medical education uses were to promote learner engagement, feedback, collaboration, and professional development (104).

EXAMPLE: *Crowdsourcing and Mobile Technology with Spaced Repetition.* Medical students used a software program to simultaneously access and edit questions related to the basic science curriculum, in the form of flashcards. In one year, more than 16,000 questions were created and refined in the database. Analysis of class performance before and after development of the flashcards showed overall higher exam performance after introduction of the flashcards. This database was subsequently developed into a mobile application that used push spaced repetition to facilitate long-term recall (105).

- *Gaming.* Although gamification is a rapidly developing field and holds promise for the future of education, it is still unattainable in most educational settings due to expense and the time investment required for game production. Once produced, however, there are unique advantages to the use of gaming. Gaming invariably contains elements of competition, fun, entertainment, and feedback that encourage players to continue use. Access to games is available to learners through computers, smartphones, or video game systems, and on their preferred schedule. The value in gaming, as some researchers advocate, is in the freedom it offers: freedom to fail, experiment, fashion identities, and focus effort—that is, the freedom to personalize learning structure (106). Gaming typically follows the structure of deliberate practice and seems appropriate for development of expertise (107). A *serious game* is an interactive computer application that has a challenging goal, includes some scoring mechanism, and supplies the user with knowledge, skills, or attitudes that would be useful in reality (107).

  In medical education, gaming has been explored as a method of training in psychomotor skills and as a tool for development of team skills and complex decision making. A recent systematic review of serious games in medical education found that half were used for team training in critical care and triage and half for training in laparoscopic skills (107). Once it was noted that video gaming was associated with enhanced visuospatial skills and hand-eye coordination, video gaming was explored as a method to enhance surgical skills. Several studies show that video gamers had better basic surgical skills and that interventions of video games improved subsequent laparoscopic simulator performance (108).

  > **EXAMPLE:** *Gaming for Complex Decision Making.* A serious game, GeriatriX, was developed to train medical students in complex geriatric decision making, including weighing patient preferences and appropriateness and costs of care. As a supplement to the geriatric education program, use of the game resulted in a positive increase in self-perceived competence in these topics for the intervention group and better performance in cost-consciousness (109).

- *Learning and Assessment Analytics. Learning and assessment analytics* refers to the digital capture of educational or clinical data that can be displayed visually in real time (110). At the program and course levels, learning analytics can identify students' degrees of participation in curricular offerings, predict the likelihood of students' success or failure, and identify opportunities for early intervention, at both the student and instructor levels (111). Analytics also has the potential to personalize and adapt instruction to each learner's needs. Furthermore, there is the potential to integrate data from both educational program and clinical datasets to provide feedback and instructional guidance. Software systems for learning analytics are designed to present the information visually, affording the user a friendlier and accessible format for the information needed (112).

- *Integrating New Educational Technology.* Rapidly evolving technology can be disruptive and calls for curriculum developers and educators to be thoughtful and purposeful about its inclusion in curriculum planning. The SAMR model is a frequently cited model that describes a hierarchy of goals for inclusion of technology in educational practice and can be used to understand the rationale for introduction of technology into an educational environment (113). In this model, technology tools can be used as:

Substitution, with no functional change
Augmentation as a substitute, with functional improvement
Modification, allowing significant task redesign
Redefinition, allowing creation of new tasks, previously inconceivable; transformational

Before adopting new technology, then, curriculum planners should consider:

- Will this technology supplement or replace a current educational method? If it is a supplement, will all learners be able to access it? Is there sufficient protected time for its use?
- If introducing a new technology, have plans for faculty development and ongoing support been specified? Is there capacity for a transient drop in performance as the technology is implemented?
- What is the evidence that this technology results in improved learning outcomes, is cost-effective, or saves other resources (such as faculty time)? If evidence is lacking, can this be a focus of educational research as the technology is introduced?
- If the technology is collecting data on individuals, such as hours of usage and learning outcomes, have privacy concerns been adequately addressed? Who has access to the data? (See Chapter 7, Evaluation and Feedback).

Staying abreast of available educational technology is challenging. One extremely useful resource is the annual New Media Consortium's "Horizon Report" for higher education (114). Often, educational technology is introduced in other areas of the university or health system, and partnering with those resources can be an effective strategy for health professional schools and clinical sites.

CONCLUSION

The challenge of Step 4 is to devise educational strategies that achieve the curricular objectives set out in Step 3, within the resource constraints of available time, space, money, clinical material, and faculty. The need to promote learner-centeredness and professional development and to address the newly defined competencies, milestones, and EPAs may be additional considerations that are consistent with initiatives in the overall training program or school or the educational philosophy of the curriculum developers themselves. Creativity in the development of educational strategies is an opportunity for facilitating meaningful, enduring learning and for scholarship, particularly if the curriculum is carefully evaluated, as we shall see in Chapters 7 and 9.

QUESTIONS

For the curriculum you are coordinating, planning, or would like to be planning, please answer or think about the following questions:

1. In the table below, write one important, specific measurable objective in each of the following domains: cognitive, affective, and psychomotor.

2. Choose educational methods from Table 5.3 to achieve each of your educational objectives.

3. Is each educational method congruent with the domain of its objective?

4. Are you concerned that there will be decay over time in the achievement of any of your objectives?

5. From Tables 5.2 and 5.3, choose an additional method for each objective that would most likely prevent decay after its achievement.

6. Identify the resources that you will need to implement your educational methods. Consider available teachers in your institution, costs for simulations or clinical experiences, time in the training program or elective, and space. Are your methods feasible?

	Cognitive (Knowledge)	Affective (Attitudinal)	Psychomotor (Skill or Performance)
Specific measurable objectives			
Educational method to achieve			
Educational method to prevent decay			
Resources required			

7. Have you included any methods that are learner-centered or that promote self-directed learning? If yes, what are they?

8. Will your curriculum include educational strategies that promote practice-based learning and improvement or systems-based practice? Why or why not? If yes, what are these strategies?

9. Will your curriculum include educational strategies that promote professionalism, interprofessionalism, or professional formation? Why or why not? If yes, what are these strategies?

10. Have the methods you suggested in your answers to Questions 7 through 9 affected your need for resources? How? Are your methods feasible?

GENERAL REFERENCES

Bransford JD, Brown AL, Cocking RR, eds. *How People Learn: Brain, Mind, Experience, and School.* Washington, D.C.: National Academies Press; 2000.
A very readable text developed by the two National Research Council entities—the Commission on Behavioral and Social Sciences and Education and the Committee on Learning Research and Educational Practice—with a goal toward synthesizing findings of learning research and facilitating the application of research to classroom teaching and education. 374 pages.

Brookfield S. Adult learning: an overview. In: Tuinjman A, ed. *International Encyclopedia of Education*, 2nd ed. Oxford: Pergamon Press; 1996.
A short but comprehensive summary that covers four major research areas underlying adult learning (self-directed learning, critical reflection, experiential learning, and learning to learn) and three emerging trends (cross-cultural adult learning, practical theorizing, and distance learning) and identifies 10 areas for further research. Available at www.ict.mic.ul.ie/adult_ed/overview.htm.

Clark RC, Mayer RE. *e-Learning and the Science of Instruction: Proven Guidelines for Consumers and Designers of Multimedia Learning*, 3rd ed. San Francisco: Pfeiffer; 2011.
An introductory text on web-based instruction for the adult learner. It reviews adult learning theory and concepts relevant to multimedia formats, basing recommendations on proven strategies. Many examples are given throughout the book, and while these are mainly geared toward corporate human resources training, they are helpful for the medical educator interested in e-learning applications. 502 pages.

Cooke M, Irby DM, O'Brien BC. *Educating Physicians: A Call for Reform of Medical School and Residency*. San Francisco: Jossey-Bass; 2010.
This report, commissioned by the Carnegie Foundation for the Advancement of Teaching on the hundredth anniversary of the Flexner Report, takes a comprehensive look at current medical education, its strengths and limitations, and calls for four new goals of medical education: 1) standardization of learning outcomes and individualization of the learning process; 2) integration of formal knowledge and clinical experience; 3) development of habits of inquiry and innovation; and 4) focus on professional identity formation. The text is peppered with examples of best practices and innovative approaches. 304 pages.

Cross KP. *Adults as Learners: Increasing Participation and Facilitating Learning*. San Francisco: Jossey-Bass; 1992.
Classic text, written for educators and trainers of adult learners in any discipline or profession. The author describes research findings and synthesizes them into two explanatory models: one for understanding motivations of adult learners and the other for organizing knowledge about their characteristics. There is also a chapter on facilitation. 336 pages.

Dent JA, Harden RM, eds. *A Practical Guide for Medical Teachers*, 4th ed. New York: Churchill Livingstone/Elsevier; 2014.
Includes 73 international authors and provides global perspectives on curriculum development and instructional design. 436 pages.

Dick W, Carey L, Carey JO. *The Systematic Design of Instruction*, 7th ed. Boston: Pearson Allyn & Bacon; 2009.
The authors present a framework for instructional design similar to that proposed in this chapter. The book places particular emphasis on behavioral objectives, preinstructional activities, student participation, and testing. Chapters 8 and 9 address the development of instructional strategy and selection of instructional materials. Specific (non-health-related) examples are detailed in the text. 396 pages.

Ende J, Atkins E. Conceptualizing curriculum for graduate medical education. *Acad Med*. 1992;67:528–34.
Discusses limitations of objective-driven curricula and how to structure educational programs to maximize learning from experience. (See also discussion at the end of Chapter 4, Goals and Objectives.)

Ericsson KA, Charness N, Feltovich PJ, Hoffman RR. *The Cambridge Handbook of Expertise and Expert Performance.* New York: Cambridge University Press; 2006.
A comprehensive compendium of the research on expert performance. One section is devoted to research on professional expertise, including a short chapter on expertise in medicine. 901 pages.

Green LW, Kreuter MW, Deeds SG, Partridge KB. Selection of educational strategies. In: Green LW, Kreuter MW, Deeds SG, Partridge KB. *Health Education Planning: A Diagnostic Approach.* Palo Alto, Calif.: Mayfield Publishing; 1980. Pp. 86–115.
Classic text that uses a conceptual framework for planning and implementing health programs. The framework includes epidemiological diagnosis/health problem definition, behavioral and educational diagnosis, social/community/target group factors, and administrative diagnosis. Chapter 6 discusses the selection of educational strategies in the context of this framework. The book is oriented to educational interventions for communities and patient populations, but the concepts are also applicable to educational programs targeted at health professionals. 306 pages.

Grunwald T, Corsbie-Massey C. Guidelines for cognitively efficient multimedia learning tools: educational strategies, cognitive load, and interface design. *Acad Med.* 2006;81:213–23.
This narrative review summarizes existing research in the use of multimedia, including how educational theories and design should be considered in crafting effective multimedia.

Knowles MS, Swanson RA, Holton EF. *The Adult Learner: The Definitive Classic in Adult Education and Human Resource Development*, 7th ed. Burlington, MA: Elsevier Science; 2011.
Classic work by Malcolm Knowles, updated posthumously by two professors of education, Elwood Holton II and Richard Swanson. The book covers adult learning theory, recent advances, and application. 626 pages.

Lee VS, ed. *Teaching and Learning through Inquiry: A Guidebook for Institutions and Instructors.* Sterling, VA: Stylus Publishing; 2004.
Written from the perspective of one undergraduate program's initiative to incorporate the inquiry method, this is a nice resource to better understand the method's theoretical grounding and practical applications. Includes classroom examples, faculty development, and service learning. 288 pages.

Mezirow J. *Transformative Dimensions of Adult Learning.* San Francisco: Jossey-Bass; 1991.
Classic book that describes transformational learning as learning that affects how learners interpret or construct meaning out of experience and their beliefs, attitudes, and emotions. Such learning is influenced by past and new experiences, culture, communication with others, and critical reflection. The interpretive lens through which a person views experiences influences his or her behavior. The book integrates perspectives on learning from many disciplines, including education, psychology, sociology, and philosophy, to develop this theory of transformative learning. 247 pages.

Michaelsen LK, Knight AB, Fink LD. *Team-Based Learning: A Transformative Use of Small Groups in College Teaching.* Sterling, Va.: Stylus Publishing; 2004.
Detailed guide for implementing team-based learning teaching strategies, written by the originator, Larry Michaelsen. 286 pages.

Michaelsen LK, Parmelee DX, McMahon KK, Levine RE. *Team-Based Learning for Health Professions Education: A Guide to Using Small Groups for Improving Learning.* Sterling, Va.: Stylus Publishing; 2007.
This book provides an introduction to team-based learning for health educators; it covers theory, structure, models, and details of implementation, including performance feedback and evaluation. 256 pages.

Rogers CR. Significant learning in therapy and education. In: Rogers R. *On Becoming a Person: A Therapist's View of Psychotherapy.* Boston: Houghton Mifflin; 1961. Pp. 279–96.
Chapter in a classic book by Carl Rogers describing conditions that promote transformational learning: genuineness and congruence of the teacher; empathetic understanding and acceptance

of the learner; contact with problems; provision of resources; and a safe, supportive learning environment.

Rubenstein W, Talbot Y. *Medical Teaching in Ambulatory Care: A Practical Guide*, 2nd ed. New York: Springer Publishing Co.; 2003.
    A short, practical, useful text on office-based precepting that includes a section on challenging learning situations. 152 pages.

Schon DA. *Educating the Reflective Practitioner*. San Francisco: Jossey-Bass; 1987.
    Classic book on the critical role of reflection, in as well as on action, in professional education. 355 pages.

Whitman N, Schwenk TL. *The Physician as Teacher*, 2nd ed. Salt Lake City, Utah: Whitman Associates; 1997.
    This book discusses teaching as a form of communication and relationship, as well as specific teaching responsibilities: lectures, group discussions, teaching rounds and morning report, bedside teaching, and teaching in the ambulatory setting. 275 pages.

Whitman NA, Schwenk TL. *Preceptors as Teachers: A Guide to Clinical Teaching*, 2nd ed. Salt Lake City, Utah: University of Utah School of Medicine; 1995.
    An excellent practical, pithy text that covers the essentials of clinical teaching. 30 pages.

SPECIFIC REFERENCES

1. Bransford JD, Brown AL, Cocking RR, eds. *How People Learn: Brain, Mind, Experience, and School*. Washington, D.C.: National Academies Press; 2000.
2. Simkins S, Maier M, eds. *Just in Time Teaching: Across the Disciplines and across the Academy*. Sterling, Va.: Stylus Publishing; 2009.
3. Kruse GD, Bruer JT, Gardner H, et al. Learning and learning styles. In: Parkay FW, Anctil EJ, Hass G, eds. *Curriculum Planning: A Contemporary Approach*, 8th ed. New York: Pearson; 2006. Pp. 165–218.
4. Grunwald T, Corsbie-Massay C. Guidelines for cognitively efficient multimedia learning tools: educational strategies, cognitive load, and interface design. *Acad Med*. 2006;81:213–23.
5. Price GE. Diagnosing learning styles. In: Smith RM, ed. *Helping Adults Learn How to Learn*. San Francisco: Jossey-Bass; 1983. Pp. 49–55.
6. Rohrer D, Pashler H. Learning styles: where's the evidence? *Med Educ*. 2012;46:34–35.
7. Bennett CJ, Sackett KD, Haynes RB, et al. A controlled trial of teaching critical appraisal of the clinical literature to medical students. *JAMA*. 1987;257:2451–54.
8. Issa N, Schuller M, Santacaterina S, et al. Applying multimedia design principles enhances learning in medical education. *Med Educ*. 2011;45:818–26.
9. Westberg J, Jason H. *Making Presentations: A Guide Book for Health Professions Teachers*. Boulder, Colo.: Center for Instructional Support; 1991. Pp. 1–89.
10. Bourne PE. Ten simple rules for making good oral presentations. *PLoS Comput Biol*. 2007;3(4):e77. doi:10.1371/journal.pcbi.0030077.
11. Walters MR. Problem based learning within endocrine physiology lectures. *Adv Physiol Educ*. 2001;25:225–27.
12. Dong C, Goh PS. Twelve tips for the effective use of videos in medical education. *Med Teach*. 2015;37:140–45.
13. Wiley D. Connecting learning objects to instructional design theory: a definition, a metaphor and a taxonomy. In: Wiley D, ed. *The Instructional Use of Learning Objects*. Available at http://reusability.org/read.
14. Windle R, McCormick D, Dadrea J, Wharrad H. The characteristics of reusable learning

objects that enhance learning: a case-study in health-science education. *Br J Educ Technol*. 2010;42 (5):811–23.

15. Khan S. *The One World School House: Education Reimagined*. New York: Twelve; 2000.

16. Prober CG, Khan S. Medical education reimagined: a call to action. *Acad Med*. 2013;88: 1407–10.

17. KhanAcademy.org Health and Medicine: Respiratory System [Internet]. Available at www .khanacademy.org/science/health-and-medicine/respiratory-system.

18. Sisson SD, Hughes MT, Levine D, Brancati FL. Effect of an Internet-based curriculum on postgraduate education: a multicenter intervention. *J Gen Intern Med*. 2004;19:505–9.

19. Karpicke JD, Roediger HL. Repeated retrieval during learning is the key to long-term retention. *J Mem Lang*. 2007;57:151–62. doi:10.1016/j.jml.2006.09.004.

20. Shaw T, Long A, Chopra S, Kerfoot BP. Impact on clinical behavior of face-to-face continuing medical education blended with online spaced education: a randomized controlled trial. *J Cont Educ Health Prof*. 2011;31(2):103–8.

21. Whitman NE, Schwenk TL. *A Handbook for Group Discussion Leaders: Alternatives to Lecturing Medical Students to Death*. Salt Lake City, Utah: University of Utah School of Medicine; 1983. Pp. 1–38.

22. Whitman N, Schwenk TL. *The Physician as Teacher*, 2nd ed. Salt Lake City, Utah: Whitman Associates; 1997. Pp. 131–46.

23. Tiberius RG. *Small Group Teaching: A Trouble-Shooting Guide*. Toronto: Ontario Institute for Studies in Education Press; 1990. Pp. 1–194.

24. Westburg J, Jason H. *Fostering Learning in Small Groups: A Practical Guide*. New York: Springer Publishing Co.; 1996. Pp. 1–267.

25. Triola M, Djukic M. NUY3T: Teaching, Technology, Teamwork [Internet]. NYULMC Division of Educational Informatics. Available at http://dei.med.nyu.edu/research/nyu3t.

26. Djukic M, Fulmer T, Adams JG, Lee S, Triola M. NYU3T: Teaching, technology, teamwork: a model for interprofessional education scalability and sustainability. *Nurs Clin N Am*. 2012;47:333–46.

27. Dolmans DH, DeGrave W, Wolfhagen IH, van der Vleuten CP. Problem-based learning: future challenges for educational practice and research. *Med Educ*. 2005;39(7):732–41.

28. Distlehorst LH, Dawson E, Robbs RS, Barrows HS. Problem-based learning outcomes: the glass half-full. *Acad Med*. 2005;80(3):294–99.

29. Mamede S, Schmidt HG, Norman GR. Innovations in problem-based learning: what can we learn from recent studies? *Adv Health Sci Educ*. 2006;11:403–22.

30. Lee VS. What is inquiry-guided learning? *New Dir Teach Learn*. 2012;29:5–14.

31. Justice C, Rice J, Warry W, et al. Inquiry in higher education: reflections and directions on course design and teaching methods. *Innov High Educ*. 2007;31:201–14.

32. Wolpaw TM, Hull AL, Wilson-Delfosse AL, et al. Case Western Reserve University School of Medicine and Cleveland Clinic. *Acad Med*. 2010;85:S439–45.

33. Ornt DB, Aron DC, King NB, et al. Population medicine in a curricular revision at Case Western Reserve. *Acad Med*. 2008;83:327–31.

34. Johnson EO, Charchanti AV, Troupis TG. Modernization of an anatomy class: from conceptualization to implementation. *Anat Sci Educ*. 2012;5(6):354–66.

35. ten Cate O, Durning S. Peer teaching in medical education: twelve reasons to move from theory to practice. *Med Teach*. 2007;29:591–99.

36. Henerson ME, Morris LL, Fitz-Gibbon CT. *How to Measure Attitudes*. Book 6 in: Herman JL, ed. *Program Evaluation Kit*. Newbury Park, Calif.: SAGE Publications; 1987. Pp. 9–13.

37. Dick W, Carey L, Carey JO. *The Systematic Design of Instruction*, 6th ed. Boston: Pearson Allyn & Bacon; 2005. Pp. 205–6, 210–11.

38. Charon R. *Narrative Medicine: Honoring the Stories of Illness*. New York: Oxford, 2006.

39. Wald HS, Reis SP. Beyond the margins: reflective writing and development of reflective capacity in medical education. *J Gen Intern Med*. 2010;25:746–49.

40. Bentley TJ. *Facilitation: Providing Opportunities for Learning*. Berkshire, U.K.: McGraw-Hill Publishing; 1994. Pp. 25–60.
41. Brookfield SD. *Understanding and Facilitating Adult Learning*. San Francisco: Jossey-Bass; 1987. Pp. 123–26.
42. Rogers CR. Significant learning in therapy and education. In: Rogers CR. *On Becoming a Person: A Therapist's View of Psychotherapy*. Boston: Houghton Mifflin; 1961. Pp. 279–96.
43. Wright S, Wong A, Newill C. The impact of role models on medical students. *J Gen Intern Med*. 1997;12:53–56.
44. Wright S. Examining what residents look for in their role models. *Acad Med*. 1996;71:290–92.
45. Patterson N, Hulton LJ. Enhancing nursing students' understanding of poverty through simulation. *Public Health Nurs*. 2011;29(2):143–51.
46. Horn J, Masunaga H. A merging theory of expertise and intelligence. In: Ericsson KA, Charness N, Feltovich PJ, Hoffman RR, eds. *The Cambridge Handbook of Expertise and Expert Performance*. New York: Cambridge University Press; 2006. Pp. 600–601.
47. Ende J. Feedback in clinical medical education. *JAMA*. 1983;250(6):777–81.
48. McGaghie WC, Issenberg SB, Petrusa ER, Scalese RJ. Effect of practice on standardized learning outcomes in simulation-based medical education. *Med Educ*. 2006;40:792–97.
49. McGaghie WC. Simulation in professional competence assessment: basic considerations. In: Tekian A, McGuire CH, McGaghie WC, eds. *Innovative Simulations for Assessing Professional Competence: From Paper and Pencil to Virtual Reality*. Chicago: University of Illinois at Chicago; 1999.
50. Issenberg SB, Petrusa ER, McGaghie WC, et al. Effectiveness of a computer-based system to teach bedside cardiology. *Acad Med*. 1999;74:S93–95.
51. Andreatta P, Saxton E, Thompson M, Annich G. Simulation-based mock codes significantly correlate with improved pediatric cardiorespiratory arrest survival rates. *Pediatr Crit Care Med*. 2011;12:33–38.
52. McGaghie WC, Issenberg SB, Petrusa ER, Scalese RJ. A critical review of simulation-based medical education research: 2003–2009. *Med Educ*. 2010;44:50–63.
53. Salas E, Klein C, King H, Salisbury M. Debriefing medical teams: 12 evidence-based practices and tips. *Jt Comm J Qual Patient Saf*. 2008;34:518–27.
54. Nestel D, Tierney T. Role-play for medical students learning about communication: guidelines for maximising benefits. *BMC Med Educ*. 2007;7:3.
55. Lane C, Rollnick S. The use of simulated patients and role-play in communication skills training: a review of the literature to August, 2005. *Patient Educ Couns*. 2007;67:13–20.
56. Singer PA, Robb A, Cohen R, Norman G, Turnbull J. Performance-based assessment of clinical ethics using an objective structured clinical examination. *Acad Med*. 1996;71: 495–98.
57. Stillman PL, Swanson D, Regan B, et al. Assessment of clinical skills of residents utilizing standardized patients. *Ann Intern Med*. 1991;114:393–401.
58. Edwards A, Tzelepis A, Klingbeil C, et al. Fifteen years of a videotape review program for internal medicine and medicine-pediatrics residents. *Acad Med*. 1996;71:744–48.
59. Guerlain S, Adams RB, Turentine FB, et al. Assessing team performance in the operating room: development and use of a "black-box" recorder and other tools for the intraoperative environment. *J Am Coll Surg*. 2005;200:29–37.
60. Palter VN, Grantcharov TP. Individualized deliberate practice on a virtual reality simulator improves technical performance of surgical novices in the operating room: a randomized controlled trial. *Ann Surg*. 2014;259(3):443–48.
61. The Pediatric Milestone Project: A Joint Initiative of the Accreditation Council for Graduate Medical Education and the American Board of Pediatrics [Internet]. 2015. Available at http://acgme.org/acgmeweb/Portals/0/PDFs/Milestones/PediatricsMilestones.pdf.
62. Farnan JM, Raro JAM, Rodriguez RM, et al. Hand-off education and evaluation: piloting the Observed Simulated Hand-off Experience (OSHE). *J Gen Intern Med*. 2010;25:129–34.

63. Bloom BS. Learning for mastery. *Eval Comment.* 1968;9(2):1–12 (ERIC Document Repro-duction No. ED053419).

64. Guskey TR. Closing achievement gaps: revising Benjamin S. Bloom's "Learning for Mastery." *J Adv Acad.* 2007;19(1):8–31.

65. Harden RM, Snowden S, Dunn WR. Educational strategies in curriculum development: the SPICES model. *Med Educ.* 1984;18:284–97.

66. Englander R, Cameron T, Ballard AJ, et al. Toward a common taxonomy of competency domains for the health professions and competencies for physicians. *Acad Med.* 2013;88:1088–94.

67. Brookfield S, ed. *Self-Directed Learning: From Theory to Practice.* San Francisco: Jossey-Bass; 1985.

68. Knowles MS. *Self-Directed Learning: A Guide for Learners and Teachers.* New York: Association Press; 1975.

69. Challis M. AMEE medical education guide no. 11 (revised): portfolio-based learning and assessment in medical education. *Med Teach.* 1999;4:370–86.

70. Kjaer NK, Maagaard R, Wied S. Using an online portfolio in postgraduate training. *Med Teach.* 2006;28:708–12.

71. Knowles MS. *Using Learning Contracts.* San Francisco: Jossey-Bass; 1986. Pp. 3–8.

72. Duffy FD, Lynn LA, Diduralt, et al. Self-assessment of practice performance: development of the ABIM Practice Improvement Module (PIM^SM). *J Contin Educ Health Prof.* 2008;28(1):38–46.

73. Leape LL, Cullen DJ, Clapp MD, et al. Pharmacist participation on physician rounds and adverse drug events in the intensive care unit. *JAMA.* 1999;282:267–70.

74. Bingham JW, Quinn DC, Richardson MG, Miles PV, Gabbe SG. Using a healthcare matrix to assess patient care in terms of aims for improvement and core competencies. *Jt Comm J Qual Patient Saf.* 2005;31:98–105.

75. Helms AS, Perez TE, Baltz J, et al. Use of appreciative inquiry approach to improve resident sign-out in an era of multiple shift changes. *J Gen Intern Med.* 2011;27(3):287–91.

76. Baker DP, Salas E, King H, Battles J, Barach P. The role of teamwork in the professional edu-cation of physicians: current status and assessment recommendations. *Jt Comm J Qual Patient Saf.* 2005;31(4):185–202.

77. Clancy CM, Tornberg DN. TeamSTEPPS: assuring optimal teamwork in clinical settings. *Am J Med Qual.* 2007;22:214–17.

78. Mayer CM, Cluff L, Wei-Ting L, et al. Evaluating efforts to optimize TeamSTEPPS implementa-tion in surgical and pediatric intensive care units. *Jt Com J Qual Patient Saf.* 2011;37(8):365–74.

79. Robertson B, Kaplan B, Atallah H, et al. The use of simulation and a modified TeamSTEPPS curriculum for medical and nursing student team training. *Simul Healthc.* 2010;5:332–37.

80. Interprofessional Education Collaborative Expert Panel. *Core Competencies for Interprofessional Collaborative Practice: Report of an Expert Panel.* Washington, D.C.: Interprofessional Education Collaborative; 2011.

81. Nelson S, Tassone M, Hodges BD. *Creating the Health Care Team of the Future: The Toronto Model for Interprofessional Education and Practice.* Ithaca, N.Y.: Cornell University Press; 2014.

82. Wang T, Bhakta H. A new model for interprofessional collaboration at a student-run free clinic. *J Interprof Care.* 2013;4:339–40.

83. ABIM Foundation, American Board of Internal Medicine, ACP-ASIM Foundation, American College of Physicians–American Society of Internal Medicine, European Federation of Internal Medicine. Medical professionalism in the new millennium: a physician charter. *Ann Intern Med.* 2002;136:243–46.

84. Blank L, Kimball HABIM Foundation, ACP Foundation, et al. Medical professionalism in the new millennium: a physician charter 15 months later. *Ann Intern Med.* 2003;138:839–41.

85. Cook M, Irby DM, O'Brien BC. *Educating Physicians: A Call for Reform of Medical School and Residency.* Stanford, Calif.: Jossey-Bass, 2010. Pp. 60–65.

86. Holden M, Buck E, Clark M, Szauter K, Trumble J. Professional identity formation in medical education: the convergence of multiple domains. *HEC Forum.* 2012;24:245–55. doi:10.1007/s10730-012-9197-6.

87. Inui TS. *A Flag in the Wind: Educating for Professionalism in Medicine.* Washington, D.C.: Association of American Medical Colleges; 2003.

88. Ratanawongsa N, Bolen S, Howell EE, et al. Resident's perceptions of professionalism in training and practice: barriers, promoters, and duty hour requirements. *J Gen Intern Med.* 2006;21:758–63.

89. Goldstein EA, Maestas RR, Fryer-Edwards K, et al. Professionalism in medical education: an institutional challenge. *Acad Med.* 2006;81:871–76.

90. Branch WT, Kern D, Haidet P, et al. Teaching the human dimensions of care in clinical settings. *JAMA.* 2001;286:1067–74.

91. Quaintance JL, Arnold L, Thompson GS. What students learn about professionalism from faculty stories: an "appreciative inquiry" approach. *Acad Med.* 2010;85:118–23.

92. Suchman AT, Williamson PR, Litzelman DK, et al. Toward an informal curriculum that teaches professionalism: transforming the social environment of a medical school. *J Gen Intern Med.* 2004;19:501–4.

93. Hafferty FW. Beyond curriculum reform: confronting medicine's hidden curriculum. *Acad Med.* 1998;73:403–7.

94. Hundert EM, Hafferty FW, Christakis D. Characteristics of the informal curriculum and trainees' ethical choices. *Acad Med.* 1996;71:624–33.

95. O'Toole TP, Kathuria N, Mishra M, Schukart D. Teaching professionalism within a community context: perspectives from a national demonstration project. *Acad Med.* 2005;80:339–43.

96. Cook D, Hatala R, Brydges R, et al. Technology-enhanced simulation for health professions education: a systematic review and meta-analysis. *JAMA.* 2011;306(9):978–88.

97. Health Workforce Information Center. Technology in health professions education [Internet]. Available at http://ruralhealth.und.edu/projects/hwic/pdf/educational-technology.pdf.

98. Teeley KH. Multimedia in the classroom: creating learning experiences with technology. In: Bradshaw M, Lowenstein A, eds. *Innovative Teaching Strategies in Nursing and Related Health Professions*, 6th ed. Burlington, Mass.: Jones & Bartlett; 2014.

99. Lowenstein A. Blended learning. In: Bradshaw M, Lowenstein A, eds. *Innovative Teaching Strategies in Nursing and Related Health Professions*, 6th ed. Burlington, Mass.: Jones & Bartlett; 2014.

100. Cosper SM, Jaffe L. Synchronous distance education: bringing everyone together. In: Bradshaw M, Lowenstein A, eds. *Innovative Teaching Strategies in Nursing and Related Health Professions,* 6th ed. Burlington, Mass.: Jones & Bartlett; 2014.

101. Liyanagunawardena TR, Williams SA. Massive open online courses on health and medicine: review. *J Med Internet Res.* 2014;16(8):e191.

102. Sopczyk D, Doyle N, Jacobs K. Technology in education. In: Bastable S, Gramet P, Jacobs K, Sopczyck D, eds. *Health Professional as Educator: Principles of Teaching and Learning.* Salisbury, Mass.: Jones & Bartlett; 2011.

103. West DM. Mobile Learning: Transforming Education, Engaging Students, and Improving Outcomes [Internet]. Center for Technology Innovation at Brookings. 2013. Available at www.brookings.edu/research/papers/2013/09/17-mobile-learning-education-engaging-students-west.

104. Cheston CC, Flickinger TE, Chisolm MS. Social media use in medical education: a systematic review. *Acad Med.* 2013;88(6):893–901.

105. Bow HC, Dattilo JR, Jonas AM, Lehmann C. A crowdsourcing model for creating preclinical medical education study tools. *Acad Med.* 2013;88(6):766–70.

106. Klopfer E, Osterweil S, Salen K. Moving Learning Games Forward: Obstacles, Opportunities

& Openness [Internet]. The Education Arcade at MIT. Boston, MA: The Creative Commons. 2009. Available at http://education.mit.edu/wp-content/uploads/2015/01/Moving LearningGamesForward_EdArcade.pdf.

107. Graafland M, Schraagen JM, Schijven MP. Systematic review of serious games for medical education and surgical skills training. *Br J Surg.* 2012;99:1322–30.

108. Jalink MB, Goris J, Heineman E, et al. The effects of video games on laparoscopic simulator skills. *Am J Surg.* 2014;208:151–56.

109. Lagro J, van de Pol MH, Laan A, et al. A randomized controlled trial on teaching geriatric medical decision making and cost consciousness with the serious game GeriatriX. *J Am Med Dir Assoc.* 2014 Jun 6, pii:S1525–8610(14)00229–1. doi:10.1016/j.jamda.2014.04.011.

110. Ellaway RH, Pusic MV, Galbraith RM, Cameron T. Developing the role of big data and analytics in health professional education. *Med Teach.* 2014;36:216–22.

111. Baepler P, Murdoch CJ. Academic analytics and data mining in higher education. *Int J Schol Teach Learn.* 2010;4(2):1–9.

112. Brown M. Learning Analytics: Moving from Concept to Practice [Internet]. EDUCAUSE Learning Initiative Briefing. 2012. Available at http://net.educause.edu/ir/library/pdf /ELIB1203.pdf.

113. Puentedura RR. SAMR: getting to transformation [Internet]. Available at www.hippasus.com /rrpweblog/archives/2013/04/16/SAMRGettingToTransformation.pdf.

114. Johnson L, Adams Becker S, Estrada V, Freeman A. (2015). NMC Horizon Report: 2015 Higher Education Edition. Austin, Texas: The New Media Consortium. Available at http:// cdn.nmc.org/media/2015-nmc-horizon-report-HE-EN.pdf.

CHAPTER SIX

Step 5
Implementation

. . . making the curriculum a reality

Mark T. Hughes, MD, MA

IMPORTANCE

For a curriculum to achieve its potential, careful attention must be paid to issues of implementation. The curriculum developer must ensure that sufficient resources, political and financial support, and administrative structures have been developed to successfully implement the curriculum (Table 6.1).

Table 6.1.   Checklist for Implementation

____ Identify resources
   ____ Personnel: faculty, audiovisual, computing, information technology, secretarial and other support staff, patients
   ____ Time: curriculum director, faculty, support staff, learners
   ____ Facilities: space, clinical sites, clinical equipment, educational equipment, virtual space (servers, content management software)
   ____ Funding/costs: direct financial costs, hidden or opportunity costs, faculty compensation, costs of scholarship

____ Obtain support
   ____ Internal
      from: those with administrative authority (dean's office, hospital administration, department chair, program director, division director, etc.), faculty, learners, other stakeholders
      for: curricular time, personnel, resources, political support
   ____ External
      from: government, professional societies, philanthropic organizations or foundations, accreditation bodies, other entities (e.g., managed care organizations), individual donors
      for: funding, political support, external requirements, curricular or faculty development resources

____ Develop administrative mechanisms to support the curriculum
   ____ Administrative structure: to delineate responsibilities and decision making
   ____ Communication
      content: rationale; goals and objectives; information about the curriculum, learners, faculty, facilities and equipment, scheduling; changes in the curriculum; evaluation results; etc.
      mechanisms: websites, social media, memos, meetings, syllabus materials, site visits, reports, etc.
   ____ Operations: preparation and distribution of schedules and curricular materials; collection, collation, and distribution of evaluation data; curricular revisions and changes, etc.
   ____ Scholarship: plans for presenting and publishing about curriculum; human subjects protection considerations; IRB approval, if necessary

____ Anticipate and address barriers
   ____ Financial and other resources
   ____ Competing demands
   ____ People: attitudes, job/role security, power and authority, etc.

____ Pilot
   ____ Phase-in
   ____ Full implementation

____ Plan for curriculum enhancement and maintenance

In many respects, Step 5 requires that the curriculum developer become a project manager, overseeing the people and operations that will successfully implement the curriculum. Implementation can be viewed as a developmental process with four stages: generating support, planning for change, operationalizing implementation, and ensuring viability (1). These four stages correspond to the six steps of curriculum development. Stage 1, generating support, requires developing the leadership for the curriculum and enlisting stakeholder support through problem identification and the general and targeted needs assessments (see Chapters 2 and 3). Stage 2, planning for change, involves creation of goals, objectives, and educational strategies that are clearly articulated to stakeholders (Chapters 4 and 5). Stage 3, operationalizing implementation, is the actual implementation of all steps and is primarily addressed in this chapter, with special attention to promptly responding to operational issues so that curriculum developers, learners, faculty, and support staff remain invested in the curriculum. Stage 4, ensuring viability, consists of establishing procedures for evaluation and feedback, obtaining ongoing financial and administrative support, and planning for curriculum maintenance and enhancement (Chapters 7 and 8).

IDENTIFICATION OF RESOURCES

The curriculum developer must realistically assess the resources that will be required to implement the educational strategies (Chapter 5) and the evaluation (Chapter 7) planned for the curriculum. Resources include personnel, time, facilities, and funding.

Personnel

Personnel includes curriculum directors, curriculum faculty, instructors, and support staff. The curriculum developers often become the *curriculum directors* and need to have sufficient time blocked in their schedules to oversee implementation of the curriculum. Ideally, *faculty* and *instructors* will be available and skilled in both teaching and content. If there are insufficient numbers of skilled faculty, one must contemplate hiring new faculty or developing existing faculty.

EXAMPLE: *Hiring New Faculty in Response to Accreditation Mandate.* To meet new educational requirements for interprofessional education for students in medicine, nursing, and pharmacy, three faculty members, representing each school, were enlisted as curriculum developers. The needs assessment identified small group sessions as the best educational strategy for the professional students to achieve the learning objectives. Consequently, multiple faculty from each professional school needed to be recruited to serve as small group co-facilitators. To ensure that new faculty were knowledgeable about principles of interprofessionalism and the particular learning goals, objectives, and educational methods to be employed in the curriculum, a series of orientation workshops were conducted.

EXAMPLE: *Faculty Development before the Start of the Curriculum.* A module on ectoparasites was developed in a course on parasitology at the Kilimanjaro Christian Medical University College (KCMUC), utilizing team-based learning (TBL) as its main educational method. The medical school faculty were relatively inexperienced in this method of teaching. Two faculty members attended a one-week intensive course on TBL at the Duke–National University of Singapore Graduate Medical School (Duke-NUS). A targeted three-day faculty development program on TBL was then presented at KCMUC by visiting faculty. Following delivery of the parasitology curriculum, three of the faculty members who, historically, had taught the ectoparasite module didactically reported enhanced job satisfaction with this new method of teaching (2).

EXAMPLE: *Faculty Development in Response to Evaluation.* Evaluations from an existing clinical skills course for second-year medical students revealed some deficiencies in preceptors' provision of feedback. The course director asked other faculty from the same institution, who were experts in faculty development, to develop a two-and-a-half hour workshop on feedback skills that could be integrated into the orientation session for course preceptors. After two years of workshops, evaluations reflected an improved performance in this area.

For large curricula involving many learners or extending over a long period of time, curriculum developers may need to hire a dedicated *curriculum administrator. Administrative assistants and other support staff* are usually needed to prepare budgets, curricular materials, and evaluation reports; coordinate and communicate schedules; collect evaluation data; and support learning activities. Institutional curricular support such as the scheduling of rooms, academic computing assistance, or audiovisual support must be planned.

For clinicians in training, a suitable mix of patients is also a "personnel" need that should not be overlooked.

EXAMPLE: *Case-Mix.* A musculoskeletal curriculum was developed for internal medicine residents. In a rheumatology rotation, the case-mix was concentrated on patients with inflammatory arthritis and connective tissue disease. Experiences in an orthopedic clinic involved a case-mix that included many postoperative patients. The general and targeted needs assessments found that residents needed to learn about musculoskeletal conditions commonly encountered in a primary care practice (e.g., shoulder pain, back pain, knee pain). In addition, learners wanted to practice examination maneuvers and diagnostic/therapeutic skills (e.g., arthrocentesis) that did not require specialist training. Therefore, curriculum developers created a musculoskeletal clinic for primary care patients with common joint and muscle complaints. The musculoskeletal clinic was staffed by attending general internists, who precepted residents as they saw patients referred by their usual general internal medicine provider (3).

Sometimes, standardized patients can help meet the need for a range of clinical experiences and can augment education by providing opportunities for practice and feedback (see Chapter 5).

EXAMPLE: *Identifying Standardized Patient Needs for a New Curriculum.* Evaluations from an existing course preparing fourth-year medical students for internship indicated that the informed consent lecture was not meeting students' needs. Consequently, a new skills-based curriculum was developed using standardized patients (SPs). SPs needed to be trained on the clinical scenario (informed consent for placement of a central venous access device) and on how to respond to the student's disclosure of information. To deliver the curriculum to 120 students in 12 hours over the span of the course, 10 SPs needed to be recruited and trained. Six encounters between an SP and a pair of students ran concurrently each hour. After the first set of students, modifications to the scenario were made based on student feedback, and the SPs were coached on their performances.

Time

Curriculum directors need time to coordinate management of the curriculum, which includes working with support staff to be sure that faculty are teaching, learners are participating, and process objectives are being met.

Faculty require time to prepare and teach. Generally, for each increment of contact time with a learner (in-person or asynchronous), at least several times that amount of time will be needed to develop the content and educational strategy. Time should also be budgeted for faculty to provide formative feedback to learners and summative evaluations of the learners and of the curriculum back to curriculum developers. As much as possible, curriculum directors should ease the amount of work required of faculty. If curriculum directors or their staff manage the logistics of the curriculum (scheduling, distribution of electronic or paper-based curricular materials, training of SPs, etc.), then faculty can concentrate on delivering the curriculum articulated in the goals and objectives.

For curriculum directors and faculty who have other responsibilities (e.g., meeting clinical productivity expectations), the implementation plan must include ways to compensate, reward, and/or accommodate faculty for the time they devote to the curriculum. Volunteer medical faculty may be most motivated by the personal satisfaction of giving back to the profession, but they may also appreciate opportunities for continuing education, academic appointments, awards, or other forms of recognition (4, 5). For salaried faculty, educational relative value units (RVUs) can be one way to acknowledge their time commitment to educational endeavors (see below).

Learners require time not only to attend scheduled learning activities but also to read, reflect, do independent learning, and apply what they have learned. As part of the targeted needs assessment (Chapter 3), curriculum developers should become familiar with the learners' schedule and understand what barriers exist for participation in the curriculum. For instance, postgraduate medical trainees may have to meet expectations on regulatory work hour limits.

Support staff members need time to perform their functions. Clearly delineating their responsibilities can help to budget the amount of time they require for curriculum implementation.

If educational research is to be performed as part of the targeted needs assessment (see Chapter 3) or curriculum evaluation (see Chapter 7), curriculum developers may need to budget time for review and approval of the research plans by an institutional review board (IRB).

Facilities

Curricula require facilities, such as space and equipment. The simplest curriculum may require only a room in which to meet or lecture. Clinical curricula often require access to patients and must provide learners with clinical facilities and equipment. A curriculum that addresses acquisition of clinical knowledge or skills may need a clinical site that can accommodate learners and provide the appropriate volume and mix of patients to ensure a valuable clinical experience.

> **EXAMPLE:** *Access to Patients in the Community and Clinical Equipment.* The curriculum developers of a home care curriculum wanted residents to have the experience of making home visits as part of their ambulatory rotation. The support of key stakeholders needed to be garnered in order to ensure that residents could visit housebound elderly patients in an existing home care program and discuss their visits with faculty preceptors. Evaluation instruments were developed to facilitate preceptors giving feedback to residents on their geriatric clinical skills (6, 7). A "travel kit" that served as the "doctor's black bag" was created to guarantee that the resident had the supplies and equipment necessary to evaluate the patient in his or her home.

Other curricula may need special educational resources, such as audio or video equipment, computers, software, online learning platforms, or artificial models to teach clinical skills. Appendix A provides an example of a curriculum on resuscitation skills for second-year medical students, detailing the extensive resources needed, including a simulation center, human patient simulators, durable medical equipment, and consumable medical supplies.

EXAMPLE: *Use of Simulation.* A curriculum was developed to teach surgical residents basic laparoscopic skills. In addition to watching video clips reviewing proper technique in maneuvering a laparoscope, a skills lab using a laparoscopic simulator was established. The residents' time to complete laparoscopic tasks was recorded. Faculty preceptors observed the residents' technique and rated them, using validated scales. They provided feedback and guidance on use of the instrument. Once residents achieved proficiency with the instrument in the simulation lab, they performed the same tasks in the operating room, where they also received feedback using validated scales. This feedback was then used when the residents went back to the simulation lab for more training and practice (8).

EXAMPLE: *Identification and Use of Learning Management System.* Based on accreditation standards and a targeted needs assessment, curriculum developers designed online modules to highlight key concepts in clinical teaching. They secured funding from the medical school for salary support and production of modules on the one-minute preceptor, chalk talks, and coaching. The curriculum developers worked with an instructional designer to identify an appropriate online learning platform that integrated video content and didactic and assessment methods (9).

Funding/Costs

Curriculum developers must consider both financial and opportunity costs in implementing the curriculum. Some of these costs will have been identified in the targeted needs assessment. These costs need to be accounted for in order to determine how a curriculum is to be funded.

EXAMPLE: *Financial Support and Opportunity Costs of a New Curriculum.* The Johns Hopkins Hospital Center for Innovation and Safety financially supported a two-day Patient Safety course offered to second-year medical students as preparation for their clinical clerkships. The curriculum included discussions of hospital patient safety initiatives, the strengths of high-reliability teamwork, and effective team communications. Simulation Center activities included stations dedicated to basic cardiac life support, sterile technique, infection control procedures, and isolation practices. In addition to obtaining financial support, curriculum developers had to obtain permission from faculty leaders in the medical students' pathophysiology course to block time from their course to allow students to attend the clerkship preparation course.

Sometimes, curricula can be accomplished by redeploying existing resources. If this appears to be the case, one should ask what will be given up in redeploying the resources (i.e., what is the hidden or opportunity cost of the curriculum?). When additional resources are required, they must be provided from somewhere. If additional funding is requested, it is necessary to develop and justify a budget.

As a project manager, the curriculum developer will need to itemize facility fees, equipment and supply costs, and personnel compensation. Costs for personnel, including curriculum directors, curriculum coordinators, faculty, administrative staff, and others, often represent the biggest budget item. Often, compensation will be based on the percentage of time devoted to curricular activities relative to full-time equivalents (FTEs). Researchers and consensus panels have attempted to define amount of effort and adequate compensation for various curricular roles (10–13). One important consideration for faculty support is whether they are being compensated through other funding sources—for basic science faculty, this can come in the form of research grants or school investments (14); for clinical faculty, the funding may come from billable patient care revenues (15). Educational or academic RVUs serve as a method to quantify the effort educators put toward curricular activities (16–18). Calculating educational RVUs can take into account factors such as the time required by the activity, the level of learner, the complexity of the teaching, the level of faculty expertise, and the quality of teaching (16). The curriculum developer can present a sound budget justification if these factors are considered in the implementation plan.

Curriculum developers must also be cognizant of the financial costs of conducting educational scholarship (see Chapter 9). In addition to whatever funds are needed to deliver the curriculum, funds may also be necessary to perform robust curriculum evaluation with a view toward dissemination of the curriculum. It has been shown that manuscripts reporting on well-funded curricula are of better quality and have higher rates of acceptance for publication in a peer-reviewed journal (19, 20).

OBTAINING SUPPORT FOR THE CURRICULUM

A curriculum is more likely to be successful in achieving its goals and objectives if it has broad support.

Internal Support

It is important that curriculum developers and coordinators recognize who the stakeholders are in a curriculum and foster their support. Stakeholders are those individuals who directly affect or are directly affected by a curriculum. For most curricula, stakeholders include the learners, the faculty who will deliver the curriculum, and individuals with administrative power within the institution.

Having the support of *learners* when implementing the curriculum can make or break the curriculum. Adult learners, in particular, need to be convinced that the goals and objectives are important to them and that the curriculum has the means to achieve their personal goals (Chapter 5) (21, 22). Learners' opinions can also influence those with administrative power.

> **EXAMPLE:** *Support of Learners.* Curriculum developers created a capstone course for fourth-year medical students called Transition to Residency and Internship and Preparation for Life (TRIPLE). The goal of TRIPLE was to prepare students at the start of their professional lives to acquire the knowledge, skills, and attitudes necessary to be successful physicians. The curriculum was initially offered as an elective, and the course was refined over a several-year period based on feedback from learners. Overall, students who elected to take the course rated it highly, convincing school administrators to make it a mandatory course for all fourth-year students before graduation.

Curricular faculty can devote varying amounts of their time, enthusiasm, and energy to the curriculum. Gaining broad faculty support may be important for some innovative curricula, especially when the curriculum will cross disciplines or specialties. *Other faculty* who have administrative influence or who may be competitors for curricular space or time can facilitate or create barriers for a curriculum.

> **EXAMPLE:** *Barriers from Other Faculty.* A new curriculum for a geriatrics elective in an internal medicine residency program was developed by junior faculty. Although the curriculum developers had met with key stakeholders along the way, they had not secured commitment from the director of the elective. When it came time to implement the curriculum, the director of the elective, an influential faculty member in the division, decided to continue to teach the old curriculum rather than incorporate the new one. The

curriculum developers then modified the new curriculum to make it suitable for fourth-year medical students and implemented it later that year.

Those with administrative authority (e.g., dean, hospital administrators, department chair, program director, division director) can allocate or deny the funds, space, faculty time, curricular time, and political support that are critical to a curriculum.

EXAMPLE: *Administrative Support of a New Curriculum.* A task force of university faculty from multiple specialties was convened by the dean of the school and tasked with developing curricular innovations in graduate medical education (GME). The task force identified patient handoffs as a focus area. The targeted needs assessment found that nearly half of residents felt that patient information was lost during shift changes and that unit-to-unit transfers were a source of problems. It was also recognized that duty-hour restrictions would increase the number of handoffs between residents. Consequently, the task force met regularly to discuss educational strategies. Funding did not permit direct observation and feedback of patient handoffs, but the task force obtained funding from the GME office and dean's office to develop a curriculum to be delivered during intern orientation (23).

Individuals who feel that a curriculum is important, effective, and popular, who believe that a curriculum positively affects them or their institution, and who have had input into that curriculum are more likely to support it. It is, therefore, helpful to *encourage input* from stakeholders as the curriculum is being planned, as well as to *provide* stakeholders with the appropriate *rationale* (see Chapters 2 and 3) and *evaluation data* (Chapter 7) to address their concerns.

EXAMPLE: *Early Success of Curriculum Convincing Stakeholders to Expand Program.* With philanthropic support to the Johns Hopkins Center for Innovative Medicine, an initiative was undertaken to assign one inpatient medical housestaff team half the usual patient census. Residents had more time to focus on patient-centered care activities such as enhanced communication skills to know patients better, help with transitions of care, and more attention to medication adherence. The program demonstrated decreased readmission rates for congestive heart failure. Higher satisfaction rates among patients and housestaff were observed compared with standard housestaff teams (24). Due to the early success of the initiative, hospital and residency program administrators supported incorporation of the patient-centered housestaff team as an important component in the overall residency curriculum. Additional grant support from two nonprofit organizations allowed the initiative to concentrate even further on involvement of patients in the discharge planning process.

Curriculum developers may need to *negotiate* with key stakeholders to obtain the political support and resources required to implement their curriculum successfully. Development of skills related to negotiation can therefore be useful. There are five generally recognized modes for conflict management (25, 26). A *collaborative* or principled negotiation style that focuses on interests, not positions, is most frequently useful (27). When negotiating with those who have power or influence, this model would advise the curriculum developer to find areas of common ground, to understand the needs of the other party, and to focus on mutual interests, rather than negotiating from fixed positions. Most of the examples provided in this section have ingredients of a collaborative approach, in which the goal is a win-win solution. Sometimes one must settle for a *compromise* (less than ideal, better than nothing) solution. Occasionally, the curriculum developer may need to *compete* for resources and support, which creates the possibility of either winning or losing. At other times, *avoidance* or *accommodation* (see the Example "Barriers from Other Faculty," above) may be the most reasonable approach, at least for certain aspects of the curriculum implementation. By engaging stakeholders, addressing their needs, providing a strong rationale, providing needs assessment and evaluation data, and building broad-based political support, curriculum developers put themselves in an advantageous bargaining position.

In some situations, the curriculum developer must be a change agent to champion curricular innovation at an institution. It helps if a new curriculum is consistent with the institution's mission, goals, and culture and if the institution is open to educational innovation (28). When these factors are not in place, the curriculum developer must become an agent of change (29–34). (See Chapter 10.)

> **EXAMPLE:** *Becoming an Organizational Change Agent.* A junior faculty member identified as his academic focus improving the systems of care within health care organizations through quality improvement and educational interventions. Over several years, he assumed increasing responsibility in positions of clinical care leadership, quality improvement, and patient safety at his academic medical center. In 1995, he introduced into the internal medicine residency training program a novel, collaborative multidisciplinary conference on patient care that examined systems issues, including use of resources (35). In 2001, he introduced a multidisciplinary Patient Safety and Quality of Care Conference into the residency training program. Two years later, because of the conference's popularity and unique approach, it replaced the traditional monthly morbidity and mortality conferences during Grand Rounds (36). This innovative morbidity and mortality conference used both systems and individual perspectives in a problem-solving manner without assigning blame. It evolved to include a matrix to examine cases from both quality-of-care and core competencies perspectives (37–39). The conference stimulated systems improvements in areas such as triage of patients into intensive care units, the placement and maintenance of intravenous lines, and management of patients with acute abdominal pain and vascular compromise. Organizational change occurred, as evidenced by the promotion of a collaborative, multidisciplinary, systems-based approach to the clinical and educational programs at the institution.

Organizational change can occur when the curriculum developer is intentional about creating a vision but also flexible in how the vision comes to fruition (29, 30).

External Support

Sometimes there are insufficient institutional resources to support part or all of a curriculum or to support its further development or expansion. In these situations, developing a sound budget and seeking a source of external support are critical.

Potential sources of *external funding* (see Appendix B) include government agencies, professional societies, philanthropic organizations or foundations, corporate entities, and individual donors. Research and development grants may be available from one's own institution, and the competition may be less intense than for truly external funds. External funding may be more justifiable when the funding is legitimately not available from internal sources. Funding for student summer jobs (usually by universities, professional schools, or professional societies) is another resource that may be available to support needed curricular or evaluation activities. External funds are more likely to be obtained when there has been a request for proposals by a funding source, such as the Josiah Macy Jr. Foundation's grant priorities on Interprofessional Education and Teamwork (40) (see Appendix B). Curriculum developers may also find success with external funding when support is requested for an innovative or particularly needed curriculum.

> **EXAMPLE:** *Combination of Internal and External Support.* The Urban Health Residency Primary Care Track of the Johns Hopkins Hospital Osler Medical Housestaff Training Program was developed to help train physician primary care leaders whose focus would be on the medical and social issues affecting underserved and vulnerable populations in urban settings. The school of medicine program partnered

with the schools of nursing and public health, the university's Urban Health Institute, the county health department, community-based organizations, and multiple community-based health centers to provide this novel training experience. In addition to hospital and departmental financial support, initial funding came from a university-based foundation, the Osler Center for Clinical Excellence, and a nonprofit organization devoted to advancing the education of health professionals, the Josiah Macy Jr. Foundation. Subsequent funding came from federal grants through the Affordable Care Act to cover the costs of resident salaries and insurance and other residency-related expenditures (41, 42).

A period of external funding can be used to build a level of internal support that may sustain the curriculum after cessation of the external funding.

EXAMPLE: *Foundation Support for Faculty Leading to Internal Support.* Bioethics faculty who were designing clinical ethics curricula in postgraduate education obtained philanthropic support from two foundations for their work. The salary support lasted several years, during which time the faculty members successfully implemented curricula for residency programs in medicine, pediatrics, surgery, obstetrics-gynecology, and neurology. The funding also allowed them time to publish educational research about their work. The success of their curricular program led to institutional financial support as an annual line-item in the budget, permitting the faculty to sustain and expand their curricular efforts once one of the foundational grants expired.

Government, professional societies, and other entities may have *influence*, through their political or funding power, that can affect the degree of internal support for a curriculum. The curriculum developer may want to bring guidelines or requirements of such bodies to the attention of stakeholders within their own institution.

EXAMPLE: *Accreditation Standards.* In May 2011, an expert panel published *Core Competencies for Interprofessional Collaborative Practice* (43). The report was sponsored by the Interprofessional Education Collaborative (IPEC), which has representation from nursing, pharmacy, dentistry, public health, and osteopathic and allopathic medicine. The report advocated for "a coordinated effort across the health professions to embed essential content in all health professions education curricula." In March 2014, the Liaison Committee on Medical Education (LCME) adopted standards on Interprofessional Collaborative Skills, which entailed, effective July 2015, that medical school "curricular experiences include practitioners and/or students from the other health professions" (44). The guidelines promulgated by these organizations provide a strong impetus for health professional schools to work together in delivering mutually advantageous, collaborative, interprofessional curricula.

Accrediting bodies may also be a source of support for innovative curricula, such as with demonstration projects.

Finally, professional societies or other institutions may have *curricular or faculty development resources* that can be used by curriculum developers (see Appendix B).

ADMINISTRATION OF THE CURRICULUM

Administrative Structure

A curriculum does not operate by itself. It requires an administrative structure to assume responsibility, to maintain communication, and to make operational and policy decisions. Often these functions are those of the curriculum director. Some types of decisions can be delegated to a curriculum administrator for segments of the curriculum. Major policy changes may best be made with the help of a core faculty group or after even broader input. In any case, a structure for efficient communication and decision making should be established and made clear to faculty, learners, and support staff.

Communication

As implied above, the rationale, goals, and objectives of the curriculum, evaluation results, and changes in the curriculum need to be communicated in appropriate detail to all involved stakeholders. Lines of communication need to be open to and from stakeholders. Therefore, the curriculum coordinator needs to establish *mechanisms for communication*, such as a website, periodic meetings, memos, syllabi, presentations, site visits or observations, and a policy regarding one's accessibility.

Operations

Mechanisms need to be developed to ensure that important functions that support the curriculum are performed. Such functions include preparing and distributing schedules and curricular materials, collecting and collating evaluation data, and supporting the communication function of the curriculum director. The operations component of the curriculum implementation is where decisions by the curriculum director or administrators are put into action (e.g., Whom should one talk to about a problem with the curriculum? When should syllabus material be distributed? When and where will evaluation data be collected? Should there be a midpoint change in curricular content? Should a learner be assigned to a different faculty member?) Large curricula usually have support staff to whom these functions can be delegated and who need to be supervised in their performance.

> **EXAMPLE:** *Operation of a School-wide Curriculum.* A course on research ethics for principal investigators and members of the research team in a medical school is coordinated through the combined efforts of the Office of Research Administration and the Office of Continuing Medical Education. An overall course director delegates operational functions to support staff from both offices, while serving as a point person for learners and faculty. Support staff in the Office of Research Administration administer the online curricular materials, while a course administrator in the Office of Continuing Medical Education communicates with learners and coordinates the logistics of the in-person component (registration of learners, printing and distributing syllabus materials, scheduling classroom space, confirming faculty availability, collection and analysis of evaluations, annual certification of the course, etc.).

Scholarship

As discussed in Chapter 9, curriculum developers may wish to disseminate, through presentation or publication, information related to their curricula, such as the needs assessment, curricular methods, or curricular evaluations. When dissemination is a goal, additional resources and administration may be required for more rigorous needs assessments, educational methodology, evaluation designs, data collection and analysis, and/or assessment instruments.

Curriculum developers also have to address ethical issues related to research (Chapter 7). Issues such as informed consent of learners, confidentiality, and the use of incentives to encourage participation in a curriculum all need to be considered (45, 46). An important consideration is whether learners are to be classified as human research subjects. Federal regulations governing research in the United States categorize many educational research projects as exempt from the regulations if the research involves the study of normal educational practices or records information about learners in such a way that they cannot be identified (47). However, IRBs may differ in their interpretation of what is exempt under the regulations (48, 49). Or some IRBs may want to ensure additional safeguards for learners besides those that the regulations require. It is, therefore, prudent for curriculum developers to seek guidance from their IRBs about how best to protect the rights and interests of learners who are also research subjects (50–52). Failure to consult one's IRB before implementation of the curriculum can have adverse consequences for the curriculum developer who later tries to publish research about the curriculum (53).

ANTICIPATING BARRIERS

Before initiating a new curriculum or making changes in an old curriculum, it is helpful to anticipate and address any potential barriers to their accomplishment. Barriers can relate to finances, other resources, or people (e.g., competing demands for resources; nonsupportive attitudes; issues of job or role security, credit, and political power) (54). Time can also pose a barrier, such as carving out curricular time when medical students are dispersed at different clinical sites or residents are not available to attend teaching sessions because of duty-hour restrictions.

EXAMPLE: *Competition.* In planning the ambulatory component of the internal medicine clerkship for third-year medical students, the curriculum developer anticipated resistance from the inpatient clerkship director, based on loss of curricular time and responsibility/power. The curriculum developer built a well-reasoned argument for the ambulatory component based on external recommendations and current needs. She ensured student support for the change and the support of critical faculty. She gained support from the dean's office and was granted additional curricular time for the ambulatory component, which addressed some of the inpatient director's concerns about loss of curricular time for training on the inpatient services. She invited the inpatient coordinator to be on the planning committee for the ambulatory component, to increase his understanding of needs, to promote his sense of ownership and responsibility for the ambulatory component, and to promote coordination of learning and educational methodology between the inpatient and ambulatory components.

EXAMPLE: *Resistance.* The developers of a tool to evaluate the surgical skills of residents anticipated resistance from faculty in completing an evaluation after each surgery. They therefore had to make the evaluation tool user-friendly and readily accessible. Knowing that collection and collation of paper-based forms would be cumbersome and difficult, the curriculum developers created an online instrument. Because the evaluation would be completed postoperatively, when there were still patient care issues to address, the developers also anticipated the need to make the instrument brief enough to be completed in a couple of minutes (55).

INTRODUCING THE CURRICULUM

Piloting

It is important to pilot critical segments of a new curriculum on friendly or convenient audiences before formally introducing it. Critical segments might include needs assessment and evaluation instruments, as well as educational methods. Piloting enables curriculum developers to receive critical feedback and to make important revisions that increase the likelihood of successful implementation.

EXAMPLE: *Piloting a Course during Faculty Orientation.* For a new course on research ethics for all faculty conducting human subjects research in the school of medicine, course developers first piloted the curriculum in an abbreviated fashion during the orientation for new faculty. The pilot mainly involved the use of small group workshops in which participants commented on the ethical issues involved in a mock research protocol. Piloting the curriculum on new faculty allowed curriculum developers to get a fresh perspective from learners not yet familiar with institutional culture. Feedback was obtained from learners and course faculty to aid in shaping the eventual curriculum that was rolled out to the entire faculty in the subsequent year.

Phasing In

Phasing in a complex curriculum one part at a time or the entire curriculum on a segment of the targeted learners permits a focusing of initial efforts, as faculty and staff learn new procedures. When the curriculum represents a cultural shift in an institution or requires attitudinal changes in the stakeholders, introducing the curriculum one step at a time, rather than all at once, can lessen resistance and increase acceptance, particularly if the stakeholders are involved in the process (29). Like piloting, phasing in affords the opportunity to have a cycle of experience, feedback, evaluation, and response before full implementation.

> **EXAMPLE:** *Phasing in a New Interprofessional Curriculum.* Curriculum developers designing a curriculum in spiritual care for medical residents and chaplain trainees viewed involvement of the chaplain trainees in medical rounds as a key educational strategy. This strategy was introduced on a medical service dedicated to a more holistic approach to patient care. Two successive groups of chaplain trainees rotated through the medical service attending rounds with the resident team before the entire curriculum was fully implemented in the following year (56).

> **EXAMPLE:** *An Anticipated Phase-in.* Curriculum developers of a new Master of Education in the Health Professions (MEHP) degree program planned to deliver the first year of the curriculum during in-person sessions, then to transition to an exclusively online curriculum. This approach allowed the curricular content and educational strategies to be refined based on feedback from a small, invested group of learners before being made available to larger audiences via the Internet. Evaluation and feedback from faculty and learners in the first year of the program were used to improve the overall curriculum.

Both the piloting and phasing-in approaches to implementing a curriculum advertise it as a curriculum in development, increase participants' tolerance and desire to help, decrease faculty resistance to negative feedback, and increase the chance for success on full implementation.

Full Implementation

In general, full implementation should follow a piloting and/or phasing-in experience. Sometimes, however, the demand for a full curriculum for all learners is so pressing, or a curriculum is so limited in scope, that immediate full implementation is preferable. In this case, the first cycle of the curriculum can be considered a "pilot" cycle. Evaluation data on educational outcomes (i.e., achievement of goals and objectives) and processes (i.e., milestones of curriculum delivery) from initial cycles of a curriculum can then be used to refine the implementation of subsequent cycles (see Chapter 7). Of course, a successful curriculum should always be in a stage of continuous improvement, as described in Chapter 8.

> **EXAMPLE:** *Full Implementation in Response to Curricular Change.* When an entirely new overall medical school curriculum was introduced in 2009, a systems-based elective on the principles of patient safety, in existence since 2004, was made mandatory. The original course was delivered in 6 to 10 hours over a three- to five-week period and was given to first-year students. The new course was delivered during

a three-day concentration to second-year students. The course was modified in response to a targeted needs assessment and evaluation from the previous course. The new course served as an anchor for other safety and quality educational initiatives throughout the medical school curriculum (57).

INTERACTION WITH OTHER STEPS

When thinking through what is required to implement a curriculum as it has initially been conceived, one often discovers that there are insufficient resources and administrative structures to support such a curriculum. The curriculum developer should not become discouraged. With insight about the targeted learners and their learning environment, further prioritization and focusing of curricular objectives, educational strategies, and/or evaluation are required. For this reason, it is usually wise to be thinking of Step 5 (Implementation) in conjunction with Step 2 (Targeted Needs Assessment), Step 3 (Goals and Objectives), Step 4 (Educational Strategies), and Step 6 (Evaluation and Feedback).

It is better to anticipate problems than to discover them too late. Curriculum development is an interactive, cyclical process, and each step affects the others. It may be more prudent to start small and build on a curriculum's success than to aim too high and watch the curriculum fail due to unachievable goals, insufficient resources, or inadequate support. *Implementation is the step that converts a mental exercise to reality.*

QUESTIONS

For the curriculum you are coordinating, planning, or would like to be planning, please answer or think about the questions below. If your thoughts about a curriculum are just beginning, you may wish to answer these questions in the context of a few educational strategies, such as the ones you identified in your answers to the questions at the end of Chapter 5.

1. What *resources* are required for the curriculum you envision, in terms of personnel, time, and facilities? Will your faculty need specialized training before implementation? Did you remember to think of patients as well as faculty and support staff? What are the internal costs of this curriculum? Is there a need for external resources or funding? If there is a need for external funding, construct a budget. Finally, are your curricular plans feasible in terms of the required resources?

2. What is the degree of *support* within your institution for the curriculum? Where will the resistance come from? How could you increase support and decrease resistance? How likely is it that you will get the support necessary? Will external support be necessary? If so, what are some possible sources and what is the nature of the support that is required (e.g., funds, resource materials, accreditation requirements, political support)?

3. What sort of *administration*, in terms of *administrative structure, communications, operations, and scholarship*, is necessary to implement and maintain the curriculum? Think of how decisions will be made, how communication will take place, and what operations are necessary for the smooth functioning of the curriculum (e.g., prep-

aration and distribution of schedules, curricular and evaluation materials, evaluation reports). Are IRB review and approval of an educational research project needed?

4. What *barriers* do you anticipate to implementing the curriculum? Develop plans for addressing them.

5. Develop plans to *introduce* the curriculum. What are the most critical segments of the curriculum that would be a priority for *piloting*? On whom would you pilot it? Can the curriculum be *phased in*, or must it be implemented all at once on all learners? How will you learn from piloting and phasing in the curriculum and apply this learning to the curriculum? If you are planning on full implementation, what structures are in place to provide feedback to the curriculum for further improvements?

6. Given your answers to Questions 1 through 5, is your curriculum likely to be feasible and successful? Do you need to go back to the drawing board and alter your approach to some of the steps?

GENERAL REFERENCES

Glanz K, Rimer BK, Viswanath K, eds. *Health Behavior and Health Education: Theory, Research, and Practice*, 4th ed. San Francisco: Jossey-Bass; 2008.
This book reviews theories and models for behavioral change important in delivering health education. Health education involves an awareness of the impact of communication, interpersonal relationships, and community on those who are targeted for behavioral change. For the curriculum developer, the chapters on diffusion of innovations and organizational change are particularly relevant. Chapter 14 (pp. 313–34) describes diffusion as a multilevel change process, with success achieved not just by demonstrating efficacy and effectiveness but also by actively implementing strategies to ensure sustainability. Chapter 15 (pp. 335–62) advances the idea that establishment of an education program often involves some degree of organizational change. The chapter reviews the history and characteristics of organizational development theory and includes two health care application examples. 592 pages.

Heagney J. *Fundamentals of Project Management*, 4th ed. New York: American Management Association; 2012.
An introduction to the principles and practice of project management, offering a step-by-step approach and useful tips in planning and executing a project. The suggestions on how to function as a project leader can be helpful for the curriculum developer to enable successful implementation of a curriculum. 202 pages.

Knowles MS, Holton EF, Swanson RA. *The Adult Learner: The Definitive Classic in Adult Education and Human Resource Development*, 8th ed. London: Routledge; 2014.
The classic text that reviews learning theory, with emphasis on andragogy and the key principles in adult learning, including the learner's need to know, the learner's self-concept of autonomy, the importance of prior experience, the learner's readiness to learn, the learner's problem-based orientation to learning, and the learner's motivation to learn derived from the intrinsic value and personal payoff from learning. Includes suggestions on how to put andragogy into practice. 288 pages.

Kotter JP. *Leading Change*. Boston: Harvard Business Review Press; 2012.
An excellent book on leadership, differentiating between leadership and management and outlining the qualities of a good leader. The author discusses eight steps critical to creating major change in an organization: 1) establishing a sense of urgency, 2) creating the guiding coalition, 3) developing a vision and strategy, 4) communicating the change vision, 5) empowering employ-

ees for broad-based action, 6) generating short-term wins, 7) consolidating gains and producing more change, and 8) anchoring new approaches in the culture. 208 pages.

Larson EW, Gray CF. *Project Management: The Managerial Process*, 6th ed. New York: McGraw-Hill/Irwin; 2013.
A book written for the professional or student business manager but of interest to anyone overseeing the planning and implementation of a project. It guides the reader through the steps in project management, from defining the problem and planning an intervention to executing the project and overseeing its impact. 686 pages.

Rogers EM. *Diffusion of Innovations*, 5th ed. New York: Free Press; 2003.
Classic text describing all aspects and stages of the process whereby new phenomena are adopted and diffused throughout social systems. The book contains a discussion of the elements of diffusion, the history and status of diffusion research, the generation of innovations, the innovation-decision process, attributes of innovations and their rate of adoption, innovativeness and adopter categories, opinion leadership and diffusion networks, the change agent, innovations in organizations, and consequences of innovations. Among many other disciplines, education, public health, and medical sociology have made practical use of the theory with empirical research of Rogers's work. Implementation is addressed specifically in several pages (pp. 179–88, 430–32), highlighting the great importance of implementation to the diffusion process. 551 pages.

Westley F, Zimmerman B, Patton MQ. *Getting to Maybe: How the World Is Changed*. Toronto: Random House Canada; 2006.
Richly illustrated with real-world examples, this book focuses on complex organizations and social change. Change can come from the bottom up as well as from the top down. The authors contend that an agent of change needs to have intentionality and flexibility, must recognize that achieving success can have peaks and valleys, should understand that relationships are key to engaging in social intervention, and must have a mindset framed by inquiry rather than certitude. With this framework, the book outlines the steps necessary to achieve change for complex problems. 258 pages.

Whitman N, Weiss E. *Executive Skills for Medical Faculty*, 3rd ed. Pacific Grove, Calif.: Whitman Associates; 2006.
Many of the skills needed by health care leaders are also important for successful development and implementation of curricula, such as improving communication skills, becoming a leader, working through others, negotiating, implementing change, strategic planning, getting things done, team building and coaching, and planning a career strategy. 195 pages.

SPECIFIC REFERENCES

1. Lemon M, Greer T, Siegel B. Implementation issues in generalist education. *J Gen Intern Med.* 1994;9(Suppl 1):S98–104.
2. Nyindo M, Kitau J, Lisasi E, et al. Introduction of team-based learning (TBL) at Kilimanjaro Christian Medical University College: experience with the ectoparasites module. *Med Teach.* 2014;36(4):308–13.
3. Houston TK, Connors RL, Cutler N, Nidiry MA. A primary care musculoskeletal clinic for residents: success and sustainability. *J Gen Intern Med.* 2004;19(5 Pt 2):524–29.
4. Kumar A, Loomba D, Rahangdale RY, Kallen DJ. Rewards and incentives for nonsalaried clinical faculty who teach medical students. *J Gen Intern Med.* 1999;14(6):370–72.
5. Kumar A, Kallen DJ, Mathew T. Volunteer faculty: what rewards or incentives do they prefer? *Teach Learn Med.* 2002;14(2):119–23.
6. Hayashi JL, Phillips KA, Arbaje A, et al. A curriculum to teach internal medicine residents to perform house calls for older adults. *J Am Geriatr Soc.* 2007;55(8):1287–94.

7. Hayashi J, Christmas C, Durso SC. Educational outcomes from a novel house call curriculum for internal medicine residents: report of a 3-year experience. *J Am Geriatr Soc.* 2011; 59(7):1340–49.
8. Example adapted with permission from the curricular project of Kimberly Steele, MD, and Yvette Young, MD, for the Johns Hopkins Longitudinal Program in Faculty Development, cohort 20, 2006–2007.
9. Example adapted with permission from the curricular projects of Michael Melia, MD, Lauren Block, MD, MPH, Lorrel Brown, MD, and Deepa Rangachari, MD, for the Johns Hopkins Longitudinal Program in Faculty Development, cohort 26, 2012–2013, and cohort 27, 2013–2014.
10. Rouan GW, Wones RG, Tsevat J, et al. Rewarding teaching faculty with a reimbursement plan. *J Gen Intern Med.* 1999;14(6):327–32.
11. Yeh MM, Cahill DF. Quantifying physician teaching productivity using clinical relative value units. *J Gen Intern Med.* 1999;14(10):617–21.
12. Mallon WT, Jones RF. How do medical schools use measurement systems to track faculty activity and productivity in teaching? *Acad Med.* 2002 Feb;77(2):115–23.
13. Sainté M, Kanter SL, Muller D. Mission-based budgeting for education: ready for prime time? *Mt Sinai J Med.* 2009;76(4):381–86.
14. Dorsey ER, Van Wuyckhuyse BC, Beck CA, Passalacqua WP, Guzick DS. The economics of new faculty hires in basic science. *Acad Med.* 2009;84(1):26–31.
15. Geraci SA, Devine DR, Babbott SF, et al. AAIM report on master teachers and clinician educators. Part 3: Finances and resourcing. *Am J Med.* 2010;123(10):963–67.
16. Stites S, Vansaghi L, Pingleton S, Cox G, Paolo A. Aligning compensation with education: design and implementation of the educational value unit (EVU) system in an academic internal medicine department. *Acad Med.* 2005;80(12):1100–1106.
17. Mezrich R, Nagy PG. The academic RVU: a system for measuring academic productivity. *J Am Coll Radiol.* 2007;4(7):471–78.
18. Clyburn EB, Wood C, Moran W, Feussner JR. Valuing the education mission: implementing an educational value units system. *Am J Med.* 2011;124(6):567–72.
19. Reed DA, Cook DA, Beckman TJ, et al. Association between funding and quality of published medical education research. *JAMA.* 2007;298:1002–9.
20. Reed DA, Beckman TJ, Wright SM, et al. Predictive validity evidence for medical education research study quality instrument scores: quality of submissions to JGIM's Medical Education Special Issue. *J Gen Intern Med.* 2008;23(7):903–7.
21. Knowles MS, Holton EF, Swanson RA. *The Adult Learner: The Definitive Classic in Adult Education and Human Resource Development*, 8th ed. London: Routledge; 2014.
22. Brookfield S. *Powerful Techniques for Teaching Adults*. San Francisco: Jossey-Bass; 2013.
23. Allen S, Caton C, Cluver J, Mainous AG 3rd, Clyburn B. Targeting improvements in patient safety at a large academic center: an institutional handoff curriculum for graduate medical education. *Acad Med.* 2014 Oct;89(10):1366–69.
24. Ratanawongsa N, Federowicz MA, Christmas C, et al. Effects of a focused patient-centered care curriculum on the experiences of internal medicine residents and their patients. *J Gen Intern Med.* 2012;27(4):473–77.
25. Thomas KW. *Introduction to Conflict Management: Improving Performance Using the TKI.* Mountain View, Calif.: CPP; 2002.
26. Thomas KW, Kilmann RH. An Overview of the Thomas-Kilmann Conflict Mode Instrument (TKI) [Internet]. Available at www.kilmanndiagnostics.com/overview-thomas-kilmann-conflict-mode-instrument-tki.
27. Fisher R, Ury W, Patton B. *Getting to Yes: Negotiating Agreement without Giving In*, 3rd ed. New York: Penguin Books; 2011.
28. Bland CJ, Starnaman S, Wersal L, et al. Curricular change in medical schools: how to succeed. *Acad Med.* 2000;75(6):575–94.

29. Kotter JP. *Leading Change*. Boston: Harvard Business Review Press; 2012.
30. Westley F, Zimmerman B, Patton MQ. *Getting to Maybe: How the World Is Changed.* Toronto: Random House Canada; 2006.
31. Cameron KS, Quinn RE. *Diagnosing and Changing Organizational Culture: Based on the Competing Values Framework*, 3rd ed. San Francisco: Jossey-Bass; 2011.
32. de Caluwé L, Vermaak H. *Learning to Change: A Guide for Organization Change Agents.* Thousand Oaks, Calif.: SAGE Publications; 2003.
33. Meyerson D. *Tempered Radicals: How People Use Differences to Inspire Change at Work.* Boston: Harvard Business School Press; 2001.
34. Shepard HA. Rules of thumb for change agents. In French WL, Bell C, Zawacki RA, eds. *Organization Development and Transformation: Managing Effective Change*, 6th ed. New York: McGraw-Hill/Irwin; 2005. Pp. 336–41.
35. Kravet SJ, Wright, SW, Carrese JA. Teaching resource and information management using an innovative case-based conference. *J Gen Intern Med.* 2001;16(6):399–403.
36. Kravet SJ, Wright SM. Morbidity and mortality conference, grand rounds, and the ACGME's core competencies. *J Gen Intern Med.* 2006;21(11):1192–94.
37. Institute of Medicine. *Crossing the Quality Chasm: A New Health System for the 21st Century.* Report of the Committee on Quality of Health Care in America. Washington, D.C.: National Academies Press; 2001.
38. Quinn DC, Bingham JW, Shourbaji NA, Jarquin-Valdivia AA. Medical students learn to assess care using the healthcare matrix. *Med Teach.* 2007;29(7):660–65.
39. Accreditation Council for Graduate Medical Education [Internet]. Available at www.acgme .org.
40. The Josiah Macy Jr. Foundation [Internet]. Available at http://macyfoundation.org/priorities.
41. Pelletier SG. Hopkins Pilots Residency Program in Urban Health [Internet]. *AAMC Reporter*, March 2011. Available at https://www.aamc.org/newsroom/reporter/march11/180244/hop kins_pilots_residency_program_in_urban_health.html.
42. Stewart R, Feldman L, Bitzel D, Gibbons MC, McGuire M. Urban health and primary care at Johns Hopkins: urban primary care medical home resident training programs. *J Health Care Poor Underserved.* 2012;23(3 Suppl):103–13.
43. Interprofessional Education Collaborative Expert Panel. *Core Competencies for Interprofessional Collaborative Practice: Report of an Expert Panel.* Washington, D.C.: Interprofessional Education Collaborative; 2011. Available at https://ipecollaborative.org /uploads/IPEC-Core-Competencies.pdf.
44. Liaison Committee on Medical Education. *Functions and Structure of a Medical School: Standards for Accreditation of Medical Education Programs Leading to the M.D. Degree.* March 2014 Standards and Elements Effective July 1, 2015. Available at www.lcme.org /connections.htm.
45. Roberts LW, Geppert C, Connor R, Nguyen K, Warner TD. An invitation for medical educators to focus on ethical and policy issues in research and scholarly practice. *Acad Med.* 2001;76(9):876–85.
46. Keune JD, Brunsvold ME, Hohmann E, et al. The ethics of conducting graduate medical education research on residents. *Acad Med.* 2013 Apr;88(4):449–53. doi:10.1097/ACM .0b013e3182854bef.
47. Miser WF. Educational research—to IRB, or not to IRB? *Fam Med.* 2005;37(3):168–73.
48. Sarpel U, Hopkins MA, More F, et al. Medical students as human subjects in educational research. *Med Educ Online.* 2013, Feb 25;18:1–6. doi:10.3402/meo.v18i0.19524.
49. Dyrbye LN, Thomas MR, Mechaber AJ, et al. Medical education research and IRB review: an analysis and comparison of the IRB review process at six institutions. *Acad Med.* 2007;82(7):654–60.
50. Henry RC, Wright DE. When do medical students become human subjects of research? The case of program evaluation. *Acad Med.* 2001;76(9):871–75.

51. Dyrbye LN, Thomas MR, Papp KK, Durning SJ. Clinician educators' experiences with institutional review boards: results of a national survey. *Acad Med.* 2008 Jun;83(6):590–95.
52. Sullivan GM. Education research and human subject protection: crossing the IRB quagmire. *J Grad Med Educ.* 2011;3(1):1–4.
53. Tomkowiak JM, Gunderson AJ. To IRB or not to IRB? *Acad Med.* 2004 Jul;79(7):628–32.
54. Whitman N. Implementing change. In: Whitman N, Weiss E, eds. *Executive Skills for Medical Faculty*, 3rd ed. Pacific Grove, Calif.: Whitman Associates; 2006. Pp. 71–87.
55. Example adapted with permission from the curricular project of JP Dunn, MD, Kristina Altman, MD, and John Caccamese Jr, DMD, MD, FACS, for the Johns Hopkins Longitudinal Program in Faculty Development, cohort 19, 2005–2006.
56. Example adapted with permission from the curricular project of Tahara Akmal, MA, Ty Crowe, MDiv, Patrick Hemming, MD, MPH, Tommy Rogers, MDiv, Emmanuel Saidi, PhD, Monica Sandoval, MD, and Paula Teague, DMin, MBA, for the Johns Hopkins Longitudinal Program in Faculty Development, cohort 26, 2012–2013.
57. Aboumatar HJ, Thompson D, Wu A, et al. Development and evaluation of a 3-day patient safety curriculum to advance knowledge, self-efficacy and system thinking among medical students. *BMJ Qual Saf.* 2012;21(5):416–22.

CHAPTER SEVEN

Step 6
Evaluation and Feedback

*. . . assessing the achievement of objectives and stimulating
continuous improvement*

Brenessa M. Lindeman, MD, MEHP, and
Pamela A. Lipsett, MD, MHPE

DEFINITIONS

Evaluation, for the purposes of this book, is defined as the identification, clarification, and application of criteria to determine the merit or worth of what is being evaluated (1). While often used interchangeably, *assessment* is sometimes used to connote characterizations and measurements, while *evaluation* is used to connote appraisal or judgment. In education, assessment is often of an individual student, while evaluation is of a program; for the most part, we follow this convention in this chapter. Feedback is defined as the provision of information on an individual's or curriculum's performance to learners, faculty, and other stakeholders in the curriculum.

IMPORTANCE

Step 6, Evaluation and Feedback, closes the loop in the curriculum development cycle. The evaluation process helps those who have a stake in the curriculum make a decision or judgment about the curriculum. The evaluation step helps curriculum developers ask and answer the critical question: Were the goals and objectives of the curriculum met? Evaluation provides information that can be used to guide individuals and the curriculum in cycles of ongoing improvement. Evaluation results can also be used to maintain and garner support for a curriculum, to assess student achievement, to satisfy external requirements, to document the accomplishments of curriculum developers, and to serve as a basis for presentations and publications.

It is helpful to be methodical in designing the evaluation for a curriculum, to ensure that important questions are answered and relevant needs met. This chapter outlines a 10-task approach that begins with consideration of the potential users and uses of an evaluation, moves to the identification of evaluation questions and methods, proceeds to the collection of data, and ends with data analysis and reporting of results.

TASK I: IDENTIFY USERS

The first step in planning the evaluation for a curriculum is to identify the likely users of the evaluation. *Participants* in the curriculum have an interest in the assessment of their own performance and the performance of the curriculum. Evaluation can provide feedback and motivation for continued improvement for *learners*, *faculty*, and *curriculum developers*.

Other stakeholders who have administrative responsibility for, allocate resources to, or are otherwise affected by the curriculum will also be interested in evaluation results. These might include individuals in the *dean's office*, *hospital administrators*, the *department chair*, the *program director* for the residency program or medical student education, the *division director*, *other faculty* who have contributed political support or who might be in competition for limited resources, and *individuals, granting agencies, or other organizations that have contributed funds or other resources* to the curriculum. Individuals who need to make decisions about whether or not to participate in the curriculum, such as *future learners or faculty*, may also be interested in evaluation results.

To the extent that a curriculum innovatively addresses an important need or tests new educational strategies, evaluation results may also be of interest to *educators from other institutions* and serve as a basis for publications/presentations. As society is often the intended beneficiary of a medical care curriculum, society members are also stakeholders in this process.

Finally, evaluation results can document the achievements of *curriculum developers*. Promotion committees and department chairs assign a high degree of importance to clinician-educators' accomplishments in curriculum development (2, 3), and these accomplishments can be included in the educational portfolios that are increasingly being used to support applications for promotion (4–6).

TASK II: IDENTIFY USES

Generic Uses

In designing an evaluation strategy for a curriculum, the curriculum developer should be aware of the generic uses of an evaluation. These generic uses can be classified along two axes, as shown in Table 7.1. The first axis refers to whether the evaluation is used to appraise the performance of *individuals*, the performance of the entire *program*, or both. The assessment of an individual usually involves determining whether he or she has achieved the cognitive, affective, or psychomotor or competency objectives of a curriculum (see Chapter 4). Program evaluation usually determines the aggregate achievements of all individuals, clinical or other outcomes, the actual processes of a curriculum, or the perceptions of learners and faculty. The second axis in Table 7.1 refers to whether an evaluation is used for *formative* purposes (to improve performance), for *summative* purposes (to judge performance and make decisions about its future or adoption), or for both purposes (7). From the discussion and examples below, the reader may surmise that *some evaluations can be used for both summative and formative purposes.*

One emerging educational framework that can be informative for both formative and summative assessment is the use of entrustable professional activities, or EPAs. EPAs are units of professional practice and have been defined as tasks or responsibilities that trainees are entrusted to perform without supervision, once they have attained sufficient competence (8). EPAs are related to competencies (such as the competency framework used in GME training from the Accreditation Council for Graduate Medical Education [ACGME]), in that performance of an EPA requires integration of competencies, often across multiple domains of competence (9). While the EPA framework was initially formulated for the transition from residency to independent practice, this concept has recently been extended to develop EPAs for the transition from medical school to residency (10), and some medical schools have developed EPAs for their students. (See also Chapter 4.)

Table 7.1.   Evaluation Types: Levels and Uses

Use	Level	
	Individual	Program
Formative	Evaluation of an individual learner or faculty member that is used to help the individual improve performance: ▪ identification of areas for improvement ▪ specific suggestions for improvement	Evaluation of a program that is used to improve program performance: ▪ identification of areas for improvement ▪ specific suggestions for improvement
Summative	Evaluation of an individual learner or faculty member that is used for judgments or decisions about the individual: ▪ verification of achievement for individual ▪ motivation of individual to maintain or improve performance ▪ certification of performance for others ▪ grades ▪ promotion	Evaluation of a program that is used for judgments or decisions about the program or program developers: ▪ judgments regarding success, efficacy ▪ decisions regarding allocation of resources ▪ motivation/recruitment of learners and faculty ▪ influencing attitudes regarding value of curriculum ▪ satisfying external requirements ▪ prestige, power, influence, promotion ▪ dissemination: presentations, publications

Specific Uses

Having identified the likely users of the evaluation and understood the generic uses of curriculum evaluation, the curriculum developer should consider the specific needs of different users (stakeholders) and the specific ways in which they will put the evaluation to use (7). Specific uses for evaluation results might include the following:

▪ *Feedback on and improvement of individual performance:* Both learners and faculty can use the results of timely feedback (formative individual assessment) to direct improvements in their own performances. This type of assessment identifies areas for improvement and provides specific suggestions for improvement (feedback). It, therefore, also serves as an educational method (see Chapter 5).

EXAMPLE: *Formative Individual Assessment.* During a women's health clerkship, students are assessed on their ability to perform the Core EPA for Entering Residency, "Provide an oral presentation of a clinical encounter" (10), after interviewing a standardized patient with a breast mass, and are given specific verbal feedback about the presentation to improve their performance.

▪ *Judgments regarding individual performance:* The accomplishments of individual learners may need to be documented (summative individual assessment) to assign grades, to demonstrate mastery in a particular area or achievement of certain curricular objectives, or to satisfy the demands of external bodies, such as specialty boards. In these instances, it is important to clarify criteria for the achievement of objectives or competency before the evaluation. Assessment of individual faculty can be used to make decisions about their continuation as curriculum faculty, as material for their promotion portfolios, and as data for teaching awards. Used in this manner, assessments become evaluations.

EXAMPLE: *Summative Individual Assessment.* At the conclusion of the women's health clerkship, a multistation Objective Structured Clinical Examination (OSCE) is conducted in which each student gives an oral presentation after an interview with a standardized patient with a breast mass. Students are assessed using a checklist form developed from the oral presentation EPA milestones (10), from which a passing score in each station determines mastery of giving an oral presentation of a clinical encounter.

- *Feedback on and improvement of program performance:* Curriculum coordinators can use evaluation results (formative program evaluation) to identify parts of the curriculum that are effective and parts that are in need of improvement. Evaluation results may also provide suggestions about how parts of the curriculum could be improved.

   Such formative program evaluation usually takes the form of surveys (see Chapter 3) of learners to obtain feedback about and suggestions for improving a curriculum. Quantitative information, such as ratings of various aspects of the curriculum, can help identify areas that need revision. Qualitative information, such as responses to open-ended questions about program strengths, program weaknesses, and suggestions for change, provides feedback in areas that may not have been anticipated and ideas for improvement. Information can also be obtained from faculty or other observers, such as nurses and patients. Aggregates of formative and summative individual assessments can be used for formative program evaluation as well, to identify specific areas of the curriculum in need of revision.

EXAMPLE: *Formative Program Evaluation.* At the midpoint of a surgery clinical clerkship, students met with the clerkship director for a discussion of experiences to date. Several students wanted additional elective clinic experiences. The clerkship director reviewed this information with surgery faculty and team leaders, and a two-week selective in ambulatory surgical clinics was implemented in the following term (11).

EXAMPLE: *Formative Program Evaluation.* After each didactic lecture of the radiology residency curriculum, residents were asked to complete a "Minute Paper" in which they briefly noted either the most important thing they had learned during the lecture or the muddiest point in the lecture, as well as an important question that remained unanswered (12). This technique allowed the instructor to know what knowledge students were gaining from the lecture (or not) and provided information about where to make future refinements.

- *Judgments regarding program success:* Summative program evaluation provides information on the degree to which a curriculum has met its various objectives and expectations, under what specific conditions, and at what cost. It can also document the curriculum's success in engaging, motivating, and pleasing its learners and faculty. In addition to quantitative data, summative program evaluation may include qualitative information about unintended barriers, unanticipated factors encountered in the program implementation, or unintended consequences of the curriculum. It may identify aspects of the hidden curriculum (13, 14). The results of summative program evaluations are often reported to others to obtain or maintain curricular time, funding, and other resources.

EXAMPLE: *Summative Program Evaluation.* At the conclusion of a psychiatry clinical clerkship, 90% of students received a passing grade in the performance of a standardized patient history and mental status examination: assessing 10 cognitive and 6 skill objectives in the areas of history, physical and mental status examination, diagnosis, management, and counseling.

EXAMPLE: *Summative Program Evaluation Leading to Further Investigation and Change.* One curricular objective of a trauma and acute care surgery rotation stated that surgery residents would correctly prescribe twice-daily prophylaxis for venous thromboembolism (VTE) in eligible trauma patients. The use of twice-daily VTE prophylaxis over the academic year was examined and compared with the use of other VTE prophylaxis. Examination of the reasons why twice-daily VTE prophylaxis had not been used revealed a misalignment of the electronic order-entry system with the clinical guideline. Review of this information with department administrators led to changes in the electronic order-entry system (15).

EXAMPLE: *Summative Program Evaluation Leading to Curricular Expansion.* Summative evaluation of all 13 Core EPAs for Entering Residency (10) among fourth-year students at one medical school revealed gaps in students' abilities to identify system failures and contribute to a culture of safety. As a result, the curriculum for intersessions between clinical clerkships was expanded to include discussions of the importance of error prevention to individual patients and to systems, a mock Root Cause Analysis exercise, and resources for reporting of real or potential errors within the institution.

- *Justification for the allocation of resources:* Those with administrative authority can use evaluation results (summative program evaluation) to guide and justify decisions about the allocation of resources for a curriculum. They may be more likely to allocate limited resources to a curriculum if the evaluation provides evidence of success or if revisions are planned to a curriculum that presently demonstrates evidence of deficiency in an accreditation standard. In the above Example, assessment of newly defined program outcomes identified deficiencies in student preparation, leading to expanded allocation of resources for the curriculum.
- *Motivation and recruitment:* Feedback on individual and program success and the identification of areas for future improvement can be motivational to faculty (formative and summative individual assessment and program evaluation). Evidence of programs' responsiveness to formative program evaluation can be attractive to future learners, just as evidence of programs' success through summative evaluation can also help in the recruitment of both learners and faculty.
- *Attitude change:* Evidence that significant change has occurred in learners (summative program evaluation) with the use of an unfamiliar method, such as participation in quality improvement projects, or in a previously unknown content area, such as systems-based practice, can significantly alter attitudes about the importance of such methods and content.

EXAMPLE: *Summative Program Evaluation Leading to Attitude Change.* A group quality improvement curriculum and project were added to the annual requirements for pediatrics residents. The pre-curriculum needs assessment revealed that 38% of residents agreed that physicians play an important role in quality improvement efforts. However, after participation in the curriculum and project, 96% of residents agreed with the same statement.

- *Satisfaction of external and internal requirements:* Summative individual and program evaluation results can be used to satisfy the requirements of regulatory bodies, such as the Liaison Committee on Medical Education or the Residency Review and Graduate Medical Education Committees. These evaluations, therefore, may be necessary for program accreditation and will be welcomed by those who have administrative responsibility for an overall program.

- *Demonstration of popularity:* Evidence that learners and faculty truly enjoyed and valued their experience (summative program evaluation) and evidence of other stakeholder support (patients, benefactors) may be important to educational and other administrative leaders, who want to meet the needs of existing trainees, faculty, and other stakeholders and to recruit new ones. A high degree of learner, faculty, and stakeholder support provides strong political support for a curriculum.

- *Prestige, power, promotion, and influence:* A successful program (summative program evaluation) reflects positively on its institution, department chair, division chief, overall program director, curriculum coordinator, and faculty, thereby conveying a certain degree of prestige, power, and influence. Summative program and individual assessment data can be used as evidence of accomplishment in one's promotion portfolio.

- *Presentations, publications, and adoption of curricular components by others:* To the degree that an evaluation (summative program evaluation) provides evidence of the success (or failure) of an innovative or insufficiently studied educational program or method, it will be of interest to educators at other institutions and to publishers (see Chapter 9).

TASK III: IDENTIFY RESOURCES

The most carefully planned evaluation will fail if the resources are not available to accomplish it (16). Limits in resources may require a prioritization of evaluation questions and changes in evaluation methods. For this reason, curriculum developers should *consider resource needs early in the planning of the evaluation process*, including *time*, *personnel*, *equipment*, *facilities*, and *funds*. Appropriate *time* should be allocated for the collection, analysis, and reporting of evaluation results. *Personnel* needs often include staff to help in the collection and collation of data and distribution of reports, as well as people with statistical or computer expertise to help verify and analyze the data. *Equipment and facilities* might include the appropriate computer hardware and software. *Funding* from internal or external sources is required for resources that are not otherwise available, in which case a budget and budget justification may have to be developed.

Formal funding may often be challenging to obtain, but informal networking can reveal potential assistance locally, such as computer programmers or biostatisticians interested in measurements pertinent to the curriculum, or quality improvement personnel in a hospital interested in measuring patient outcomes. Survey instruments can be adopted from other residency programs or clerkships within an institution or can be shared among institutions. Medical schools and residency programs often have summative assessments in place for students and residents, in the form of subject, specialty board, and in-service training examinations. Specific information on learner performance in the knowledge areas addressed by these tests can be readily accessed through the department chair, with little cost to the curriculum.

> **EXAMPLE:** *Use of an Existing Resource for Curricular Evaluation.* An objective of the acute neurological event curriculum for emergency medicine residents is the appropriate administration of thrombolytic therapy within 60 minutes of the patient's hospital arrival with symptoms of acute ischemic stroke. The evaluation plan included the need for a follow-up audit of this practice, but resources were not available for an independent audit. The information was then added to the comprehensive electronic medical

record maintained by the emergency department staff, which provided both measures of individual residents' performance and overall program success in the timely administration of thrombolytics.

An additional source of peer-reviewed assessment tools is the Directory and Repository of Educational Assessment Measures (DREAM), part of the Association of American Medical Colleges (AAMC) MedEdPORTAL (17).

EXAMPLE: *Use of a Publicly Accessible Resource for Curricular Evaluation.* One objective of the neurology clerkship curriculum is students' demonstration of understanding when to apply specific aspects of the neurological exam. The Hypothesis-Driven Physical Exam (HDPE) instrument available in DREAM, from MedEdPORTAL (17), was added to the clerkship OSCE to assess students' skill in the neurological exam, as well as their diagnostic reasoning around the exam.

TASK IV: IDENTIFY EVALUATION QUESTIONS

Evaluation questions direct the evaluation. They are to curriculum evaluation as research questions are to research projects. *Most evaluation questions* (18, 19) *should relate to the specific measurable learner, process, or clinical outcome objectives of a curriculum* (see Chapter 4). As described in Chapter 4, specific measurable objectives should state who will do how much (how well) of what by when. The "who" may refer to learners or instructors, or to the program itself, if one is evaluating program activities. "How much (how well) of what by when" provides a standard of acceptability that is measurable. Often, in the process of writing evaluation questions and thinking through what designs and methods might be able to answer a question, it becomes clear that a curricular objective needs further clarification.

EXAMPLE: *Clarifying an Objective for the Purpose of Evaluation.* The initial draft of one curricular objective stated: "By the end of the curriculum, all residents will be proficient in obtaining informed consent." In formulating the evaluation question and thinking through the evaluation methodology, it became clear to the curriculum developers that "proficient" needed to be defined operationally. Also, they determined that an increase of 25% or more of learners that demonstrated proficiency in obtaining informed consent, for a total of at least 90%, would define success for the curriculum. After appropriate revisions in the objective, the curricular evaluation questions became: "By the end of the curriculum, what percent of residents have achieved a passing score on the proficiency checklist for informed consent, as assessed using standardized patients?" and "Has there been a statistically and quantitatively (>25%) significant increase in the number of proficient residents, as defined above, from the beginning to the end of the curriculum?"

The curriculum developer should also make sure that the evaluation question is *congruent* with the related curricular objective.

EXAMPLE: *Congruence between an Objective and the Evaluation Question.* An objective of a resident teaching skills workshop is that participants will demonstrate the five microskills of clinical teaching in a role-play exercise (a skill objective). The evaluation question "What percentage of residents express confidence in their ability to provide effective teaching?" is not congruent with the objective because the evaluation question addressed an affective objective, not a skill objective (see Chapter 4). A congruent evaluation question would be: "What percentage of residents demonstrated application of at least four of five teaching microskills during workshop role-playing exercises?" If curriculum developers wanted to include an affective objective, then an expanded curriculum that addressed residents' sense of the importance of and their responsibility for teaching, as well as barriers to that practice, would be necessary.

Often, resources will limit the number of objectives for which accomplishment can be assessed. In this situation it is necessary to *prioritize and select key evaluation questions*, based on the needs of the users and the feasibility of the related evaluation methodology. Sometimes, several objectives can be grouped efficiently into a single evaluation question.

> **EXAMPLE:** *Prioritizing Which Objective to Evaluate.* A curriculum on endotracheal intubation for anesthesia residents has cognitive, attitudinal, skill, and behavioral objectives. The curriculum developers decided that what mattered most was post-curricular behavior or performance and that effective performance required achievement of the appropriate cognitive, attitudinal, and skill objectives. Setup, placement, maintenance, and evaluation of an endotracheal intubation are all critical for success in securing a patient's airway. Their evaluation question and evaluation methodology, therefore, assessed post-curricular behaviors, rather than knowledge, attitudes, or technical skill mastery. It was assumed that if the performance objectives were met, there would be sufficient accomplishment of the knowledge, attitude, and skill objectives. If performance objectives were not met, the curriculum developers would need to reconsider specific assessment of cognitive, attitudinal, and/or skill objectives.

Not all evaluation questions need to relate to explicit, written learner objectives. Some curricular objectives are implicitly understood, but not written down, to prevent a curriculum document from becoming unwieldy. Most curriculum developers, for example, will want to *include evaluation questions that relate to the effectiveness of specific curricular components or faculty*, even when the related objectives are implicit rather than explicit.

> **EXAMPLE:** *Evaluation Question Directed toward Curricular Processes.* What was the perceived effectiveness of the curriculum's online modules, small group discussions, simulated patients, clinical experiences, and required case presentations?

Sometimes there are unexpected strengths and weaknesses in a curriculum. Sometimes the curriculum on paper may differ from the curriculum as delivered. Therefore, it is almost always helpful to *include some evaluation questions that do not relate to specific curricular objectives and that are open-ended in nature.*

> **EXAMPLES:** *Use of Open-Ended Questions Related to Curricular Processes.* What do learners perceive as the major strengths and weaknesses of the curriculum? What did learners identify as the most important take-away and least understood point from each session (Minute Paper/Muddiest Point technique [12])? How could the curriculum be improved?

TASK V: CHOOSE EVALUATION DESIGNS

Once the evaluation questions have been identified and prioritized, the curriculum developer should *consider which evaluation designs (19–25) are most appropriate to answer the evaluation questions and most feasible in terms of resources.*

An evaluation is said to possess *internal validity* (22) if it accurately assesses the impact of a specific intervention on specific subjects in a specific setting. An internally valid evaluation that is generalizable to other populations and other settings is said to possess *external validity* (22). Usually, a curriculum's targeted learners and setting are predetermined for the curriculum developer. To the extent that their uniqueness can be minimized and their representativeness maximized, the external validity (or generalizability) of the evaluation will be strengthened.

The choice of evaluation design directly affects the internal validity and indirectly affects the external validity of an evaluation (an evaluation cannot have external validity if it does not have internal validity). In choosing an evaluation design, one must be aware of each design's strengths and limitations with respect to *factors that could threaten the internal validity of the evaluation*. These factors include subject characteristics (selection bias), loss of subjects (mortality, attrition), location, instrumentation, testing, history, maturation, attitude of subjects, statistical regression, and implementation (19, 21–25). The term *subject characteristics* refers to the differences between individuals or groups. If present systematically, they may lead to selection bias. *Selection bias* occurs when subjects in an intervention or comparison group possess characteristics that affect the results of the evaluation by affecting the measurements of interest or the response of subjects to the intervention. For example, studying only volunteers who are excited to learn about a particular subject may yield different results than studying all students in a cohort. If subjects are lost from or fail to complete an evaluation process, this can be a *mortality* threat. This is common because many evaluations are designed to occur over time. When subjects who drop out are different from those who complete the evaluation, the evaluation will no longer be representative of all subjects. *Location* refers to the fact that the particular place where data are collected or where an intervention has occurred may affect results. For example, an intervention in one intensive care unit that is modern and well-resourced with a large amount of technology may provide different effects from the same intervention in another intensive care unit with fewer resources. *Instrumentation* refers to the effects that changes in raters or measurement methods, or lack of precision in the measurement instrument, might have on obtained measurements. For example, administering a survey about curriculum satisfaction with a three-point Likert scale may yield very different results than the same survey given with a seven- or nine-point *Likert scale*. *Testing* refers to the effects of an initial test on subjects' performance on subsequent tests. *History* refers to events or other interventions that affect subjects during the period of an evaluation. *Maturation* refers to changes within subjects that occur as a result of the passage of time, rather than as a result of discrete external interventions. The *attitude of the subjects* or the manner in which evaluation subjects view an intervention and their participation can affect the evaluation outcome. This is also known as the Hawthorne effect. *Statistical regression* can occur when subjects have been selected on the basis of low or high pre-intervention performance. Because of temporal variations in the performance of individuals, and because of characteristics of the test itself that result in imperfect test-retest reliability (see Task VI), subsequent scores on the performance assessment are likely to be less extreme, whether or not an educational intervention takes place. An *implementation threat* occurs when the results of an evaluation differ because the people who administer the evaluation differ in ways that are related to the outcome, such as one exam proctor who keeps time precisely and another who may allow test takers a few extra minutes. It may not be possible or feasible, in the choice of evaluation design, to prevent all of the above factors from affecting a given evaluation. However, the curriculum developer should be aware of the potential effects of these factors when choosing an evaluation design and when interpreting the results.

The most commonly used *evaluation designs* are posttest only, pretest-posttest, nonrandomized controlled pretest-posttest, randomized controlled posttest only, and randomized controlled pretest-posttest (20–24). *As the designs increase in methodological rigor, they also increase in the amount of resources required to execute them.*

A *single-group, posttest-only* design can be diagrammed as follows:

$$X - - - O$$

where X represents the curriculum or educational intervention, and O represents observations or measurements. This design permits assessment of what learners have achieved after the educational intervention, but the achievements could have been present before the intervention (selection bias), occurred as part of a natural maturation process during the period prior to the evaluation (maturation), or resulted from other interventions that took place prior to the evaluation (history). Because of these limitations, the conclusions of single-group, posttest-only studies are nearly always tentative. The design is acceptable when the most important evaluation question is the certification of proficiency. The design is also well suited to assess participants' perceptions of the curriculum, to solicit suggestions for improvement in the curriculum, and to solicit feedback on and ratings of student or faculty performance.

A *single-group, pretest-posttest* design can be diagrammed as

$$O_1 - - - X - - - O_2$$

where O_1 represents the first observations or measurements, in this case before the educational intervention, and O_2 the second observations or measurements, in this case after the educational intervention. This design can demonstrate that changes in proficiency have occurred in learners during the course of the curriculum. However, the changes could have occurred because of factors other than the curriculum (e.g., history, maturation, testing, and instrumentation).

The addition of a *control group* helps confirm that an observed change occurred because of the curriculum, rather than because of history, maturation, or testing, particularly if the control group was *randomized*, which also helps to eliminate selection bias. A *pretest-posttest controlled evaluation design* can be diagrammed as

$$
\begin{array}{ccc}
 & E & O_1 - - - X - - - O_2 \\
R & & \\
 & C & O_1 - - - - - - - O_2
\end{array}
$$

where E represents the experimental or intervention group, C represents the control or comparison group, and R (if present) indicates that subjects were randomized between the intervention and control groups, and time is represented on the x axis.

A *posttest-only randomized controlled design* requires fewer resources, especially when the observations or measurements are difficult and resource-intensive. It cannot, however, demonstrate changes in learners. Furthermore, the success of the randomization process in achieving comparability between the intervention and control groups before the curriculum cannot be assessed. This design can be diagrammed as follows:

$$
\begin{array}{ccc}
 & E & X - - - O_1 \\
R & & \\
 & C & - - - O_1
\end{array}
$$

Evaluation designs are sometimes classified as pre-experimental, quasi-experimental, and true experimental (21–25). *Pre-experimental designs* usually lack controls. *Quasi-experimental designs* usually include controls but lack random assignment. *True experimental designs* include both random assignment to experimental and control groups and concurrent observations or measurements in the experimental and control groups.

The advantages and disadvantages of each of the discussed evaluation designs are displayed in Table 7.2. Additional designs are possible (see General References).

Political or ethical considerations may prohibit withholding a curriculum from some learners. This obstacle to a controlled evaluation can sometimes be overcome by delaying administration of the curriculum to the control group until after data collection has been completed for a randomized controlled evaluation. This can be accomplished without interference when, for other reasons, the curriculum can be administered to only a portion of targeted learners at the same time.

EXAMPLE: *Controlled Evaluation without Denying the Curriculum to the Control Group.* The design for such an evaluation might be diagrammed as follows:

$$E \quad O_1 - - -X - - - O_2 \qquad\qquad (- - -O_3)$$
$$R$$
$$C \quad O_1 - - - - - - -O_2 - - - - -X \qquad (- - -O_3)$$

When one uses this evaluation design, a randomized controlled evaluation is accomplished without denying the curriculum to any learner. Inclusion of additional observation points, as indicated in the parentheses, is more resource-intensive but permits inclusion of all (not just half) of the learners in a noncontrolled pretest-posttest evaluation.

It is important to realize that formative assessment and feedback may occur in an ongoing fashion during a curriculum and could be diagrammed as follows:

$$O_1 - - - X - - - O_2 - - - X - - - O_3 - - - X - - - O_4$$

In this situation, a formative assessment and feedback strategy is also an educational strategy for the curriculum.

A common concern related to the efficacy of a curricular intervention is whether the desired achievements are maintained in the learners over time. This concern can be addressed by repeating post-curricular measurements after an appropriate interval:

$$O_1 - - - X - - - O_2 - - - - - - - - - - - - - - O_3$$

Whenever publication is a goal of a curricular evaluation, it is desirable to use the strongest evaluation design feasible (see Chapter 9, Table 9.4).

TASK VI: CHOOSE MEASUREMENT METHODS AND CONSTRUCT INSTRUMENTS

The choice of assessment or measurement methods and construction of measurement instruments are critical steps in the evaluation process because they determine the data that will be collected, determine how they will be collected (Task VIII), and make certain implications about how the data will be analyzed (Task IX). Formal measurement methods are discussed in this section. Table 8.2 lists additional, often informal, methods for determining how a curriculum is functioning (see Chapter 8).

Table 7.2.   Advantages and Disadvantages of Commonly Used Evaluation Designs

Design	Diagram	Advantages	Disadvantages
Single group, posttest only (pre-experimental)	X - - - O	Simple Economical Can document proficiency Can document process (what happened) Can ascertain learner and faculty perceptions of efficacy and value Can elicit suggestions for improvement	Accomplishments may have been preexisting Accomplishments may be the result of natural maturation Accomplishments may be due to factors other than the curriculum
Single group, pretest-posttest (pre-experimental)	O_1 - - - X - - - O_2	Intermediate in complexity and cost Can demonstrate pre-post changes in cognitive, affective, and psychomotor attributes	Accomplishments may be the result of natural maturation Accomplishments may be due to factors other than the curriculum Accomplishments could result from learning from the first test or evaluation rather than from the curriculum
Controlled pretest-posttest (quasi-experimental)	E O_1 - - - X - - - O_2 C O_1 - - - - - - O_2	Controls for maturation, if control group equivalent Controls for the effects of measured factors, other than the curriculum Controls for learning from the test or evaluation	Complex Resource intensive Control group may not be equivalent to the experimental group and changes could be due to differences in unmeasured factors Curriculum denied to some (see text)
Randomized controlled posttest only (true experimental)	E X - - - O_1 R C - - - O_1	Controls for maturation Controls for effects of measured and unmeasured factors Less resource intensive than a randomized controlled pretest-posttest design, while preserving the benefits of randomization	Complex Resource intensive Does not demonstrate changes in learners Totally dependent on the success of the randomization process in eliminating pretest differences in independent and dependent variables Curriculum denied to some (see text)

Table 7.2.   *(continued)*

Design	Diagram	Advantages	Disadvantages
Randomized controlled pretest-posttest (true experimental)	E O_1 ---X--- O_2 R C O_1 ------ O_2	Controls for maturation Controls for effects of measured and unmeasured factors Controls for the effects of testing If randomization is successful, controls for selection bias	Most complex Most resource intensive Curriculum denied to some (see text) Depends on success of the randomization process in eliminating pretest differences in unmeasured independent and dependent variables

Note: O = observation or measurement; X = curriculum or educational intervention; E = experimental or intervention group; C = control or comparison group; R = random allocation to experimental and control groups.

Choice of Measurement Methods

Measurement methods commonly used to evaluate individuals and programs include written or electronic rating forms, self-assessment forms, essays, written or computer-interactive tests, oral examinations, questionnaires (Chapter 3), individual interviews (Chapter 3), group interviews/discussions (see Chapter 3 discussion of focus groups), direct observation (real life or simulation), performance audits, and portfolios (26–29). The uses, strengths, and limitations of each of these measurement methods are shown in Table 7.3.

As with the choice of evaluation design, it is important to *choose a measurement method that is congruent with the evaluation question* (25–28). Multiple-choice and direct-response written tests are appropriate methods for assessing knowledge acquisition. Higher-level cognitive ability can be assessed through essay-type and case-based computer-interactive tests. Script concordance tests, in which learners' performance is compared with performance by a sample of expert clinicians, are another type of written assessment that can be used to assess higher-level reasoning abilities (30). Direct observation (real life or simulation) using agreed-upon standards is an appropriate method for assessing skill attainment. Chart audit and unobtrusive observations are appropriate methods for assessing real-life performance.

It is desirable to choose measurement methods that have *optimal accuracy (reliability and validity, as discussed below), credibility*, and *importance*. Generally speaking, patient/health care outcomes are considered most important, followed by behaviors/performance, skills, knowledge or attitudes, and satisfaction or perceptions, in that order (31, 32). Objective measurements are preferred to subjective ratings. Curricular evaluations that incorporate measurement methods at the higher end of this hierarchy are more likely to be disseminated or published (see Chapter 9). However, it is more important for what is measured to be congruent with the program or learning objectives than to aspire to measure the "highest" level in the outcome hierarchy (33).

It is also necessary to choose measurement methods that are *feasible in terms of available resources*. Curriculum developers usually have to make difficult decisions

Table 7.3.   Uses, Strengths, and Limitations of Commonly Used Evaluation Methods

Method	Uses	Strengths	Limitations
Global rating forms (separated in time from observation)	Cognitive, affective, or psychomotor attributes; real-life performance	Economical Can evaluate anything Open-ended questions can provide information for formative purposes	Subjective Rater biases Inter- and intrarater reliability Raters frequently have insufficient data on which to base ratings
Self-assessment forms	Cognitive, affective, psychomotor attributes; real-life performance	Economical Can evaluate anything Promotes self-assessment Useful for formative evaluation	Subjective Rater biases Often little agreement with objective measurements Limited acceptance as method of summative evaluation
Essays on respondent's experience	Attitudes, feelings, description of respondent experiences, perceived impact	Rich in texture Provides unanticipated as well as anticipated information Respondent-centered	Subjective Rater biases Requires qualitative evaluation methods to analyze Focus varies from respondent to respondent
Written or computer-interactive tests	Knowledge; higher level cognitive ability	Often economical Objective Multiple choice exams can achieve high internal consistency reliability, broad sampling Good psychometric properties, low cost, low faculty time, easy to score Widely accepted Essay-type questions or computer-interactive tests can assess higher level cognitive ability, encourage students to integrate knowledge, reflect problem solving	Constructing tests of higher level cognitive ability, or computer-interactive tests, can be resource intensive Reliability and validity vary with quality of test (e.g., questions that are not carefully constructed can be interpreted differently by different respondents, there may be an insufficient number of questions to validly test a domain)

Table 7.3.   *(continued)*

Method	Uses	Strengths	Limitations
Oral examinations	Knowledge; higher level cognitive ability; indirect measure of affective attributes	Flexible, can follow-up and explore understanding Learner-centered Can be integrated into case discussions	Subjective scoring Inter- and intrarater reliability Reliability and validity vary with quality of test (e.g., questions that are not carefully constructed can be interpreted differently by different respondents, there may be an insufficient number of questions to validly test a domain) Faculty intensive Can be costly
Questionnaires	Attitudes; perceptions; suggestions for improvement	Economical	Subjective Constructing reliable and valid measures of attitudes requires time and skill
Individual interviews	Attitudes; perceptions; suggestions for improvement	Flexible, can follow-up and clarify responses Respondent-centered	Subjective Rater biases Constructing reliable and valid measures of attitudes requires time and skill Requires interviewers
Group interviews/discussions	Attitudes; perceptions; suggestions for improvement	Flexible, can follow-up and develop/explore responses Respondent-centered Efficient means of interviewing several at once Group interaction can enrich or deepen information Can be integrated into teaching sessions	Subjective Requires skilled interviewer or facilitator to control group interaction and minimize facilitator influence on responses Does not yield quantitative information Information may not be representative of all participants

Method	Uses	Strengths	Limitations
Direct observation using checklists or virtual reality simulators (observing real-life or simulated performance)	Skills; real-life behaviors	First-hand data Can provide immediate feedback to observed Development of standards, use of observation checklists, and training of observers can increase reliability and validity. The Objective Structured Clinical Examination (OSCE) (63, 64) and Objective Structured Assessment of Technical Skills (OSATS) (65) combine direct observation with structured checklists to increase reliability and validity. High-fidelity / virtual reality simulators offer the potential for automated assessment of skills (66)	Rater biases Inter- and intrarater reliability Personnel intensive Unless observation covert, assesses capability rather than real-life behaviors/ performance
Performance audits	Record keeping; provision of recorded care (e.g., tests ordered, provision of preventive care measures, prescribed treatments)	Objective Reliability and accuracy can be measured and enhanced by the use of standards and the training of raters Unobtrusive	Dependent on what is reliably recorded; much care is not documented Dependent on available, organized records or data sources
Portfolios	Comprehensive; can assess all aspects of competence, especially practice-based learning and improvement	Unobtrusive Actively involves learner, documents accomplishments, promotes reflection, and fosters development of learning plans	Selective, time-consuming Requires faculty resources to provide ongoing feedback to learner

on how to spread limited resources among problem identification, needs assessment, educational intervention, and assessment and evaluation. Global rating forms used by faculty supervisors, which assess proficiency in a number of general areas (e.g., knowledge, patient care, professionalism), and self-assessment questionnaires completed by learners can provide indirect, inexpensive measures of ability and real-life performance; however, they are subject to numerous rating biases. Direct observation (real life or simulation) and audits using trained raters and agreed-upon standards are more reliable and have more validity evidence for measuring skills and performance than global rating forms, but they also require more resources. There is little point in using the latter measurement methods, however, if their use would drain resources that are critically important for achieving a well-conceived educational intervention.

Construction of Measurement Instruments

Most evaluations will require the construction of curriculum-specific measurement instruments such as tests, rating forms, interview schedules, or questionnaires.

The *methodological rigor* with which the instruments are constructed and administered affects the reliability and validity of the scores and, unfortunately, the cost of the evaluation. Formative individual assessments and program evaluations generally require the least rigor, summative individual assessments and program evaluations for internal use an intermediate level of rigor, and summative individual assessments and program evaluations for external use (e.g., certification of mastery or publication of evaluation results) the most rigor. When a high degree of methodological rigor is required, it is worth exploring whether there is an *already existing measurement instrument* (17, 34–38) that is appropriate in terms of content, reliability, validity, feasibility, and cost. When a methodologically rigorous instrument must be constructed specifically for a curriculum, it is wise to seek *advice or mentorship from individuals with expertise in designing such instruments.*

One of the most frequent measurement instruments is the written knowledge test. Constructing knowledge tests that are reliable and valid requires attention to format and interpretation of statistical tests of quality. A useful reference for faculty learning to construct written knowledge tests is the online manual developed by the National Board of Medical Examiners (39).

A useful first step in constructing measurement instruments is to determine the desired *content*. For assessments of curricular impact, this involves the identification of independent variables and dependent variables. *Independent variables* are factors that could explain or predict the curriculum's outcomes (e.g., the curriculum itself, previous or concurrent training, environmental factors). *Dependent variables* are program outcomes (e.g., knowledge or skill attainment, real-life performance, clinical outcomes). To keep the measurement instruments from becoming unwieldy, it is prudent to focus on a few dependent variables that are most relevant to the main evaluation questions and, similarly, to focus on the independent variables that are most likely to be related to the curriculum's outcomes.

Next, attention must be devoted to the *format* of the instruments (38, 39). In determining the acceptable *length* for a measurement instrument, methodological concerns and the desire to be comprehensive must be balanced against constraints in the amount of curricular time allotted for evaluation, imposition on respondents, and concerns about response rate. Individual items should be worded and displayed in a manner that is *clear and unambiguous*. *Response scales* (e.g., true-false; strongly disagree, disagree, neither agree nor disagree, agree, strongly agree) should make sense relative to the question asked. There is no consensus about whether it is preferable for response scales to have middle points or not (e.g., neither agree nor disagree) or to have an even or odd number of response categories. In general, four to seven response categories permit greater flexibility in data analysis than two or three. It is important for the instrument as a whole to be *user-friendly* and attractive, by organizing it in a manner that facilitates quick understanding and efficient recording of responses. It is desirable for the instrument to *engage* the interest of respondents. In general, response categories should be *precoded* to facilitate data entry and analysis. Today, *online questionnaires* can provide an easy mode of delivery and facilitate collation of data for different reports. Some institutions have created secure Internet websites for this purpose and have noted improved compliance in response rates, a decrease in administrative time, and an improvement in quality (40).

Before using an instrument for evaluation purposes, it is almost always important to *pilot* it on a convenient audience (38). Audience feedback can provide important information about the instrument: how it is likely to be perceived by respondents, acceptable length, clarity of individual items, user-friendliness of the overall format, and specific ways in which the instrument could be improved.

Reliability, Validity, and Bias

Because measurement instruments are never perfect, the data they produce are never absolutely accurate. An understanding of potential threats to accuracy is helpful to the curriculum developer in planning the evaluation and reporting of results and to the users of evaluation reports in interpreting results. In recent years, there has been an emerging consensus in the educational literature about the meaning of the terms validity and reliability (41–44). Validity is now considered a unitary concept that encompasses both reliability and validity. All validity relates to the construct that is being measured and is thus considered *construct validity*.

The emphasis on construct validity has emerged from the growing realization that an instrument's scores are usually meaningful only inasmuch as they accurately reflect an abstract concept (or construct) such as knowledge, skill, or patient satisfaction. Validity is best viewed as a hypothesis regarding the link between the instrument's scores and the intended construct. Evidence is collected from a variety of sources (see below) to support or refute this hypothesis. Validity can never be "proven," just as a scientific hypothesis can never be proven; it can be supported (or refuted) only as evidence accrues.

It is also important to note that validity and reliability refer to an instrument's scores and not the instrument itself. Instruments are not "validated"; they can merely have evidence to demonstrate high levels of validity (or reliability) in one context or for one purpose, but may be ill-suited for another context (see examples in reference 44).

The construct validity of an instrument's scores can be supported by various types of evidence. The *Standards for Educational and Psychological Testing* published as a joint effort from the American Educational Research Association, American Psychological Association, and National Council on Measurement in Education (41) identifies five discrete sources of validity evidence:

1. *Internal structure evidence*, which relates to the psychometric characteristics of the measurement instrument; it includes categories previously considered "reliability," including inter-rater and intra-rater reliability, test-retest reliability, alternate-form reliability, and internal consistency. Evidence of internal structure validity also refers to other psychometric properties such as scale development and scoring, item analysis for difficulty and discrimination, and response characteristics in different settings and by different populations.
2. *Content evidence*, which evaluates the relationship between a test's content and the construct it is intended to measure, often presented as a detailed description of steps taken to ensure the items represent the construct. Older terms such as "face" and "surface" validity may be related to content validity evidence but are no longer appropriate.
3. *Relation to other variables evidence*, which is simply correlation with scores from another instrument with which correlation would be expected, in support of the relationship with the underlying construct.
4. *Response process evidence*, which includes evidence of data integrity, related to the instrument itself, its administration, and the data collection process, including the actions and thought processes of test takers or observers.
5. *Consequences evidence*, which relates to the impact or consequences of the assessments for examinees, faculty, patients, and society. Does the use of the instrument have intended/useful or unintended/harmful consequences?

Table 7.4 provides terminology and definitions for the components of validity evidence in assessment instruments.

Internal Structure Validity Evidence. Internal structure validity evidence relates to the psychometric characteristics of the assessment instrument and, as such, includes all forms of reliability testing, as well as other psychometrics. As noted above, it includes the concepts of inter-rater and intra-rater reliability, test-retest reliability, alternate-form reliability, and internal consistency. *Reliability* refers to the consistency or reproducibility of measurements (37, 41–44). As such, it is a necessary, but not sufficient, determinant of validity evidence. There are several different methods for assessing reliability of an assessment instrument. Reliability may be calculated using a number of statistical tests, but is usually reported as a coefficient between 0 and 1 (for more information, see reference 43). Regardless of the specific test used to calculate it, the reliability coefficient can also be thought of as the proportion of score variance explained by differences between subjects, with the remaining due to error (random and systematic). For high-stakes examinations (licensure), reliability should be greater than 0.9. For many testing situations a reliability of 0.7-0.8 may be acceptable. Ideally, measurement scores should be in agreement when repeated by the same person (*intra-rater reliability*) or made by different people (*inter-rater reliability*). Intra- or inter-rater reliability can be assessed by the percentage agreement between raters or by statistics such as kappa (44), which corrects for chance agreement. A commonly used method of estimating inter-rater reliability is the intraclass correlation coefficient, accessible in commonly available computer software, which uses analysis of variance to estimate the variance of different factors. It permits estimation of the inter-rater reliability of the *n* raters used, as well as the reliability of a single rater. It can also manage missing data (43). A sophisticated method for estimating inter-rater agreement often used in performance examinations uses *generalizability theory analysis*, in which variance for each of

Table 7.4.   Reliability and Validity: Terminology and Definitions

Construct Validity Evidence Sources	Components	Definition	Comments/Example
Internal structure validity evidence		Psychometric characteristics of the measurement	
	Item analysis measures	Item difficulty, other measures of item/test characteristics Response characteristics in different settings by different populations	
	Intra-rater reliability	Consistency of measurement results when repeated by same individual	Can be assessed by statistical methods such as kappa or phi coefficient, intraclass correlation coefficient, generalizability theory analysis. See text.
	Inter-rater reliability	Consistency of measurement results when performed by different individuals	
	Test-retest reliability/ stability	Degree to which same test produces same results when repeated under same conditions	
	Alternate-form reliability/ equivalence	Degree to which alternate forms of the same measurement instrument produce the same result	Of relevance in pretest-posttest evaluation, when each test encompasses only part of the domain being taught, and when learning, related to test taking, could be limited to the items being tested. In such situations, it is desirable to have equivalent but different tests.
	Internal consistency/ homogeneity	Extent to which various items legitimately team together to measure a single characteristic	Can be assessed with statistical methods such as Cronbach's alpha. Uni- vs. multidimensionality can be assessed by factor analysis. See text.
Content validity evidence		Degree to which a measurement instrument accurately represents represents the skill or characteristic it is designed to measure	

Table 7.4.   *(continued)*

Construct Validity Evidence Sources	Components	Definition	Comments/Example
	Literature review, expert consensus	Formal methods for consensus building, including literature review and use of topic experts	Systematic reviews of the literature, focus groups, nominal group technique, Delphi techniques, etc., can contribute to expert consensus. See text.
Relationship to other variables validity evidence		How the instrument under consideration relates to other instruments or theory	
	Criterion-related validity evidence	How well the instrument under consideration compares to related measurements	Often subdivided into concurrent and predictive validity evidence.
	Concurrent validity evidence	Degree to which a measurement instrument produces the same results as another accepted or proven instrument that measures the same characteristics at the same time	E.g., comparison with a previously developed but more resource-intensive measurement instrument.
	Predictive validity evidence	Degree to which a measurement instrument accurately predicts theoretically expected outcomes	E.g., higher scores on an instrument that assesses communication skills should predict higher patient satisfaction scores.
	Convergent and discriminant validity evidence	Whether an instrument performs as would theoretically be expected in groups that are known to possess or not possess the attribute being measured, or in comparison with tests that are known to measure the same attribute (high correlation) or a different attribute (low correlation)	E.g., an instrument that assesses clinical reasoning would be expected to distinguish novice from experienced clinicians. Scores on an instrument designed to measure communication skills would not be expected to correlate with scores on an instrument designed to measure technical proficiency in a procedure.

Construct Validity Evidence Sources	Components	Definition	Comments/Example
Response process validity evidence		Evidence of the actions and/or thought processes of test takers or observers Evidence of data integrity, related to test administration and data collection	E.g., documentation of data collection, entry, and cleaning procedures.
Consequences validity evidence		Degree to which the instrument has intended/useful vs. unintended/harmful consequences, the impact of its use	E.g., it would be a problem if results from a measurement method of limited reliability and validity were being used to make decisions about career advancement, when the intent was to use the results as feedback to stimulate and direct trainee improvement.

the variables in the evaluation can be estimated (i.e., subjects or true variance vs. raters and measurements or error variance). Changes can be made in the number of measurements or raters dependent on the variance seen in an individual variable (45).

> **EXAMPLE:** *Generalizability Theory Analysis.* Medical student performance on the surgery clerkship is assessed at the end of each rotation by asking for four items to be rated by three different faculty members. Generalizability theory analysis demonstrated that the reliability (true variance/total variance) of this assessment was only 0.4; that is, that only 40% of the total variance was due to the difference between subjects (true variance) and the rest of the variance was due to differences between the raters and/or items, and/or interactions among the three sources of variation. The reliability was improved to 0.8 by adding six items, as well as requiring evaluations from three different resident raters.

Other forms of internal structure validity evidence include stability, equivalence, and internal consistency or homogeneity. *Test-retest reliability*, or *stability*, is the degree to which the same test produces the same results when repeated under the same conditions. This is not commonly done, because of time, cost, and the possibility of contamination by intervening variables when the second test is separated in time. *Alternate-form reliability*, or *equivalence*, is the degree to which alternate forms of the same measurement instrument produce the same result. This form of internal structure validity is of particular relevance in pretest/posttest evaluations, when the test is a sample (only part) of what should have been learned and when specific learning could occur related to test taking, independent of the curricular intervention. In such circumstances, it is desirable to use equivalent but different tests or alternative forms of the same test. *Internal consistency*, or *homogeneity*, is the extent to which various items legitimately team together to measure a single characteristic, such as a desired attitude. Internal consistency can be assessed using the statistic Cronbach's (or coefficient) alpha (43), which is basically the average of the correlations of each item in a scale to the total score. A complex characteristic, however, could have several dimensions. In this situation, the technique of factor analysis (46) can be used to help separate out the different dimensions. When there is a need to assess the reliability of an important measure but a lack of statistical expertise among curricular faculty, statistical consultation is advisable.

> **EXAMPLE:** *Internal Structure Validity Evidence: Internal Consistency / Homogeneity.* The group of medical student clerkship directors at one medical school worked together to develop an integrative clinical reasoning assessment for chronic conditions at the completion of students' basic clerkships. Assessment of three cognitive areas was planned: 1) multidisciplinary factual knowledge for the appropriate management of diabetes mellitus and congestive heart failure in different settings; 2) clinical decision making for diagnostic and therapeutic strategies that incorporated the use of evidence and patient preferences; and 3) cost-effectiveness of decisions in relation to outcomes. After piloting of the test, a factor analysis was able to identify separate clinical decision-making and cost-effectiveness dimensions. However, there was not a single knowledge dimension. Knowledge split into two separate factors, each of which was specific to one of the two medical disorders. Cronbach's alpha was used to assess homogeneity among items that contributed to each of the four dimensions or factors. There were a large number of items for each dimension, so those with low correlation with the overall score for each dimension were considered for elimination.

> **EXAMPLE:** *Internal Structure Validity Evidence: Psychometrics.* All medical students must achieve a passing score on the United States Medical Licensure Examination (USMLE) to be eligible for licensure, and it is also a graduation requirement for many schools. For this high-stakes examination, the reliability coefficient determined by any means should be 0.8 or greater. That is, the reproducibility of the score must be very high. To support this, psychometric analysis of each item is routinely conducted, which includes an analysis of item difficulty (what percentage of individuals select the correct answer), item discrimination (how well the item distinguishes between those who scored in the upper tier and those who scored in the lower tier), and an analysis of who answered which options.

Content Validity Evidence. Content validity evidence is the degree to which an instrument's scores accurately represent the skill or characteristic the instrument is designed to measure, based on people's experience and available knowledge. Although "face" or "surface" validity are terms that may have been considered part of this category, they are based on the appearance of an instrument rather than on a formal content analysis or empirical testing and are thus no longer appropriate for use in the literature or vocabulary of health professions educators. Content validity can be enhanced by conducting an appropriate literature review to identify the most relevant content, using topic experts, and revising the instrument until a reasonable degree of consensus about its content is achieved among knowledgeable reviewers. Formal processes such as focus groups, nominal group technique, Delphi technique, use of daily diaries, observation by work sampling, time and motion studies, critical incident reviews, and reviews of ideal performance cases can also contribute (see Chapter 2).

> **EXAMPLE:** *Content Validity Evidence.* During the design of an ethics curriculum for obstetrics and gynecology residents, a group of experts in maternal-fetal medicine, genetics, neonatology, and biomedical ethics participated in a Delphi process to reach a consensus on the primary content areas to be covered during the curriculum, along with ensuring appropriate alignment of all assessment tools with the target content areas.

Relationship to Other Variables Validity Evidence. This form of validity refers to how the instrument under consideration relates to other instruments or theory. It includes the concepts of criterion-related, concurrent, and predictive validity. *Criterion-related validity evidence* encompasses concurrent validity and predictive validity evidence. *Concurrent validity evidence* demonstrates the degree to which a measurement instrument produces the same results as another accepted or proven instrument that measures the same parameters. *Predictive validity evidence* demonstrates the degree to which an instrument's scores accurately predict theoretically expected outcomes (e.g., scores from a measure of attitudes toward preventive care should correlate significantly with preventive care behaviors).

> **EXAMPLE:** *Relationship to Other Variables Validity / Concurrent Validity Evidence.* An internal medicine residency program currently uses a standardized patient OSCE to evaluate the patient care and interpersonal communication skills competencies of its interns, but is looking for an alternative assessment that may be more cost-effective. A pilot study of mini-CEX evaluations along with the OSCE is performed over the next academic year. Scores on the two measures are found to correlate highly (0.9), and the program elects to continue using only the mini-CEX evaluations.

> **EXAMPLE:** *Relationship to Other Variables Validity / Concurrent Validity Evidence.* Educators for a medical student psychiatry clerkship have created a computer-interactive psychiatry knowledge assessment to be given at the end of the clerkship. Scores on this examination are found to demonstrate a positive correlation with performance on the National Board of Medical Examiners Psychiatry Subject Examination, with clerkship grades, and with performance on the Clinical Knowledge examination of the United States Medical Licensing Examination (USMLE), Step II.

> **EXAMPLE:** *Relationship to Other Variables Validity / Predictive Validity Evidence.* For board certification in general surgery, the American Board of Surgery requires candidates to achieve passing scores on both a written Qualifying Examination (QE) and an oral Certifying Examination (CE). Many surgical residency programs use mock oral examinations to prepare their residents for the CE, as mock oral performance has been shown to predict performance on the CE (47).

Concurrent and predictive validity evidence are forms of *convergent validity evidence,* in which the study measure is shown to correlate positively with another measure or construct to which it theoretically relates. *Discriminant validity evidence*, on the other hand, is a form of evidence in which the study measure is shown to not correlate or to correlate negatively with measures or constructs to which it, theoretically, is not or is negatively related.

> **EXAMPLE:** *Relationship to Other Variables / Convergent and Discriminant Validity Evidence.* Scores from an instrument that measures clinical reasoning ability would be expected to distinguish between individuals rated by faculty as high or low in clinical reasoning and judgment (convergent validity evidence). Scores on the instrument would be expected to correlate significantly with grades on an evidence-based case presentation (convergent validity evidence), but not with measures of compassion (discriminant validity evidence).

Response Process Validity Evidence. Response process validity evidence includes evidence about the integrity of instrument administration and data collection so that these sources of error are controlled or eliminated. It could include information about quality control processes, use of properly trained raters, documentation of procedures used to ensure accuracy in data collection, evidence that students are familiar with test formats, or evidence that a test of clinical reasoning actually invokes higher-order thinking in test takers.

EXAMPLE: *Response Process Validity Evidence.* Use of a standardized orientation script, trained proc-tors at testing centers, documentation of their policies and procedures, and strict adherence to time limitations are sources of response process validity evidence for the USMLE, a high-stakes licensure exam.

Consequences Validity Evidence. This is a relatively new concept and may be the most controversial area of validity. It refers to the consequences of an assessment for examinees, faculty, patients, and society. It answers the question: What outcomes (good and bad) have occurred as a result of the assessment and related decisions? If the consequences are intended or useful, this evidence supports the ongoing use of the instrument. If the consequences are unintended and harmful, educators may think twice before using the instrument for the same purpose in the future. Consequence validity could also include the method or process to determine the cut scores, as well as the statistical properties of passing scores.

EXAMPLE: *Consequences Validity Evidence.* Before completion of medical school, students are re-quired to take a series of high-stakes examinations for licensure. Validity evidence related to the conse-quences of these examinations would include the method by which cut score or pass/fail decisions have been made, the percentage of examinees that pass versus fail, how this percentage compares with other examinations, and the ultimate outcomes of the individuals in each category (residency comple-tion, board certification, etc.).

EXAMPLE: *Consequences Validity Evidence.* Suppose that, in a hypothetical medical school, a manda-tory comprehensive assessment was implemented at the end of the first year. Students who scored below a certain mark were provided one-on-one counseling and remediation. If board scores improved and the number of students failing to graduate dropped, this would provide consequences evidence in support of the mandatory assessment (i.e., the assessment had a positive impact on students). If, how-ever, students identified for remediation dropped out at a higher than normal rate, this might suggest an unintended harm from the assessment (negative consequences evidence).

Threats to Validity. Another way to look at validity, complementary to the above perspective, is to consider the potential threats to validity (i.e., negative validity evi-dence). Bias related to insufficient sampling of trainee attributes or cases, variations in the testing environment, and inadequately trained raters can threaten validity (48). Threats to validity have been classified into two general categories: construct under-representation and construct-irrelevant variance (49). These errors interfere with the interpretation of the assessment. *Construct underrepresentation* represents inadequate sampling of the domain to be assessed, biased sampling, or a mismatch of the testing sample to the domain (49).

EXAMPLE: *Construct Underrepresentation Variance.* An instructor has just begun to design a written examination for students at the end of their cardiopulmonary physiology module. She "doesn't believe in" multiple-choice exams and plans on using one clinical scenario as an essay prompt. A majority of students' grades will be based on this examination. Unfortunately, this exam is likely to demonstrate construct underrepresentation variance because the number of questions is too few to represent the entire domain of cardiopulmonary knowledge expected.

Construct-irrelevant variance refers to systematic (as opposed to random) error that is introduced into the assessment and does not have a relationship to the construct being measured. It includes flawed or biased test items, inappropriately easy or difficult test items, indefensible passing scores, poorly trained standardized patients, and rater bias. Rating biases are particularly likely to occur when global rating forms are being used by untrained raters to assess learner or faculty performance. Rating biases can affect both an instrument's reliability and evidence of validity (48). *Errors of leniency or harshness* occur when raters consistently rate higher than is accurate (as in Garrison Keillor's Lake Wobegon, where "all the women are strong, all the men are good looking, and all the children are above average") or lower than is accurate (e.g., judging junior generalist physicians against standards appropriate to senior specialist physicians). The *error of central tendency* refers to the tendency of raters to avoid extremes. The *halo effect* occurs when individuals who perform well in one area or relate particularly well to other people are rated inappropriately high in other, often unobserved, areas of performance. *Attribution error* occurs when raters make inferences about why individuals behave as they do and then rate them in areas that are unobserved, based on these inferences.

> **EXAMPLE:** *Construct-Irrelevant Variance: Attribution Error.* An individual who consistently arrives late and does not contribute actively to group discussions is assumed to be lazy and unreliable. She is rated low on motivation. The individual has a problem with child care and is quiet, but she has done all the required reading, has been active in defining her own learning needs, and has independently pursued learning resources beyond those provided in the course syllabus.

Rater biases may be reduced and inter- and intra-rater reliability improved by training those who are performing the ratings. Because not all training is effective, it is important to confirm the efficacy of training by assessing the reliability of raters and the accuracy of their ratings.

Internal and external validity are discussed above in reference to evaluation designs (Task V). It is worth noting here that the reliability and validity of the scores for each instrument used in an evaluation affect the internal validity of the overall evaluation and, additionally, would have implications for any external validity of an evaluation.

It is also worth noting here that the reliability and validity of an instrument's scores affect the utility, feasibility, and propriety of the overall evaluation. Many of the threats to validity can be minimized once considered. Thus, open discussion of these issues should occur in the planning stages of the evaluation. Areas of validity evidence relatively easy to collect include internal structure and content validity evidence. Including some evidence of the validity of one's measurement methods increases the likelihood that a curriculum-related manuscript will be accepted for publication (see Chapter 9, Table 9.4).

Reliability and Validity in Qualitative Measurement. The above discussion of reliability and validity pertains to quantitative measurements. Frequently, *qualitative information* is also gathered to enrich and help explain the quantitative data that have been obtained. *Qualitative evaluation methods* are also used to explore the processes and impact of a curriculum, deepen understanding, generate novel insights, and develop hypotheses about both how a curriculum works and its effects.

> **EXAMPLE:** *Qualitative Evaluation Methods.* A "boot camp" curriculum for students preparing to enter a surgical residency includes an "exit interview" in the form of a focus group. During this session, students are asked structured questions about the curriculum's strengths, weaknesses, and projected impact, and suggestions for improvement. Their responses are recorded for further analysis and use in ongoing curriculum refinement.

When qualitative measurements are used as methods of evaluating a curriculum, there may be concern about their accuracy and about the interpretation of conclusions that are drawn from the data. Many of the methods for assessing reliability and validity described above pertain to quantitative measurements. The concepts of identifying evidence to support the validity of an assessment instrument's internal structure, content, relation to other variables, response process, and consequences also pertain to qualitative measurements. While a detailed discussion of the accuracy of qualitative measurement methods is beyond the scope of this book, it is worth noting that there are concepts in qualitative research that parallel the quantitative research concepts of reliability and validity (50–53). *Objectivity* refers to investigators revealing their theoretical perspectives and background characteristics/experiences that may influence their interpretation of observations. *Reflexivity* refers to investigators reflecting on and accounting for these factors (i.e., attempting to remain as free from biases as possible when interpreting data). *Confirmability* provides assurances that the conclusions that are drawn about what is studied would be reached if another investigator undertook the same analysis of the same data or used a different measurement method. Frequently, in qualitative analysis of the same dataset, two or more investigators review and abstract themes and then have a process for reaching consensus. *Triangulation* can be used to enhance the validity of study methods (use of more than one method to study a phenomenon) or of study results (pointing out how results match or differ from those of other studies). *Dependability* refers to consistency and reproducibility of the research method over time and across research subjects and contexts. There may be quality checks on how questions are asked or the data are coded. There should be an *audit trail* or record of the study's methods and procedures, so that others can replicate what was done. *Internal validity / credibility / authenticity* refers to how much the results of the qualitative inquiry ring true. Study subjects can be asked to confirm, refute, or otherwise comment on the themes and explanations that emerge from qualitative data analysis (*respondent validation* or *member checks*). The investigators should study / account for *exceptions* to the themes that emerge from the qualitative data analysis. They should consider and discuss alternative explanations. There should be a representative, rich or *thick* description of the data, including examples, sufficient to support the investigators' interpretations. The data collection methods should be adequate to address the evaluation question. *All* of the above contribute to the *trustworthiness* of the evaluation/ research. As with quantitative research methodologies, *external validity / transferability* deals with the applicability of findings more broadly. Do the results apply to other cases or settings and resonate with stakeholders in those settings? Did the investigators describe their study subjects and setting in sufficient detail? Did they compare their results with those from other studies and with empirically derived theory (*triangulation of findings*)? The reader is referred to this chapter's General References, Qualitative Evaluation, for a more detailed discussion of these concepts.

Conclusions

Because all measurement instruments are subject to threats to their reliability and validity, the ideal evaluation strategy will employ *multiple measurements using several different measurement methods and several different raters.* When all results are similar, the findings are said to be *robust*, and one can feel reasonably comfortable about their validity. This point cannot be overemphasized, as multiple concordant pieces of evidence, each individually weak, can collectively provide strong evidence to inform a program evaluation.

TASK VII: ADDRESS ETHICAL CONCERNS

Propriety Standards

More than any other step in the curriculum development process, evaluation is likely to raise ethical and what are formally called propriety concerns (19, 54). This can be broken down into seven categories (19) (Table 7.5). Major concerns relate to: concern for human rights and human interactions, which usually involve issues of confidentiality, access, and consent; resource allocation; and potential impact of the evaluation. It is wise for curriculum developers to anticipate these ethical concerns and address them in planning the evaluation. In addressing important ethical concerns, it can be helpful to obtain input both from the involved parties, such as learners and faculty, and from those with administrative oversight for the overall program. Institutional policies and procedures, external guidelines, and consultation with uninvolved parties, including those in the community, can also provide assistance.

Confidentiality, Access, and Consent

Concerns about confidentiality, access, and consent usually relate to those being evaluated. Decisions about confidentiality must be made regarding who should have access to an individual's assessments. Concerns are magnified when feasibility considerations have resulted in the use of measurement methods of limited reliability and validity, and when there is a need for those reviewing the assessments to understand these limitations.

The decision also has to be made about whether any evaluators should be granted confidentiality (the evaluator is unknown to the evaluated but can be identified by someone else) or anonymity (the evaluator is known to no one). This concern usually pertains to individuals in subordinate positions (e.g., students, employees) who have been asked to evaluate those in authority over them, and who might be subject to retaliation for an unflattering assessment. Anonymous raters may be more open and honest, but they may also be less responsible in criticizing the person being rated.

Finally, it is necessary to decide whether those being assessed need to provide informed consent for the assessment process. Even if a separate formal consent for the evaluation is not required, decisions need to be made regarding the extent to which those being assessed will be informed: about the assessment methods being used; about the strengths and limitations of the assessment methods; about the potential users of the assessments (e.g., deans, program directors, board review committees); about the uses to which assessment results will be put (e.g., formative purposes, grades, certification of proficiency for external bodies); about the location of assessment results, their confidentiality, and methods for ensuring confidentiality; and, finally, about the assessment results themselves. Which assessment results will be shared with whom, and how will that sharing take place? Will collated or individual results be shared? Will individual results be shared with those being assessed? If so, how? Each of these issues should be addressed and answered during the planning stage of the evaluation process. The "need to know" principle should be widely applied. Publication of evaluation results beyond one's institution constitutes educational research. When publication or other forms of dissemination are contemplated (see Chapter 9), curriculum developers should consult their institutional review board in the planning stages of the evaluation, before data are collected (see Chapters 6 and 9).

Table 7.5. Ethical-Propriety Concerns Related to Evaluation

Issue	Recommendation
Responsive and inclusive orientation	Place the needs of program participants and stakeholders in the center. Elicit suggestions for program improvement.
Formal policy/agreements	Have a formal policy or agreement regarding: the purpose and questions of the evaluation, the release of reports, confidentiality and anonymity of data.
Rights of human subjects	Clearly establish the protection of the rights of human subjects. Clarify intended uses of the evaluation. Ensure informed consent. Follow due process. Respect diversity. Keep stakeholders informed. Understand participant values. Follow stated protocol. Honor confidentiality and anonymity agreements. Do no harm.
Clarity and fairness	Assess and report a balance of the strengths and weaknesses and unintended outcomes. Acknowledge limitations of the evaluation.
Transparency and disclosure	Define right-to-know audiences (i.e., stakeholders). Clearly report the findings and the basis for conclusions. Disclose limitations. Assure that reports reach their intended audiences.
Conflict of interest	Identify real and perceived conflicts of interest. Assure protection against conflicts of interest. Use independent parties or reporting agencies as needed to avoid conflicts of interest.
Fiscal responsibility	Consider and specify budgetary needs. Keep some flexibility. Be frugal. Include a statement of use of funds. Consider evaluation process in the context of entire program budget.

Source: Adapted from Yarbrough et al. (19)

Resource Allocation

The use of resources for one purpose may mean that fewer resources are available for other purposes. The curriculum developer may need to ask whether the allocation of resources for a curriculum is fair and whether the allocation is likely to result in the most overall good. A strong evaluation could drain resources from other curriculum development steps. Therefore, it is appropriate to think about the impact of resource allocation on learners, faculty, curriculum coordinators, and other stakeholders in the curriculum.

A controlled evaluation design, for example, may deny an educational intervention to some learners. This consequence may be justified if the efficacy of the intervention is widely perceived as questionable and if there is consensus about the need to resolve the question through a controlled evaluation.

On the other hand, allocation of resources to an evaluation effort that is important for a faculty member's academic advancement, but that diverts needed resources from learners or other faculty, is ethically problematic.

There may also be concerns about the allocation of resources for different evaluation purposes. How much should be allocated for formative purposes, to help learners and the curriculum improve, and how much for summative purposes, to ensure trainees' competence for the public or to develop evidence of programmatic success for the curriculum developers, one's institution, or those beyond one's institution? It is important to plan for these considerations during the development process, before implementation of the curriculum (Chapter 6).

Potential Impact/Consequences

The evaluation may have an impact on learners, faculty, curriculum developers, other stakeholders, and the curriculum itself. It is helpful to think through the potential uses to which an evaluation might be put, and whether the evaluation is likely to result in more good than harm. An evaluation that lacks methodological rigor due to resource limitations could lead to false conclusions, improper interpretation, and harmful use. It is therefore important to ensure that the uses to which an evaluation is put are appropriate for its degree of methodological rigor, to ensure that the necessary degree of methodological rigor is maintained over time, and to inform users of an evaluation's methodological limitations as well as its strengths.

EXAMPLE: *Inability to Conduct Sufficiently Accurate Individual Summative Assessments.* The director for the internal medicine clerkship wants to evaluate the overall progress of students in the competencies of medical knowledge and patient care at the midpoint of the clerkship; however, she does not have sufficient resources to develop individual summative assessments of high accuracy. She instead elects to obtain individual observational assessments from one faculty member and one resident for each student. Because the assessments lack sufficient inter-rater reliability and validity evidence, they are used for formative purposes and discussed in an interactive way with learners, with suggestions for how to improve their skills. The results of these assessments are kept only until the end of the clerkship to evaluate longitudinal progress, and they are not used for summative assessment purposes or entered into the student's record where others could have access to them.

EXAMPLE: *Inability to Conduct a Sufficiently Accurate Summative Program Evaluation.* As a pilot program, a medical school designed and implemented a longitudinal third- and fourth-year curriculum around the Core EPAs for Entering Residency (10). After four months, the curriculum committee requested a report about whether the third-year students demonstrated "entrustability" yet, as proof of measurable benefits of the new curriculum. Curriculum developers had planned an evaluation at the end of one year, based on sample size, cost of the simulation-heavy evaluation, and reliability and validity evidence of the assessment tools. Given the possibility that a false conclusion could be drawn on the outcome of the curriculum after four months, and that more harm than good could result from the evaluation, the curriculum developers instead reported formative evaluation results of student and faculty satisfaction and engagement with the curriculum.

EXAMPLE: *Informing Users of Methodological Limitations of an Evaluation Method.* In a surgery residency program, multiple types of assessment data are used to rate residents' performance against the milestones that have been mapped to each of the ACGME Core Competencies to satisfy requirements for the Next Accreditation System. A listing of the limitations of and validity evidence for each instrument used in milestone assessment is included in each resident's record, along with advice about how to interpret each of the measures.

TASK VIII: COLLECT DATA

Sufficient data must be collected to ensure a useful analysis. Failure to collect important evaluation data that match the evaluation questions or low response rates can seriously compromise the value of an evaluation. While it may be tempting to cast a wide net in data collection, doing so excessively or inefficiently can consume valuable resources and lead to fatigue in respondents.

Response Rates and Efficiency

While the evaluation data design dictates when data should be collected relative to an intervention, curriculum coordinators usually have flexibility with respect to the precise time, place, and manner of data collection. Data collection can therefore be planned to maximize response rates, feasibility, and efficiency. Today, secure web-based Internet assessment and evaluation tools may allow efficiency in the collection and analysis of data (40).

Response rates can be boosted and the need for follow-up reduced when data collection is built into scheduled learner and faculty activities. This may be further facilitated through the use of asynchronous and online learning activities, for which electronic platforms may offer mechanisms for built-in evaluation. Response rates can also be increased if a learner's completion of an evaluation is required to achieve needed credit.

> **EXAMPLE:** *Integrating Data Collection into the Curriculum.* A 15-question evaluation was embedded on the last page of an interactive online learning module on the pediatrics clerkship. Students were required to complete both the module and its evaluation to receive credit, and all 30 students completed the evaluation without need for follow-up.

Sometimes an evaluation method can be designed to serve simultaneously as an educational method. This strategy reduces imposition on the learner and uses curriculum personnel efficiently.

> **EXAMPLE:** *A Method Used for both Teaching and Evaluation.* Interactions between faculty participants and a standardized learner were videotaped at the beginning and end of a five-session faculty development workshop. The videotapes were reviewed for educational purposes with participants during the sessions. Later they were reviewed in a blinded fashion by trained raters as part of a pre-post program evaluation.

Occasionally, data collection can be incorporated into already scheduled evaluation activities.

> **EXAMPLE:** *Use of an Existing Evaluation Activity.* A multistation examination was used to assess students' accomplishments at the end of a clinical clerkship in neurology. Curriculum developers for a procedural curriculum on lumbar puncture were granted a station for a simulated patient assessment during the examination.

EXAMPLE: *Use of an Existing Evaluation Activity.* Developers of a handoff curriculum for emergency medicine residents convinced the program director to include questions about the frequency with which residents used a handoff tool and the quality of the individual's handoffs in the residents' monthly peer evaluations.

Finally, curriculum developers may be able to use existing data sources, such as electronic medical records, to collect data automatically for evaluation purposes.

EXAMPLE: *Use of Available Data.* Developers of an ambulatory primary care curriculum were able to obtain reports from electronic medical records to assess pre-post curriculum delivery of targeted preventive care measures, such as immunizations, cholesterol profiles, and breast and colon cancer screening. They were also able to track these measures longitudinally to assess post-curricular maintenance versus decay of preventive care behaviors.

Impact of Data Collection on Instrument Design

What data are collected is determined by the choice of measurement instruments (see Task VI). However, the design of measurement instruments needs to be tempered by the process of data collection. Response rates for questionnaires will fall as their length and complexity increase. The amount of time and resources that have been allocated for data collection cannot be exceeded without affecting learners, faculty, or other priorities.

EXAMPLE: *Impact of Time Constraints on Instrument Length.* If 15 minutes of curricular time is allocated for evaluation, a measurement instrument that requires 30 minutes to complete will intrude on other activities and is likely to reduce participants' cooperation.

Assignment of Responsibility

Measurement instruments must be distributed, collected, and safely stored. Non-respondents require follow-up. While different individuals may distribute or administer measurement instruments within scheduled sessions, it is usually wise to delegate overall responsibility for data collection to one person.

EXAMPLE: *Assignment of Responsibility.* A curriculum to enhance residents' skills in evidence-based medicine is being conducted at three training sites in a plastic surgery residency program. A person at each site was recruited to distribute and collect responses to the written assessment activity and evaluation, but the administrative coordinator was made responsible for oversight at all three locations, including the follow-up of nonrespondents.

TASK IX: ANALYZE DATA

After the data have been collected, they need to be analyzed (55–61). *Data analysis, however, should be planned at the same time that evaluation questions are being identified and measurement instruments developed.*

Relation to Evaluation Questions

The nature of evaluation questions will determine, in part, the type of statistical approach required to answer them. Questions related to participants' perceptions of a curriculum, or to the percentage of learners who achieved a specific objective, generally require only descriptive statistics. Questions about changes in learners generally require more sophisticated tests of statistical significance.

Statistical considerations may also influence the choice of evaluation questions. A *power analysis* (55–57) is a statistical method for estimating the ability of an evaluation to detect a statistically significant relationship between an outcome measure (dependent variable) and a potential determinant of the outcome (independent variable, such as exposure to a curriculum). The power analysis can be used to determine whether a curriculum has a sufficient number of learners over a given period of time to justify a determination of the statistical significance of its impact. Sometimes there are limitations in the evaluator's statistical expertise and in the resources available for statistical consultation. Evaluation questions can then be worded in a way that at least ensures *congruence* between the questions and the analytic methods that will be employed.

> **EXAMPLE:** *Congruence between the Evaluation Question and the Analytic Methods Required.* A curriculum developer has a rudimentary knowledge of statistics and few resources for consultation. After designing the assessment instruments, the curriculum objectives and evaluation questions were changed. "Does the curriculum result in a statistically significant improvement in the proficiency of its learners in skill X?" was changed to "What percentage of learners improve or achieve proficiency in skill X by the end of the curriculum?" so that application of tests of statistical significance could be avoided.

When the curriculum evaluation involves a large number of learners, analysis could reveal a statistically significant but an educationally meaningless impact on learners. The latter consideration might prompt curriculum evaluators to develop an evaluation question that addresses the magnitude as well as the statistical significance of any impact. *Effect size* is increasingly used to provide a measure of the size of a change, or the degree to which sample results diverge from the null hypothesis (58). Several measurements have been used to give an estimate of effect size: correlation coefficient, r, which is the measure of the relationship between variables, with the value of r^2 indicating the proportion of variance shared by variables; eta-square (η^2), which is reported in analysis of variance and is interpreted as the proportion of the variance of an outcome variable explained by the independent variable; odds ratios; risk ratios; absolute risk reduction; and Cohen's d, which is the difference between two means (e.g., pre-post scores or experimental vs. control groups) divided by the pooled standard deviation associated with that measurement. The effect size is said to be small if Cohen's d = 0.20, medium if 0.50, and large if $\geq$0.80 (57). However, measures of effect size are probably more meaningful when judging the results of several studies with similar designs and directly comparable interventions, rather than using these thresholds in absolute terms. For example, it would not be surprising to see a large Cohen's d when comparing a multimodal curriculum against no intervention, whereas the expected Cohen's d for a study comparing two active educational interventions would be much smaller. It is important to remember that educational meaningfulness is still an interpretation that rests not only on the statistical significance and size of a change but also on the nature of the change and its relation to other outcomes deemed important. Examples of such outcomes might be improvements in adherence to management plans or a reduction in risk behaviors, morbidity, or mortality.

Relation to Measurement Instruments: Data Type and Entry

The measurement instrument determines the type of data collected. The *type of data*, in turn, *helps determine the type of statistical test that is appropriate to analyze the data* (59–61) (see Table 7.6). Data are first divided into one of two types: categorical or numerical. *Categorical* data are data that fit into discrete categories. *Numerical* data are data that have meaning on a numerical scale. Numerical data can be continuous (e.g., age, weight, height) or discrete, such as count data (no fractions, only nonnegative integer values, e.g., number of procedures performed, number of sessions attended). *Within the categorical domain, data can additionally be described as either nominal or ordinal. Nominal* data are categorical data that fit into discrete, nonordered categories (e.g., sex, race, eye color, exposure or not to an intervention). *Ordinal data* are categorical data that fit into discrete but inherently ordered or hierarchical categories (e.g., grades: A, B, C, D, and F; highest educational level completed: grade school, high school, college, postcollege degree program; condition: worse, same, better). Numerical data can also be subdivided into interval and ratio data. *Interval data* are numerical data with equal intervals, distances, or differences between categories, but no zero point (e.g., year, dates on a calendar). *Ratio data* are interval data with a meaningful zero point (e.g., weight; age; number of procedures completed appropriately without assistance).

Data analysis considerations affect the design of the measurement instrument. When a computer is being used, the first step in data analysis is *data entry*. In this situation, it is helpful to construct one's measurement instruments in a way that facilitates data entry, such as the precoding of responses or using electronic evaluation software that can download data into a useable spreadsheet format. If one prefers to use a specific test for statistical significance, one needs to ensure that the appropriate types of data are collected.

Choice of Statistical Methods

The choice of statistical method depends on several factors, including the evaluation question, evaluation design, sample size, number of study groups, whether groups are matched or paired for certain characteristics, number of measures, data distribution, and the type of data collected. *Descriptive statistics* are often sufficient to answer questions about participant perceptions, distribution of characteristics and responses, and percentage change or achievement. For all types of data, a display of the percentages or proportions in each response category is an important first step in analysis. Medians and ranges are sometimes useful in characterizing ordinal as well as numerical data. Means and standard deviations are reserved for describing numerical data. Ordinal data (e.g., from Likert scales) can sometimes be treated as numerical data so that means and standard deviations (or other measures of variance) can be applied.

EXAMPLE: *Conversion of Ordinal to Numerical Data for the Purpose of Statistical Analysis.* Questions from one institution's 360° resident evaluations use a Likert scale with the following categories: strongly disagree, disagree, neutral, agree, and strongly agree. For analysis, these data were converted to numerical data so that responses could be summarized by means: strongly disagree [1], disagree [2], neutral [3], agree [4], strongly agree [5].

Statistical tests of significance are required to answer questions about the statistical significance of changes in individual learners or groups of learners, and of associations between various characteristics. *Parametric statistics*, such as *t*-tests, analysis of variance, regression, and Pearson correlation analysis, are often appropriate for numerical data. Parametric tests assume that the sample has been randomly selected from the population it represents and that the distribution of data in the population has a known underlying distribution. However, these tests are often robust enough to tolerate some deviation from this assumption. The most common distribution assumption is that the distribution is normal. Other distributions include the binomial distribution (logistic regression) and the Poisson distribution (Poisson regression). Sometimes ordinal data can be treated as numerical data (see Example above) to permit the use of parametric statistics. *Nonparametric tests*, such as chi-square, Wilcoxon rank-sum test, Spearman's correlation statistic, and nonparametric versions of analysis of variance, do not make, or make few, assumptions about the distribution of data in a population. They are often appropriate for small sample sizes, categorical data, and non-normally distributed data. Statistical software packages are available that can perform parametric and nonparametric tests on the same data. This approach can provide a check of the statistical results when numerical data do not satisfy all of the assumptions for parametric tests. One can be confident about using parametric statistics on ordinal level data when nonparametric statistics confirm decisions regarding statistical significance obtained using parametric statistics. For non-normally distributed data, it may be possible to normalize the data through transformation (e.g., log transformation) in order to use parametric rather than nonparametric statistics (which tend to be more wasteful of data and have lower power).

Curriculum developers have varying degrees of statistical expertise. Those with modest levels of expertise and limited resources (the majority) may choose to keep data analysis simple. They can consult textbooks (see General References, Statistics) on how to perform simple statistical tests, such as *t*-tests, chi-squares, and the Wilcoxon rank-sum test. These tests, especially for small sample sizes, can be performed by hand or with a calculator (online calculators are now available) and do not require access to computer programs. Sometimes, however, the needs of users will require more sophisticated approaches. Often there are individuals within or beyond one's institution who can provide statistical consultation. The curriculum developer will use the statistician's time most efficiently when the evaluation questions are clearly stated and the key independent and dependent variables are clearly defined. Some familiarity with the range and purposes of commonly used statistical methods can also facilitate communication. Table 7.6 displays the situations in which statistical methods are appropriately used, based on the type of data being analyzed, the number and type of samples, and whether correlational or multivariate analysis is desired. As indicated at the bottom of the table, count data require special consideration. One type of situation that is not captured in the table is statistical analysis of time to a desired educational outcome or event, which can be analyzed using various survival analysis techniques such as the log-rank test (bivariate analysis) or Cox regression (bivariate or multivariate analysis). Cox (or proportional hazards) regression has the advantage of providing hazard ratios (akin to odds ratios).

TASK X: REPORT RESULTS

The final step in evaluation is the reporting and distribution of results (62). In planning evaluation reports, it is helpful to think of the *needs of users*.

The *timeliness* of reports can be critical. Individual learners benefit from the immediate feedback of formative assessment results, so that the information can be processed while the learning experience is still fresh and can be used to enhance subsequent learning within the curriculum. Evaluation results are helpful to faculty and curriculum planners when they are received in time to prepare for the next curricular cycle. Important decisions, such as the allocation of educational resources for the coming year, may be influenced by the timely reporting of evaluation results to administrators in concert with budget cycles. External bodies, such as funding agencies or specialty boards, may also impose deadlines for the receipt of reports.

The *format* of a report should match the needs of its users in content, language, and length. Individual learners, faculty members, and curriculum developers may want detailed evaluation reports pertaining to their particular (or the curriculum's) performance that include all relevant quantitative and qualitative data provided by the measurement instruments. Administrators, deans, and department chairs may prefer brief reports that provide background information on the curriculum and that synthesize the evaluation information relevant to their respective needs. External bodies and publishers (see Chapter 10) may specify the format they expect for a report.

It is always desirable to *display results in a succinct and clear manner and to use plain language*; an *Executive Summary* can be helpful to the reader, particularly when it precedes detailed and/or lengthy reports. Collated results can be enhanced by the addition of descriptive statistics, such as percentage distributions, means, medians, and standard deviations. Other results can be displayed in a clear and efficient manner in tables, graphs, or figures. Specific examples can help explain and bring to life summaries of qualitative data.

CONCLUSION

Evaluation is not the final step in curriculum planning, but one that directly affects and should evolve in concert with other steps in the curriculum development process (see also Chapter 1). It provides important information that can help both individuals and programs improve their performance. It provides information that facilitates judgments and decisions about individuals and the curriculum. A stepwise approach can help ensure an evaluation that meets the needs of its users and that balances methodological rigor with feasibility.

ACKNOWLEDGMENTS

We thank Joseph Carrese, MD, MPH, for his review of and input to the section "Reliability and Validity in Qualitative Measurement." We thank Ken Kolodner, ScD, for his review of and input to the section "Task IX: Analyze Data" and Table 7.6. We also thank David A. Cook, MD, MHPE, for his thoughtful review of and suggestions for the section "Reliability, Validity, and Bias" in the second edition of this book; his input has been carried forward into the third edition.

Table 7.6. Commonly Used Statistical Methods

Tests/Methods Used for Evaluating Statistically Significant Differences or Associations

Type of Measurement (Dependent Variable)	One Sample (observed vs. expected)	Two Samples		N Samples		Correlation	Multivariate Analysis*
		Independent	Related (pre-post)	Independent	Related (pre-post)		
Nominal	Binominal Test Chi-square	Fisher exact test Chi-square	McNemar's test	Chi-square	Cochran's Q test	Contingency co-efficient	Cumulative logistic regression Discriminant functional analysis
Dichotomous	Binominal Test Chi-square	Chi-square Odds ratio Relative risk Prevalence ratio	McNemar's test	Chi-square Logistic regression (odds ratios)	Logistic regression (odds ratios)		Logistic regression (odds ratios) Generalized estimating equations (GEE) Discriminant functional analysis
Ordinal or Ordered	Kolmogorov-Smirnov one sample test One-sample runs test	Median test Mann-Whitney U Kolmogorov-Smirnov test Wald-Wolfowitz runs test	Sign test Wilcoxon matched pairs signed rank test	Kruskal-Wallis ANOVA[†] (one-way ANOVA)	Friedman's two-way ANOVA	Spearman's r Kendall's τ (tau) Kendall's w	Multiple regression Polychotomous logistic regression Generalized estimating equations (GEE) Hierarchical regression models (mixed regression)

Interval and Ratio	Confidence interval	t-test	Paired t-test Wilcoxon matched pairs signed rank test	ANOVA	Repeated-measures ANOVA Generalized estimating equations (GEE) Hierarchical regression models (mixed regression)	Pearson r	Linear regression Partial correlation Multiple correlation Multiple regression ANCOVA‡ Generalized estimating equations (GEE) Hierarchical regression models (mixed regression) Canonical correlation
Count data	Confidence interval using Poisson distribution	Poisson, negative binomial, or zero-inflated Poisson models	Poisson, negative binomial, or zero-inflated Poisson models Paired t-test Wilcoxon matched pairs signed rank test	Poisson, negative binomial. or zero-inflated Poisson models	Poisson, negative binomial, or zero-inflated Poisson models	Spearman's r, if well enough distributed	Poisson, negative binomial, or zero-inflated Poisson models

* Multivariate analysis involves analysis of more than one variable at a time and permits analysis of the relationship between one independent variable (e.g., the curriculum) and a dependent variable of interest (e.g., learner skill or behavior), while controlling for other independent variables (e.g., age, gender, level of training, previous or concurrent experiences).

† ANOVA: Analysis of variance.

‡ ANCOVA: Analysis of covariance.

QUESTIONS

For the curriculum you are coordinating, planning, or would like to be planning, please answer or think about the following questions:

1. Who will be the *users* of your curriculum?

2. What are their needs? *How will evaluation results be used?*

3. What *resources* are available for evaluation, in terms of *time*, *personnel*, *equipment*, *facilities*, *funds*, and *existing data*?

4. Identify one to three critical *evaluation questions.* Are they *congruent* with the objectives of your curriculum? Do either the objectives or the evaluation questions need to be changed?

5. Name and diagram the most appropriate *evaluation design* for each evaluation question, considering both methodological rigor and feasibility (see Table 7.2 and text).

6. Choose the most appropriate *measurement methods* for the evaluation you are designing (see Table 7.3). Are the measurement methods *congruent* with the evaluation questions (i.e., are you measuring the correct items)? Would it be *feasible* for you, given available resources, to construct and administer the required measurement instruments? If not, do you need to revise the evaluation questions or choose other evaluation methods? What issues related to reliability and validity are pertinent for your measurement instrument?

7. What *ethical issues* are likely to be raised by your evaluation in terms of confidentiality, access, consent, resource allocation, potential impact, or other concerns? Should you consult your institutional review board?

8. Consider the *data collection* process. *Who will be responsible* for data collection? How can the data be collected so that *resource use* is minimized and *response rate* is maximized? Are data collection considerations likely to influence the *design of your measurement instruments*?

9. How will the data that are collected be *analyzed*? Given your evaluation questions, are *descriptive statistics* sufficient or are *tests of statistical significance* required? Is a *power analysis* desirable? Will statistical consultation be required?

10. List the goals, content, format, and time frame of the various *evaluation reports* you envision, given the needs of the users (refer to Questions 1 and 2). How will you ensure that the reports are completed?

Congratulations! You have read and thought about six steps critical to curriculum development. At this point, rereading Chapter 1 may be worthwhile, to review briefly the six steps and reflect on how they interact.

GENERAL REFERENCES

Comprehensive

Fink A. *Evaluation Fundamentals: Insights into the Outcomes, Effectiveness, and Quality of Health Programs*, 2nd ed. Thousand Oaks, Calif.: SAGE Publications; 2005.
  Reader-friendly, basic comprehensive reference on program evaluation, with examples from the health and social science fields. 265 pages.

Fitzpatrick JL, Sanders JR, Worthen BR. *Program Evaluation: Alternative Approaches and Practical Guidelines*, 4th ed. Upper Saddle River, N.J.: Pearson Education; 2011.
  Comprehensive text on evaluation methods and systematic, detailed approach to design, implementation, and reporting of an evaluation. Excellent use of a longitudinal evaluation problem throughout the text. 560 pages.

Green LW, Lewis FM. *Measurement and Evaluation in Health Education and Health Promotion*. Palo Alto, Calif.: Mayfield Publications; 1986.
  Clearly written, comprehensive text with examples from community health and patient education programs with easy applicability to medical education programs. Both quantitative and qualitative methods are included. 411 pages.

Kalet A, Chou CL, eds. *Remediation in Medical Education: A Mid-Course Correction.* New York: Springer Publishing Co.; 2014.
  This multiauthored and pithy text brings together the array of potential learner assessment methods in the new era of competency-based education, current understanding of root causes of learner failures, and potential approaches to remediation. There are numerous examples and models that can be transferred to other institutions. 367 pages.

McGaghie WC, ed. *International Best Practices for Evaluation in the Health Professions.* London, New York: Radcliffe Publishing; 2013.
  A multiauthored text encompassing an international group of 69 educational experts. Sixteen chapters, including chapters on the need for and methodology of evaluation and chapters on specific foci of evaluation, such as clinical competence, knowledge acquisition, professionalism, team performance, continuing education, outcomes, workplace performance, leadership/management, recertification, and accreditation. The final chapter describes a new educational framework of mastery learning and deliberative practice. 377 pages.

Windsor R, Clark N, Boyd NR, Goodman RM. *Evaluation of Health Promotion, Health Education, and Disease Prevention Programs*. New York: McGraw-Hill Publishing; 2004.
  Written for health professionals who are responsible for planning, implementing, and evaluating health education or health promotion programs, with direct applicability to medical education. Especially useful are the chapters on process evaluations and cost evaluation. 292 pages.

Measurement

Case SM, Swanson DB. *Constructing Written Test Questions for the Basic and Clinical Sciences*, 3rd ed. (revised). Philadelphia: National Board of Medical Examiners; 2002.
  Written for medical school educators who need to construct and interpret flawlessly written test questions. Frequent examples. Available at www.nbme.org/publications/index.html. 180 pages.

DeVellis RF. *Scale Development: Theory and Applications*, 3rd ed. Thousand Oaks, Calif.: SAGE Publications; 2012.
  Authoritative text in the Applied Social Research Methods Series that provides an eight-step framework for creation and refinement of surveys and scales for use in social sciences research. 205 pages.

Downing SM, Haladyna TM. *Handbook of Test Development.* Mahwah, N.J.: Lawrence Erlbaum Associates; 2006.
> Definitive and current handbook on the 12 steps of test development and comprehensive review of issues around testing. 778 pages.

Fink A, ed. *The Survey Kit.* Thousand Oaks, Calif.: SAGE Publications; 2003.
> Ten user-friendly, practical handbooks about various aspects of surveys, both for the novice and for those who are more experienced but want a refresher reference. The first book is an overview of the survey method. The other handbooks are "how-to" books on asking survey questions; conducting self-administered and mail surveys; conducting interviews by telephone and in person; designing survey studies; sampling for surveys; assessing and interpreting survey psychometrics; managing, analyzing, and interpreting survey data; and reporting on surveys. Ten books, ranging from 75 to 325 pages in length.

Miller DC. *Handbook of Research Design and Social Measurement*, 6th ed. Thousand Oaks, Calif.: SAGE Publications; 2002.
> The most useful part of this textbook is Part 7 (209 pages), selected sociometric scales and indexes to measure social variables. Scales in the following areas are discussed: social status; group structure and dynamics; social indicators; measures of organizational structure; community; social participation; leadership in the work organization; morale and job satisfaction; scales of attitudes, values, and norms; personality measurements; and others. 786 pages.

Shannon S, Norman G, eds. *Evaluation Methods: A Resource Handbook*, 3rd ed. Hamilton, Ont.: Programme for Educational Research and Development, McMaster University; 1996.
> A practical, well-written handbook on evaluation methods for assessing the performance of medical students. Reliability and validity issues are discussed for each evaluation method, including summary reports and ratings; oral examinations; written tests; performance tests; self- and peer assessments; assessment of problem-solving, psychomotor, communication, and critical appraisal skills; and evaluation of bioethics and professional behavior. Available at http://fhs.mcmaster.ca/perd/evaluation_methods_handbook.html. 120 pages.

Waugh CK, Gronlund NE. *Assessment of Student Achievement*, 10th ed. Upper Saddle River, N.J.: Pearson Education; 2012.
> Basic text with review of assessment methods, validity and reliability in planning, preparing and using achievement tests, performance assessments, portfolio assessment, grading reporting, and interpretation of scores. 256 pages.

Evaluation Designs

Campbell DT, Stanley JC. *Experimental and Quasi-Experimental Designs for Research.* Chicago: Rand McNally; 1963.
> Succinct, classic text on research/evaluation designs for educational programs. More concise than the later edition, and tables more complete. Table 1 (p. 8), Table 2 (p. 40), and Table 3 (p. 56) diagram different experimental designs and the degree to which they control or don't control for threats to internal and external validity. Pages 5–6 concisely summarize threats to internal validity. Pages 16–22 discuss external validity. 84 pages.

Fraenkel JR, Wallen NE. *How to Design and Evaluate Research in Education*, 8th ed. New York: McGraw-Hill Publishing; 2011.
> Comprehensive and straightforward review of educational research methods, with step-by-step analysis of research and real case studies. 704 pages.

Qualitative Evaluation

Crabtree BF, Miller WL. *Doing Qualitative Research*, 2nd ed. Thousand Oaks, Calif.: SAGE Publications; 1999.
> Practical, user-friendly text with an emphasis on using qualitative methods in primary care research. 406 pages.

Denzin NK, Lincoln YS. *Handbook of Qualitative Research*, 4th ed. Thousand Oaks, Calif.: SAGE Publications; 2011.
  Comprehensive text, useful as a reference to look up particular topics. 784 pages.

Miles M, Huberman AM, Saldana J. *Qualitative Data Analysis: A Methods Sourcebook*, 3rd ed. Thousand Oaks, Calif.: SAGE Publications; 2014.
  Practical text and useful resource on qualitative data analysis. Chapter 11 focuses on drawing and verifying conclusions, as well as issues of reliability and validity. 408 pages.

Patton MQ. *Qualitative Research & Evaluation Methods*, 3rd ed. Thousand Oaks, Calif.: SAGE Publications; 2002.
  Readable, example-filled text emphasizing strategies for generating useful and credible qualitative information for decision making. The three sections of the book cover conceptual issues in the use of qualitative methods; qualitative designs and data collection; and analysis, interpretation, and reporting of such studies. 598 pages.

Richards L, Morse JM. *READ ME FIRST for a User's Guide to Qualitative Methods*, 3rd ed. Thousand Oaks, Calif.: SAGE Publications; 2013.
  Readable, introductory book to qualitative research methods. 336 pages.

Statistics

Kanji G. *100 Statistical Tests*, 3rd ed. Thousand Oaks, Calif.: SAGE Publications; 2006.
  A handy reference for the applied statistician and everyday user of statistics. An elementary knowledge of statistics is sufficient to allow the reader to follow the formulae given and to carry out the tests. All 100 tests are cross-referenced to several headings. Examples also included. 242 pages.

Norman GR, Streiner DL. *Biostatistics: The Bare Essentials*, 3rd ed. Shelton, Conn.: People's Medical Publishing House–USA; 2008.
  This book conveys the traditional content for a statistics book in an irreverent and humorous tone, packaged for the "do-it-yourselfer." The main sections of the book include the nature of data and statistics, analysis of variance, regression and correlation, and nonparametric statistics. Three features of the book are helpful: the computer notes at the end of each chapter, which help the reader with the three most common statistical programs; highlighted important points in the text; and sample size calculations with each chapter. 200 pages.

Norman GR, Streiner D. *PDQ Statistics*, 3rd ed. Hamilton, Ont.: B. C. Decker; 2003.
  This short, well-written book covers types of variables, descriptive statistics, parametric and nonparametric statistics, multivariate methods, and research designs. The authors assume that the reader has had some introductory exposure to statistics. The intent of the book is to help the reader understand the various approaches to analysis when reading/critiquing the results section of research articles. Useful also for planning an analysis, in order to avoid misuse and misinterpretation of statistical tests. 218 pages.

Shott S. *Statistics for Health Professionals*. Philadelphia: W. B. Saunders Co.; 1990.
  The author states that after studying this text and working the problems, the reader should be able to select appropriate statistics for most datasets, interpret results, evaluate analyses reported in the literature, and interpret SPSS and SPS output for the common statistical procedures. 418 pages.

Assessment Frameworks and Instruments

Association of American Medical Colleges (AAMC) MedEdPORTAL. Directory and Repository of Educational Assessment Measures (DREAM) [Internet]. Available at www.mededportal.org /about/initiatives/dream.
  Provides easy to locate, publicly accessible information about assessment instruments. Each entry includes a copy of the instrument, a peer-reviewed critical analysis of the instrument's validity evidence, and supplementary materials for instrument administration.

Pangaro L, ten Cate O. Frameworks for learner assessment in medicine: AMEE Guide No. 78. *Med Teach*. 2013;35:e1197–1200.

SPECIFIC REFERENCES

1. Fitzpatrick JL, Sanders JR, Worthen BR. Evaluation's basic purpose, uses, and conceptual distinctions, Chapter 1. In: Fitzpatrick JL, Sanders JR, Worthen BR. *Program Evaluation: Alternative Approaches and Practical Guidelines*, 4th ed. Boston: Pearson Education, Allyn & Bacon; 2011. Pp. 3–38.
2. Atasoylu AA, Wright SM, Beasley BW, et al. Promotion criteria for clinician-educators. *J Gen Intern Med*. 2003;18:711–16.
3. Beasley BW, Wright SM, Cofrancesco J Jr., et al. Promotion criteria for clinician-educators in the United States and Canada: a survey of promotion committee chairpersons. *JAMA*. 1997;278:723–28.
4. Fleming VM, Schindler N, Martin GJ, DaRosa DA. Separate and equitable promotion tracks for clinician-educators. *JAMA*. 2005;294:1101–4.
5. Simpson D, Fincher RE, Hafler JP, et al. Advancing educators and education by defining the components and evidence associated with educational scholarship. *Med Educ*. 2007;41:1002–9.
6. Ruiz JG, Candler CS, Qadri SS, Roos BA. e-Learning as evidence of educational scholarship: a survey of chairs of promotion and tenure committees at U.S. medical schools. *Acad Med*. 2009;84:47–57.
7. Norcini J, Anderson B, Bollela V, et al. Criteria for good assessment: consensus statement and recommendations from the Ottawa 2010 Conference. *Med Teach*. 2011;33:206–14.
8. ten Cate O. Nuts and bolts of entrustable professional activities. *J Grad Med Educ*. 2013; 5(1):157–58.
9. ten Cate O, Scheele F. Viewpoint: Competency-based postgraduate training: can we bridge the gap between theory and clinical practice? *Acad Med*. 2007;82(6):542–47.
10. Association of American Medical Colleges. Core Entrustable Professional Activities for Entering Residency (CEPAER) [Internet]. Washington, D.C. March 2014. Available at www.mededportal.org/icollaborative/resource/887.
11. Adapted with permission from a curriculum of Anne Lidor, MD, MPH, at Johns Hopkins University School of Medicine.
12. Stead DR. A review of the one-minute paper. *Active Learn High Educ*. 2005;6(2):118–31.
13. Hafferty FW, Franks R. The hidden curriculum, ethics teaching, and the structure of medical education. *Acad Med*. 1994; 69(11):861–71.
14. Hafler JP, Ownby AR, Thompson BM, et al. Decoding the learning environment of medical education: a hidden curriculum perspective for faculty development. *Acad Med*. 2011;86(4):440–44.
15. Adapted with permission from a curriculum of Pamela Lipsett, MD, MHPE, at Johns Hopkins University School of Medicine.
16. Suskie L. Supporting assessment efforts with time, infrastructure, and resources, Chapter 6. In: Suskie L. *Assessing Student Learning: A Common Sense Guide*, 2nd ed. San Francisco: Jossey-Bass; 2009. Pp. 86–97.
17. Association of American Medical Colleges (AAMC) MedEdPORTAL. Directory and Repository of Educational Assessment Measures (DREAM) [Internet]. Available at www.mededportal.org/about/initiatives/dream.
18. Waugh CK, Gronlund NE. Planning for assessment, Chapter 3. In: Waugh CK, Gronlund NE. *Assessment of Student Achievement*, 10th ed. Boston: Pearson Publications; 2013. Pp. 31–47.

19. Yarbrough DB, Shulha LM, Hopson RK, Caruthers FA (Joint Committee on Standards for Educational Evaluation). *The Program Evaluation Standards: A Guide for Evaluators and Evaluation Users*, 3rd ed. Thousand Oaks, Calif.: SAGE Publications; 2011. Propriety standards available at www.jcsee.org.
20. Fink A. Designing program evaluations, Chapter 3. In: Fink A. *Evaluation Fundamentals: Insights into the Outcomes, Effectiveness, and Quality of Health Programs*, 2nd ed. Thousand Oaks, Calif.: SAGE Publications; 2005. Pp. 71–98.
21. Fitzpatrick JL, Sanders JR, Worthen BR. Collecting evaluative information: design, sampling, and cost choices, Chapter 15. In: Fitzpatrick JL, Sanders JR, Worthen BR. *Program Evaluation. Alternative Approaches and Practical Guidelines*, 4th ed. Boston: Pearson Education, Allyn & Bacon; 2011. Pp. 380–417.
22. Fraenkel JR, Wallen NE. Internal validity, Chapter 9; Experimental research, Chapter 13. In: Fraenkel JR, Wallen NE. *How to Design and Evaluate Research in Education*, 7th ed. New York: McGraw-Hill Publishing; 2009. Pp. 165–82; 260–97.
23. Downing SM, Haladyna TM. Validity and its threats, Chapter 2. In: Downing SM, Yudkowsky R, eds. *Assessment in Health Professions Education*. New York: Taylor & Francis; 2009. Pp. 21–56.
24. Waugh CK, Gronlund NE. Validity and reliability, Chapter 4. In: Waugh CK, Gronlund NE. *Assessment of Student Achievement*, 10th ed. Boston: Pearson Publications; 2013. Pp. 48–70.
25. Windsor R, Clark N, Boyd NR, Goodman RM. Formative and impact evaluations, Chapter 6. In: Windsor R, Clark N, Boyd NR, Goodman RM. *Evaluation of Health Promotion, Health Education, and Disease Prevention Programs*. New York: McGraw Hill Publishing; 2004. Pp. 215–63.
26. Epstein RM. Assessment in medical education. *N Engl J Med.* 2007;356:387–96.
27. Middle States Commission on Higher Education. Evaluating student learning, Chapter 3. In: *Student Learning Assessment: Options and Resources*, 2nd ed. Philadelphia: Middle States Commission on Higher Education; 2007.
28. Kassebaum DG. The measurement of outcomes in the assessment of educational program effectiveness. *Acad Med.* 1990;65:293–96.
29. Waugh CK, Gronlund NE. Performance assessments, Chapter 9. In: Waugh CK, Gronlund NE. *Assessment of Student Achievement*, 10th ed. Boston: Pearson Publications; 2013. Pp. 144–74.
30. Charlin B, Brailovsky C, Roy L, Goulet F, van der Vleuten C. The Script Concordance Test: a tool to assess the reflective clinician. *Teach Learn Med.* 2000;12(4):189–95.
31. Kirkpatrick DI. *Evaluating Training Programs: The Four Levels*, 3rd ed. San Francisco: Berrett-Koehler; 2006.
32. Belfield C, Thomas H, Bullock A, Eynon R, Wall D. Measuring effectiveness for best evidence medical education: a discussion. *Med Teach.* 2001;23:164–70.
33. Yardley S, Dornan T. Kirkpatrick's levels and education "evidence." *Med Educ.* 2012;46(1): 97–106.
34. McDowell I. *Measuring Health: A Guide to Rating Scales and Questionnaires*, 3rd ed. New York: Oxford University Press; 2006.
35. Miller DC. Assessing social variables: scales and indexes. Part 7. In: Miller DC. *Handbook of Research Design and Social Measurement*, 6th ed. Thousand Oaks, Calif.: SAGE Publications; 2002. Pp. 453–660.
36. *Measurement of Nursing Outcomes*, 2nd ed. Waltz CF, Jenkins LS, eds. Vol. 1: *Measuring Nursing Performance in Practice, Education, and Research.* 2001; Strickland OL, Dilorio C, eds. Vol. 2: *Client Outcomes and Quality of Care.* 2003; Strickland OL, Dilorio C, eds. Vol. 3: *Self Care and Coping.* New York: Springer Publishing Co.; 2003.
37. Fink A. Collecting information: the right data sources, Chapter 5; Evaluation measures, Chapter 6. In: Fink A. *Evaluation Fundamentals: Insights into the Outcomes, Effectiveness,*

and Quality of Health Programs, 2nd ed. Thousand Oaks, Calif.: SAGE Publications; 2005. Pp. 117–62.

38. Waugh CK, Gronlund NE. Writing selection items: multiple choice, Chapter 6; Writing selection items: true-false, matching, and interpretive exercise, Chapter 7; Writing selection items: short answer and essay, Chapter 8. In: Waugh CK, Gronlund NE. Assessment of Student Achievement, 10th ed. Boston: Pearson Publications; 2013. Pp. 91–143.

39. Case SM, Swanson DB, eds. Constructing Written Test Questions for the Basic and Clinical Sciences, 3rd ed. (revised). Philadelphia: National Board of Medical Examiners, 2002. Available at www.nbme.org/pdf/itemwriting_2003/2003iwgwhole.pdf.

40. Afrin LB, Arana GW, Medio FJ, Ybarra AF, Clarke HS Jr. Improving oversight of the graduate medical education enterprise: one institution's strategies and tools. Acad Med. 2006;81: 419–25.

41. American Educational Research Association, American Psychological Association, National Council on Measurement in Education. Standards for Educational and Psychological Testing. Washington, D.C.: American Educational Research Association; 2014.

42. Downing SM. Validity: on the meaningful interpretation of assessment data. Med Educ. 2003;37:830–37.

43. Downing SM. Reliability: on the reproducibility of assessment data. Med Educ. 2004;38: 1006–12.

44. Cook DA, Beckman TJ. Current concepts in validity and reliability for psychometric instruments: theory and application. Am J Med. 2006;119:166.e7–166.e16.

45. Crossley J, Davies H, Humphris G, Jolly B. Generalisability: a key to unlock professional assessment. Med Educ. 2002 36:972–78.

46. Norman GR, Streiner DL. Principal components and factor analysis: fooling around with factors, Chapter 19. In: Norman GR, Streiner DL. Biostatistics: The Bare Essentials, 3rd ed. Lewiston, N.Y.: B. C. Decker; 2008. Pp. 194–209.

47. Aboulian A, Schwartz S, Kaji AH, de Virgilio C. The public mock oral: a useful tool for examinees and the audience in preparation for the American Board of Surgery Certifying Examination. J Surg Educ. 2010;67(1):33–36.

48. Williams RG, Klamen DA, McGaghie WC. Cognitive, social and environmental sources of bias in clinical performance ratings. Teach Learn Med. 2003 Fall;15(4):270–92.

49. Downing SM, Haladyna T. Validity threats: overcoming interference with proposed interpretations with assessment data. Med Educ. 2004;38:327–33.

50. Mays N, Pope, C. Qualitative research in health care: assessing quality in qualitative research. BMJ. 2000:320:50–52.

51. Barbour RS. Checklists for improving rigour in qualitative research: a case of the tail wagging the dog. BMJ. 2001;322:1115–17.

52. Giacomini MK, Cook DJ, for the Evidence-based Medicine Working Group. Users' guides to the medical literature. XXIII. Qualitative research in health care: A. Are the results of the study valid? JAMA. 2000;284:357–62.

53. Giacomini MK, Cook DJ, for the Evidence-based Medicine Working Group. Users' guides to the medical literature. XXIII. Qualitative research in health care: B. What are the results and how do they help me care for my patients? JAMA. 2000;284:478–82.

54. American Evaluation Association. Guiding Principles for Evaluators, 2004 [Internet]. Available at www.eval.org/p/cm/ld/fid=51.

55. Markert RJ. Enhancing medical education by improving statistical methodology in journal articles. Teach Learn Med. 2013;25(2):159–64.

56. Fink A. Sampling, Chapter 4. In: Fink A. Evaluation Fundamentals: Insights into the Outcomes, Effectiveness, and Quality of Health Programs, 2nd ed. Thousand Oaks, Calif.: SAGE Publications; 2005. Pp. 98–115.

57. Cohen J. Statistical Power Analysis for the Behavioral Sciences. Hillsdale, N.J.: Lawrence Erlbaum Associates; 1988.

58. Baghi H, Noorbaloochi S, Moore JB. Statistical and non-statistical significance: implications for health care researchers. *Qual Manag Health Care.* 2007;16:104–12.
59. Fraenkel JR, Wallen NE. Data analysis. Part 3. In: Fraenkel JR, Wallen NE. *How to Design and Evaluate Research in Education*, 7th ed. New York: McGraw-Hill Publishing; 2009. Pp. 183–241.
60. Fink A. Analyzing evaluation data, Chapter 8. In: Fink A. *Evaluation Fundamentals: Insights into the Outcomes, Effectiveness, and Quality of Health Programs*, 2nd ed. Thousand Oaks, Calif.: SAGE Publications; 2005. Pp. 187–217.
61. Windish DM, Diener-West M. A clinician-educator's roadmap to choosing and interpreting statistical tests. *J Gen Intern Med.* 2006;21:656–60.
62. Fink A. Evaluation reports, Chapter 9. In: Fink A. *Evaluation Fundamentals: Insights into the Outcomes, Effectiveness, and Quality of Health Programs*, 2nd ed. Thousand Oaks, Calif.: SAGE Publications; 2005. Pp. 219–46.
63. Brannick MT, Erol-KorkmazHT, Prewett M. A systematic review of the reliability of objective structured clinical examination scores. *Med Educ.* 2011;45:1181–89.
64. Patricio MF, Juliao M, Fareleira F, Carneiro AV. Is the OSCE a feasible tool to assess competencies in undergraduate medical education? *Med Teach.* 2013;35:503–14.
65. van Hove PD, Tuijthof GJM, Verdaasdonk EGG, Stassen LPS, Dankelman J. Objective assessment of technical surgical skills. *Br J Surg.* 2010;97:972–87.
66. Thijssen AS, Schijven MP. Contemporary virtual reality laparoscopy simulators: quicksand or solid grounds for assessing surgical trainees? *Am J Surg.* 2010;199:529–41.

CHAPTER EIGHT

Curriculum Maintenance and Enhancement

. . . keeping the curriculum vibrant

David E. Kern, MD, MPH, and Patricia A. Thomas, MD

THE DYNAMIC NATURE OF CURRICULA

A successful curriculum is constantly developing. A curriculum that is static gradually declines. To thrive, it must respond to evaluation results and feedback, to changes in the knowledge base and the material requiring mastery, to changes in resources (including faculty), to changes in its targeted learners, to improvements in available educational methodology, and to changes in institutional and societal values and needs. A successful curriculum requires *understanding*, *management of change*, and *sustenance* to maintain its strengths and to promote further improvement. *Innovations*, *networking* with colleagues at other institutions, and *scholarly activity* can also strengthen a curriculum.

UNDERSTANDING ONE'S CURRICULUM

To appropriately nurture a curriculum and manage change, one must understand the curriculum and appreciate its complexity. This includes not only the written curriculum but also its learners, its faculty, its support staff, the processes by which it is administered and evaluated, and the setting in which it takes place. Table 8.1 lists the various areas related to a curriculum that are in need of assessment. Table 8.2 lists some methods of assessing how a curriculum is functioning. *Program evaluation* (discussed in Chapter 7) provides objective and representative subjective feedback on some of these areas. Methods that promote informal information exchange, such as internal and external reviews, observation of curricular components, and individual or group meetings with learners, faculty, and support staff, can enrich one's understanding of a curriculum. They can also build relationships that help to maintain and further develop a curriculum.

EXAMPLE: *GME Curriculum, Preparation for Practice.* Residents in an internal medicine residency program participate in an ambulatory curriculum anchored in their continuity practice at a patient-centered medical home. All interns rotate through a series of block rotations designed specifically to train them to practice as part of a team in the outpatient setting. The first intern block, called "Immersions," is a two-week curriculum that includes daily morning report, noon conference, morning small group instructional modules, afternoon clinical practice sessions, and a required individual creative project. The resident practice medical director serves as the faculty coordinator for this block, and the module faculty members have a role in the practice as attending physician, support staff, or administrator. The Immersions Block also has an administrator who is responsible for scheduling, tracking resident attendance, and organizing materials for orientation and assessment. To ensure that the curriculum leads to desired outcomes, many types of formative feedback are gathered by the program. Interns are asked to evaluate each module for "usefulness in establishing their primary care practice," to articulate specific strengths and weaknesses of the rotation, and to self-rate their level of proficiency in key skills. In addition, there are faculty assessments, including CEXs and feedback on patient care notes. Because the faculty teaching in this unit are the same individuals who are involved in supporting the residents' ongoing outpatient practice, there is an understanding of the practice learning environment and accountability for interns' achievement of basic skills. The outcomes and feedback for the entire Immersions Block are reviewed by the faculty coordinator each year, and potential updates/changes are discussed with designated faculty and clinical preceptors who meet at least quarterly throughout the year. The updated written curriculum for the entire Immersions Block is assembled by the faculty coordinator and course administrator, who then share it with all participating faculty in late spring to ensure that the curriculum remains congruent and cohesive.

EXAMPLE: *UME Curriculum, Systems Biology.* A major revision of the four-year undergraduate medical education (UME) MD curriculum at Johns Hopkins was implemented in 2009 to emphasize systems biology, enhanced behavioral and social science, and attention to transitions (1). Oversight of the curriculum was coordinated by the Educational Policy and Curriculum Committee (EPCC), chaired by the Vice Dean for Education. Subcommittees of the EPCC included the Integration Committee, Clinical Science Committee, and Student Assessment and Program Evaluation (SAPE) Committee. The SAPE Committee collected student feedback and performance data for each course and clerkship, interviewed students and faculty, and prepared a summary report for the EPCC. The EPCC reviewed student scores on the USMLE (United States Medical Licensing Examination) Step I and Step II examinations, the AAMC (Association of American Medical Colleges) Graduation Questionnaire results, residency placements, residency program directors' surveys, faculty roster results, and alumni surveys. Institutional self-study before the Liaison Committee on Medical Education (LCME) accreditation survey in 2012 prompted collection of additional data, including comparability of clerkship outcomes, monitoring of residents-as-teachers participation, and student satisfaction.

Table 8.1.   Areas for Assessment and Potential Change

The Written or Intended Curriculum

Goals and objectives	Are they understood and accepted by all involved in the curriculum? Are they realistic? Can some be deleted? Should some be altered? Do others need to be added? Do some address new external requirements/accreditation standards, such as milestones or entrustable professional activities (EPAs) (see Chapter 4)? Are the objectives measurable?
Content	Is the amount just right, too little, or too much? Does the content still match the objectives? Can some content be deleted? Should other content be updated or added?
Curricular materials	Are they being accessed and used? How useful are the various components perceived to be? Can some be deleted? Should others be altered? Should new materials be added?
Methods	Are they well executed by faculty and well received by learners? Have they been sufficient to achieve curricular objectives? Are additional methods needed to prevent decay of learning? Do any of the methods address competencies of practice-based learning and improvement, systems-based practice/teamwork, or professionalism, interprofessional collaboration, and professional identity formation (see Chapter 5)? Should they? Are new technologies/educational methodologies available that could enhance the curriculum?
Congruence	Does the curriculum on paper match the curriculum in reality? If not, is that a problem? Does one or the other need to be changed?

The Environment/Setting of the Curriculum

Funding	How is the curriculum funded? Have funding needs changed with addition of new expectations, additional learners, and new technologies or methodologies?
Space	Is there sufficient space to support the various activities of the curriculum? Will added educational methodologies (e.g., simulation, team-based or interprofessional learning) lead to new space demands? For clinical curricula, is there sufficient space for learners to see patients, to consult references, and/or to meet with preceptors? Do the residents' clinical practices have the space to support the performance of learned skills and procedures?

Equipment and supplies	Are there sufficient equipment and supplies to support the curriculum while in progress, as well as to support and reinforce learning after completion of the curriculum? For example: Are there adequate clinical skills space and resources to support learning of interviewing skills? Are there adequate robotic simulators to support learning of surgical skills? Will new technologies / educational methodologies require additional equipment and supplies? If online learning is increasing, do learners have access to these resources? Are there sufficient, easily accessible references / electronic resources to support clinical practice experiences? Do the residents' clinical practices have the equipment to incorporate learned skills and procedures into routine practice?
Clinical experience	Is there sufficient concentrated clinical experience to support learning during the course of the curriculum? Is there sufficient clinical experience to reinforce learning after completion of the main curriculum? If there is insufficient patient volume or case mix, do alternative clinical experiences need to be found? Do alternative approaches need to be developed, such as simulation or virtual patients? Are curricular objectives and general programmatic goals (e.g., efficiency, cost-effectiveness, customer service, record keeping, communication between referring and consulting practitioners, interprofessional collaboration, and provision of needed services) supported by clinical practice operations? Do support staff members support the curriculum?
Learning climate	Is the climate cooperative or competitive? Are learners encouraged to communicate or to hide what they do not know? Is the curriculum sufficiently learner-centered and directed? Is it sufficiently teacher-centered and directed? Are learners encouraged and supported in identifying and pursuing their own learning needs and goals related to the curriculum?
Associated settings	Is learning from the curriculum supported and reinforced in the learners' prior, concomitant, and subsequent settings? If not, is there an opportunity to influence those settings?

Administration of the Curriculum

Scheduling	Are schedules understandable, accurate, realistic, and helpful? Are they put out far enough in advance? Are they adhered to? How are scheduling changes managed? Is there a plan for missed sessions?
Preparation and distribution / electronic posting of curricular materials	Is this being accomplished in a timely and consistent manner?

Table 8.1. *(continued)*

Collection, collation, and distribution of evaluation information	Is this being accomplished in a consistent and timely manner? If there are several different evaluation forms, can they be consolidated into one form or administered at one time, to decrease respondent fatigue?
Communication	Are changes in and important information about the curriculum being communicated to the appropriate individuals in a user-friendly, understandable, and timely manner?

Evaluation

Congruence	Is what is being evaluated consistent with the goals, objectives, content, and methods of the curriculum? Does the evaluation reflect the main priorities of the curriculum?
Response rate	Is it sufficient to be representative of learners, faculty, or others involved in or affected by the curriculum?
Accuracy	Is the information reliable and valid?
Usefulness	Does the evaluation provide timely, easily understandable, and useful information to learners, faculty, curriculum coordinators, and relevant others? Is it being used? How?

Faculty

Number/type	Are the number and type of faculty appropriate? Do planned revisions (e.g., interprofessional collaboration, simulation) create new needs?
Reliability/accessibility	How reliable are the faculty members in performing their curricular responsibilities? Are they devoting more or less time to the curriculum than expected? How accessible are faculty members in responding to learner questions and individual learner needs? Do faculty members schedule free time for discussion before or after sessions?
Teaching/facilitation skills	How skillful are faculty members at assessing learners' needs, imparting information, asking questions, providing feedback, promoting practice-based learning and improvement, stimulating self-directed learning, and creating a learning environment that is open, honest, exciting, and fun? Do new educational methodologies (e.g., online teaching, team-based learning, simulation) create a need for new faculty development?
Nature of the learner-faculty relationship	Is the relationship more authoritative or collaborative? Is it more teacher-centered or learner-centered? For clinical precepting, does the learner see patients on his/her own? Does the learner observe the faculty member seeing patients or in other roles? Are learners exposed to faculty members' professional life outside the curriculum, e.g., clinical practice, research, community work? Do learners get to know faculty members as people and how they balance professional, family, and personal life? Do faculty members serve as good role models?

Satisfaction	Do faculty members feel adequately recognized and rewarded for their teaching? Do they feel that their role is an important one? Are they enthusiastic? How satisfied are faculty members with clinical practice, teaching, and their professional lives in general?
Involvement	To what extent are faculty members involved in the curriculum? Do faculty members complete evaluation forms in a timely manner? Do faculty members attend scheduled meetings? Do faculty members provide useful suggestions for improving the curriculum?

Learners

Needs assessment	Have prior training, preparation, or expectations of learners changed?
Achievement of curriculum objectives	Have cognitive, affective, psychomotor, process, and outcome objectives been achieved? Are learners responsible in meeting their obligations to the curriculum?
Satisfaction	How satisfied are learners with various aspects of the curriculum?
Involvement	To what extent are learners involved in the curriculum? Do they complete evaluation forms in a timely manner? Do they attend scheduled activities and meetings? Do they provide useful suggestions for improving the curriculum?
Application	Do learners apply their learning in other settings and contexts? Do they teach what they have learned to others?

Table 8.2.   Methods of Assessing How a Curriculum Is Functioning

See program evaluation as described in Chapter 7
"Just-in-time" evaluations by learners
Learner/faculty/staff/patient questionnaires
Objective measures of skills and performance
Focus groups of learners, faculty, staff, patients
Other systematically collected data
Regular/periodic meetings with learners, faculty, staff
Special retreats and strategic planning sessions
Site visits
Informal observation of curricular components, learners, faculty, staff
Informal discussions with learners, faculty, staff
Monitoring of online forums / discussion boards / chat rooms

Electronic curriculum management systems are being used increasingly to provide coordinated information for understanding and managing both subject-focused curricula and complex educational programs, such as an entire medical school curriculum (2, 3).

MANAGEMENT OF CHANGE

Overview and Level of Decision Making

Most curricula require midcourse, end-of-cycle, and/or end-of-year changes. Changes may be prompted by informal feedback, evaluation results, accreditation standards, changes in available methods and resources, and/or the evolving needs of learners, faculty, institutions, or society. Before expending resources to make curricular changes, however, it is often wise to *establish that the need for change 1) is sufficiently important, 2) affects a significant number of people, and 3) will persist if it is not addressed.*

It is also helpful to consider *who should make the changes and at what level they should be addressed*. Minor operational changes that are necessary for the smooth functioning of a curriculum are most efficiently made at the level of the curriculum coordinator or the core group responsible for managing the curriculum. More complicated needs that require in-depth analysis and thoughtful planning may best be assigned to a carefully selected task group. Other needs may best be discussed and addressed in meetings of learners, faculty, and/or staff. Before implementing major curricular changes, it is often wise to ensure broad, representative support. It can also be helpful to pilot major or complex changes before implementing them fully.

EXAMPLE: *GME Curriculum.* A special block curriculum called "Med-Psych" was developed for a general internal medicine residency program to provide specific training in communication skills and the psychosocial domains of medicine. Individual faculty tasked with specific topics, such as "Smoking Cessation: An Introduction to Motivational Interviewing," responded to evaluation feedback annually and updated the content of their particular sessions. Clinical content was thereby kept up-to-date, and the overall format was well received by the residents. The block director noticed, however, that an increasing number of interns reported having had targeted training in communication skills in medical school. Also, planned changes in the residency organization (to a block outpatient system) meant that interns had more opportunity to practice. Therefore, the block director led a panel of faculty through a year-long curriculum revision process. Current need was reassessed, potential topics for learning were reviewed and prioritized, and correlation with outpatient practice needs was coordinated. A new one-year curriculum was then implemented in conjunction with the new block system. An example of a specific change was moving beyond motivational interviewing to shared clinical decision making.

EXAMPLE: *UME Curriculum.* In the initial years of implementation, a number of changes occurred in the four-year UME curriculum. Several innovative short courses, such as "Substance Abuse Care" and "Pain Care," required major changes in educational methods (e.g., inclusion of more clinical correlations) and assessment (e.g., reduction in reflective writing assignments). A new translational science course, "Regenerative Medicine," was added to the clinical curriculum. A course in "Restorative Medicine" was reorganized, after discussion with the Integration Committee and the EPCC, to emphasize more complementary and alternative medicine and less student wellness. A required clerkship in Chronic Disease and Disability struggled to provide active clinical experience for students, and after three SAPE review cycles, was dropped by the EPCC. The Vice Dean for Education charged faculty to strengthen Primary Care teaching, and a new Primary Care track in the curriculum is in development. The overall educational objectives of the curriculum have not changed.

Accreditation Standards

Important drivers of change in medical education curricula are the organizations charged with accreditation at each level of the continuum. In the United States, the national accrediting bodies are the Liaison Committee on Medical Education (LCME) for undergraduate medical education (4), the Accreditation Council for Graduate Medical Education (ACGME) for graduate (residency) education (5), and the Accreditation Council for Continuing Medical Education (ACCME) for continuing medical education (6). Curriculum developers should stay abreast of *changing* accreditation standards that will affect their curricula, since these standards must be explicitly addressed. It is also useful to look at expectations beyond the immediate timeline of the curriculum. For instance, a medical school curriculum must address the LCME standards, but it should also be aware of the ACGME Common Program Requirements. Adoption of the six ACGME Core Competencies and more recent emphasis on entrustable professional activities (EPAs) (7, 8) have altered many undergraduate programs' approaches to teaching and assessment (9) (see Chapter 5). Attending to these generic competencies in undergraduate, graduate, and postgraduate/continuing medical education curricula can improve coordination throughout the medical education continuum and permit reinforcement and increasing sophistication of learning at each level.

EXAMPLE: *UME Curriculum, New Accreditation Standard.* Following a number of publications noting the need for interprofessional education and interprofessional collaborative practice to improve patient safety and quality of care, the LCME introduced a new accreditation standard in 2012. The new standard states: "The core curriculum of a medical education program must prepare medical students to function collaboratively on health care teams that include other health professionals. Members of the health care teams from other health professions may be either students or practitioners" (4). Anticipating this standard, curriculum leadership worked with colleagues from other professional schools to introduce a new formal curriculum event involving students from three health professional schools (medicine, nursing, and pharmacy) in small group, case-based discussions.

Environmental Changes

Changes in the environment in which a curriculum takes place can *create new opportunities* for the curriculum, *reinforce* the learning that has occurred, and *support* its *application* by learners or create challenges for curriculum coordinators. Decisions to increase class size or open new campus sites can profoundly affect resources in UME curricula. In both UME and GME, practice development activities often affect clinical curricula. New institutional or extra-institutional resources might be used to benefit a curriculum.

EXAMPLE: *Development of Clinical Settings.* A curriculum on gynecology and women's health for internal medicine residents that included excellent lectures and small group discussions was hampered by the lack of sufficient clinical training experiences. The development of medical record systems and well-trained support staff in the residents' primary care practices promoted the provision of women's health preventive care services. In the same practices, an incentive system for the faculty that rewarded the provision of preventive services created faculty support for women's health preventive services and promoted the development of role models for residents and students.

EXAMPLE: *Development of Clinical Settings.* The development of active faculty and staff quality improvement teams as part of a hospitalist service creates opportunities for student, resident, and fellow training in systems-based practice and teamwork.

EXAMPLE: *New Resources.* The provision of electronic medical record (EMR) databases that track residents' clinical experiences creates the opportunity for assessment of and reflection on their experiences, as well as interventions when appropriate.

EXAMPLE: *UME Curriculum, Organizational Change Opportunity.* Three health professional schools (the Schools of Medicine, Nursing, and Public Health) at Johns Hopkins funded an office to coordinate volunteer and service learning opportunities for interprofessional students. After several years, this office also created faculty development programs to develop faculty with expertise in service learning (10).

EXAMPLE: *UME Curriculum, Faculty Resources.* In 2005, the School of Medicine funded a College system, in which master clinicians assume teaching of clinical skills and advising over four years. The creation and development of this faculty learning community enhanced the quality and consistency of teaching in the clinical skills course, which had previously been dependent on volunteer faculty (11).

EXAMPLE: *GME Curriculum, Organizational Change Challenge.* Within one year, the residency practice both moved to a new building with a clinical pod structure *and* adopted a new EMR. These challenges were viewed as opportunities to expand the outpatient curriculum. For example, the clinics now include experiences in conducting preclinic "huddles" (enhancing interprofessional education and experience interacting with staff proactively). The new EMR allows residents to more easily identify personal clinical correlations for didactic sessions.

Early adoption of resources must sometimes be tempered with a need to understand the context of the entire curriculum and to strategize for best utilization.

EXAMPLE: *UME Curriculum, Electronic Student Portfolios.* The curriculum developers for the new integrated curriculum recommended an electronic student portfolio to track students' development of competencies across the four-year curriculum, with inclusion of evaluations and reflective writing, as well as communications with advisors. The EPCC noted that this was the fourth secured electronic system that would be required in the curriculum, and it recommended that coordination and programming be further developed to simplify students' access and maximize use of the system.

Faculty Development

One of the most important resources for any curriculum is its faculty. As discussed in Chapter 6, a curriculum may benefit from faculty development efforts specifically targeted toward the needs of the curriculum. Institution-wide, regional, or national faculty development programs (see Appendix B) that train faculty in specific content areas or in time management, teaching, curriculum development, management, or research skills may also benefit a curriculum. Introduction of new educational technology invariably requires a plan for faculty development, if the technology is to be used effectively.

EXAMPLE: *GME Curriculum.* Faculty preceptors for residents in their continuity practices have participated in the Johns Hopkins Faculty Development Program for Clinician-Educators (12–16). This program provides training in adult learning principles, time management, feedback, precepting, small group teaching, communication, lecturing, management skills, and curriculum development. Residents receive ongoing feedback from teaching-evaluation exercises, co-precepting, and paired observations from colleagues. At quarterly preceptor meetings, new concepts, teaching methods, and tools can be introduced.

EXAMPLE: *UME Curriculum.* The inclusion of interprofessional curricular events required careful faculty development, working with School of Nursing, School of Medicine, and School of Pharmacy faculty together, to develop skills and attitudes toward interprofessionalism.

SUSTAINING THE CURRICULUM TEAM

The curriculum team includes not only the faculty but also the support staff and learners, all of whom are critical to a curriculum's success. Therefore, it is important to attend to processes that motivate, develop, and support the team. These processes include orientation, communication, involvement, faculty development and team activities, recognition, and celebration (Table 8.3).

> **EXAMPLE:** *GME Curriculum.* Within clinic, the residents are assigned to one of four groups that meet monthly during a noon conference and cover for each other during clinic absences. Each group has a faculty attending who follows the residents longitudinally. The faculty leaders also meet monthly with each other and quarterly with the larger preceptor group responsible for precepting daily clinic sessions. The interprofessional staff are included in preclinic huddles. In addition, an ambulatory chief resident coordinates the outpatient clinical experiences.

> **EXAMPLE:** *UME Curriculum.* An infrastructure of several curriculum teams maintains the UME program. This structure begins with course directors, their faculty, and administrative staff, who report to the subcommittees and, ultimately, to the EPCC. Coordination of these teams allows curricular coordination and consistency as changes are introduced and policies made, such as grading and absence policies, introduction of new technology, and awareness of innovation in related courses.

Table 8.3.   Methods of Motivating, Developing, and Supporting a Curriculum Team

Method	Mechanisms
Orientation and Communication • Goals and objectives • Guidelines/standards • Evaluation results • Program changes • Rationale for above • Learner, faculty, staff, patient experiences	• Syllabi/handouts • Meetings • Memos/e-mails • Newsletters • Web site
Involvement of Faculty, Learners, Staff • Goal and objective setting • Guideline development • Curricular changes • Determining evaluation and feedback needs • Questionnaires/interviews	• Informal one-on-one meetings • Group meetings • Online forums/discussion boards • Task group membership • Strategic planning
Faculty Development and Team Activities	• Team teaching/co-teaching • Faculty development activities • Retreats • Task groups to analyze/assess needs • Strategic planning groups
Recognition and Celebration	• Private communication • Public recognition • Rewards • Parties and other social gatherings

THE LIFE OF A CURRICULUM

A curriculum should keep pace with the needs of its learners, its faculty, its institution, patients, and society. It should adjust to changes in knowledge and practice, and it should take advantage of developments in educational methodology and technology. A vibrant curriculum keeps pace with its environment and continually changes and improves (17, 18). After a few years, it may differ markedly from its initial form. As health problems and societal needs evolve, even a well-conceived curriculum that has been carefully maintained and developed may appropriately be downscaled or come to an end.

> **EXAMPLE:** *GME Curriculum, Changing Health Care Environment.* In the 1990s, capitated (HMO) insurance was on the ascendancy in the United States, and the majority of community-based practice (CBP) patients were covered under HMO insurance. A managed care curriculum was introduced into the General Internal Medicine Residency Program. Subsequently, the prevalence of HMO-insured patients dropped in the United States as a whole and in CBPs. The course was renamed the "Medical Practice and Health Systems Curriculum." The curriculum content evolved from one with emphasis on capitated care to one that emphasizes systems-based practice, including quality improvement theory and practice, patient safety, U.S. health insurance systems, health systems finance and utilization, medical informatics, practice management, and teamwork.

> **EXAMPLE**: *UME Curriculum, Development in Educational Methodology/Technology.* In the year 1 "Molecules and Cells" course, virtual microscopy replaced slide sets and microscopes, and students had online access to the full array of slides. This increased the efficiency of learning histology and allowed the introduction of more interactive laboratories and student teaching of content.

> **EXAMPLE:** *GME and UME Curricula, Societal Needs.* With the increased attention to the Triple Aims of the Affordable Care Act, the American Board of Internal Medicine initiated an effort incorporating more than 60 medical professional societies to identify tests and procedures that incur excess cost and risk to patients, without proven benefit. Resources for both physicians and patients were made available online as the "Choosing Wisely" campaign (19). The Vice Dean for Medical Education charged the residency program directors and the Curriculum Committees to plan for incorporation of "Choosing Wisely" across GME and UME curricula.

> **EXAMPLE:** *UME Curriculum, Changing Structure of Knowledge and Practice.* In the new "Genes to Society" curriculum, basic science teaching was reorganized by teaching the science of medicine from societal and genetic perspectives, emphasizing individual variability affected by genetics, social factors, and environmental factors. The previous dichotomy of "normal" and "abnormal" was abandoned. Basic science faculty were enthused by the approach because it modeled translational research. Additional time for basic science teaching was built into the clinical biennium to bring students with an appreciation of clinical medicine back to the study of basic science and to deepen students' understanding of causality (1).

NETWORKING, INNOVATION, AND SCHOLARLY ACTIVITY

A curriculum can be strengthened not only by improvements in the existing curriculum per se, environmental changes, new resources, faculty development, and processes that support the curricular team but also by networking, ongoing innovation, and associated scholarship.

Networking

Faculty responsible for a curriculum at one institution can benefit from and be invigorated by *communication with colleagues at other institutions* (20, 21). Conceptual clarity and understanding of a curriculum are usually enhanced as it is prepared for publication or presentation. New ideas and approaches may come from the manuscript reviewers' comments or from the interchange that occurs after publication or presentation. Multi-institutional efforts can produce scholarly products (see below), such as annotated bibliographies (22), articles (23, 24), texts (25, 26), and curricula (27, 28), that improve upon or transcend the capabilities of faculty at a single institution. The opportunity for such interchange and collaboration can be provided at professional meetings and through professional organizations.

> **EXAMPLE:** *Interest Group at a Professional Organization.* Usually, one to a few internal medicine faculty are responsible for teaching perioperative medicine/medical consultation for surgical, obstetric, and psychiatric patients at any single institution. The Perioperative Medicine/Medical Consultation Interest Group of the Society of General Internal Medicine has provided the opportunity for such faculty to meet yearly, discuss issues electronically, update medical knowledge, share curricula and teaching approaches, and engage in collaborative writing and research (29).

> **EXAMPLE:** *Professional Organization.* The American Academy on Communication in Healthcare (30) serves as the professional home for researchers, educators, practitioners, and patients committed to improving communication and relationships in health care. Through courses, training programs, conferences, interest groups, and online resources, the organization provides opportunities for collaboration, support, and personal and professional development.

Innovation and Scholarly Activity

Scholarly inquiry can enrich a curriculum by increasing the breadth and depth of knowledge and understanding of its faculty, by creating a sense of excitement among faculty and learners, and by providing the opportunity for learners to engage in scholarly projects. Scholarly activities may include original research or critical reviews in the subject matter of the curriculum or in the methods of teaching and learning that subject matter. Such scholarship can result not only in publications for curriculum developers but also in other forms of dissemination (see Chapter 9). Scholarship can arise from means other than the original development, implementation, and evaluation of a curriculum. Once developed, curricula provide ongoing opportunities for innovation that can form the basis of scholarship. The need for innovation is often heralded by learner and faculty assessments, as well as by opportunities to use new educational methods. Support for innovation can come from networking and the habits of scholarly inquiry.

> **EXAMPLE:** *Mentored Scholarly Activity by Learners.* A curriculum in informatics and evidence-based medicine requires that each PGY-1 resident complete and present a critical review of a preventive, diagnostic, or treatment modality of her or his choice at the end of the one-month rotation. This project creates the opportunity for residents and their faculty mentors to apply the critical thinking, clinical decision-making, literature search, and presentation skills that are emphasized in the curriculum (31).

> **EXAMPLE:** *UME Curriculum, Enhanced Behavioral and Social Sciences.* The introduction into the new curriculum of several short courses that emphasized experiential learning in the behavioral and social sciences resulted in faculty publications (32–34).

> **EXAMPLE:** *Scholarly Activity by Faculty.* Faculty involved in a curriculum development project on domestic violence became interested in the prevalence of domestic violence and clinical characteristics

among female primary care patients. They assembled a team to conduct a study (35–37) that took place in community-based practices associated with an academic medical center. They received support from an institutional research grant and from the administration of the practices. The faculty expertise and new knowledge that resulted from this study enriched the domestic violence curriculum, which became integrated into the gynecology/women's health curriculum.

CONCLUSION

Attending to processes that maintain and enhance a curriculum helps the curriculum remain relevant and vibrant. These processes help a curriculum to evolve in a direction of continuous improvement.

QUESTIONS

For the curriculum you are coordinating, planning, or would like to be planning, please answer or think about the following questions:

1. As curriculum developer, what methods will you use (Table 8.2) to *understand* the curriculum in its complexity (Table 8.1)?

2. How will you implement minor *changes*? Major changes? What changes need to be reviewed by an oversight committee?

3. Will evolving *accreditation standards* affect your curriculum?

4. Could *environmental* or *resource changes* provide opportunities for your curriculum? Can you stimulate positive changes, or build upon new opportunities? Do environmental or resources changes present new challenges? How should you respond?

5. Is *faculty development* required or desirable?

6. What methods (Table 8.3) will you use to maintain the *motivation and involvement* of your faculty and of your support staff?

7. How could you *network* to strengthen the curriculum, as well as your own knowledge, abilities, and productivity?

8. Are there *related scholarly activities* that you could encourage, support, or engage in that would strengthen your curriculum, help others engaged in similar work, and/or improve your faculty's/your own promotion portfolio?

GENERAL REFERENCES

Baker DP, Salas E, King H, Battles J, Barach P. The role of teamwork in the professional education of physicians: current status and assessment recommendations. *Jt Comm J Qual Patient Saf*. 2005;31(4):185–202.
A review article that describes eight broad competencies of teamwork that may be relevant to sustaining a curricular team: effective leadership, shared mental models, collaborative orientation, mutual performance monitoring, backup behavior, mutual trust, adaptability, and communication.

Duerden MD, Witt PA. Assessing program implementation, what it is, why it's important, and how to do it. *J Extension.* 2012;50(1):Art. 1FEA4.
   This article discusses why assessment of program implementation is important (e.g., enhances interpretation of outcome results) and describes five main dimensions of implementation: adherence to operational expectations, dosage, quality of delivery, participants' engagement/involvement, and program differentiations (i.e., what components contributed what to the outcomes).

Dyer WG, Dyer WG Jr, Dyer JH. *Team Building: Proven Strategies for Improving Team Performance*, 5th ed. San Francisco: John Wiley & Sons; 2013.
   Practical, easy-to-read book, now in its fifth edition, written by three business professors—a father and his two sons. Useful for leaders and members of committees, task forces, and other task-oriented teams, and for anyone engaged in collaboration. 304 pages.

Saunders RP, Evans MH, Joshi P. Developing a process-evaluation plan for assessing health promotion program implementations: a how-to-guide. *Health Promot Pract.* 2005;6(2): 134–47.
   A comprehensive, systematic approach to evaluating implementation; includes a list of useful questions.

Whitman N. Managing faculty development. In: Whitman N, Weiss E, Bishop FM. *Executive Skills for Medical Faculty*, 1st ed. Salt Lake City, Utah: University of Utah School of Medicine; 1989. Pp. 99–106.
   Managing faculty development to improve teaching skills is discussed as a needed executive function. Five strategies are offered to promote education as a product of the medical school: rewards, assistance, feedback, connoisseurship (developing a taste for good teaching), and creativity. 8 pages.

SPECIFIC REFERENCES

1. Wiener CM, Thomas PA, Goodspeed E, Valle D, Nichols DG. "Genes to Society"—the logic and process of the new curriculum for the Johns Hopkins University School of Medicine. *Acad Med.* 2010;85(3):498–506.
2. Watson EG, Moloney PJ, Toohey SM, et al. Development of eMed: a comprehensive, modular curriculum-management system. *Acad Med.* 2007;82:351–60.
3. Willett TG. Current status of curriculum mapping in Canada and the UK. *Med Educ.* 2008;42:786–93.
4. Liaison Committee on Medical Education. Functions and Structure of a Medical School: Standards for Accreditation of Educational Programs Leading to the M.D. Degree (revised 2014, March) [Internet]. Available at www.lcme.org.
5. Accreditation Council for Graduate Medical Education. Common Program Requirements [Internet]. Available at www.acgme.org.
6. Accreditation Council for Continuing Medical Education. Accreditation Requirements [Internet]. Available at www.accme.org.
7. ten Cate O. Nuts and bolts of entrustable professional activities. *J Grad Med Educ.* 2013;5(1):157–58.
8. ten Cate O, Scheele F. Viewpoint: Competency-based postgraduate training: can we bridge the gap between theory and clinical practice? *Acad Med.* 2007;82(6):542–47.
9. Association of American Medical Colleges. Core Entrustable Professional Activities for Entering Residency (CEPAER) [Internet]. Washington, D.C. March 2014. Available at www.mededportal.org/icollaborative/resource/887.
10. Levin MB, Rutkow L. Infrastructure for teaching and learning in the community: Johns Hopkins University Student Outreach Resource Center (SOURCE). *J Public Health Manag Pract.* 2011;17(4):328–36.

11. Ashar B, Levine R, Magaziner J, Shochet R, Wright S. An association between paying physician-teachers for their teaching efforts and an improved educational experience for learners. *J Gen Intern Med.* 2007;22(10):1393–97.
12. Cole KA, Barker LR, Kolodner K, et al. Faculty development in teaching skills: an intensive longitudinal model. *Acad Med.* 2004;79(5):469–80.
13. Knight AM, Cole KA, Kern DE, et al. Long-term follow-up of a longitudinal faculty development program in teaching skills. *J Gen Intern Med.* 2005;20(8):721–25.
14. Knight AM, Carrese JA, Wright SM. Qualitative assessment of the long-term impact of a faculty development programme in teaching skills. *Med Educ.* 2007;41:592–600.
15. Windish DM, Gozu A, Bass EB, et al. A ten-month program in curriculum development for medical educators: 16 years of experience. *J Gen Intern Med.* 2007;22:655–61.
16. Gozu A, Windish DM, Knight AM, et al. Long-term outcomes of a ten-month program in curriculum development: a controlled study. *Med Educ.* 2008;42:684–92.
17. Institute of Medicine. *Improving Medical Education: Enhancing the Behavioral and Social Science Content of Medical School Curricula.* Washington, D.C.: National Academies Press; 2004.
18. Cooke M, Irby DM, O'Brien BC. *Educating Physicians: A Call for Reform of Medical School and Residency.* Stanford, Calif.: Jossey-Bass; 2010.
19. Choosing Wisely : An Initiative of the ABIM Foundation [Internet]. Available at www.choosing wisely.org.
20. Woods SE, Reid A, Arndt JE, Curtis P, Stritter FT. Collegial networking and faculty vitality. *Fam Med.* 1997;29(1):45–49.
21. Castiglioni A, Aagaard E, Spencer A, et al. Succeeding as a clinician educator: useful tips and resources. *J Gen Intern Med.* 2013;28(1):136–40.
22. Revere D, Stevens KC. Accelerating public health situational awareness through health information exchanges: an annotated bibliography. *J Public Health Inform* (Online). 2010;2(2). Epub 2010 Oct 29. pii:ojphi.v2i2.3212. doi:10.5210/ojphi.v2i2.3212.
23. Branch WT Jr, Frankel R, Gracey CF, et al. A good clinician and a caring person: longitudinal faculty development and the enhancement of the human dimensions of care. *Acad Med.* 2009;84(1):117–25.
24. Holmboe ES, Bown JL, Green M, et al. Reforming internal medicine residency training: a report from the Society of General Internal Medicine's Task Force for Residency Reform. *J Gen Intern Med.* 2005;20:1165–72.
25. Lipkin ML Jr, Putnam SM, Lazare A, eds. *The Medical Interview: Clinical Care, Education, and Research.* New York: Springer-Verlag; 1995.
26. Kalet A, Chou CL. *Remediation in Medical Education: A Mid-Course Correction.* New York: Springer Publishing Co.; 2014.
27. Clerkship directors in internal medicine. In: *Core Medicine Clerkship Guide: A Resource for Teachers and Learners*, 3rd ed. [Internet]. 2006. Available at http://connect.im.org/p/cm/ld /fid=385.
28. Ende J, Kelley M, Sox H. The Federated Council of Internal Medicine's resource guide for residency education: an instrument for curricular change. *Ann Intern Med.* 1997;127(6): 454–57.
29. Society of General Internal Medicine [Internet]. Available at www.sgim.org.
30. American Academy on Communication in Healthcare [Internet]. Available at www.aachonline .org.
31. Example from Evidence-Based Medicine Curriculum, Internal Medicine Residency Program, Johns Hopkins Bayview Medical Center, Scott Wright, MD, Coordinator.
32. Aboumatar HJ, Thompson D, Wu A, et al. Development and evaluation of a 3-day patient safety curriculum to advance knowledge, self-efficacy and system thinking among medical students. *BMJ Qual Saf.* 2012;21(5):416–22.
33. Neufeld KJ, Alvanzo A, King VL, et al. A collaborative approach to teaching medical students

how to screen, intervene and treat substance use disorders. *Subst Abuse*. 2012;33(3): 286–91.

34. Goldner BW, Bollinger RC. Global health education for medical students: new learning opportunities and strategies. *Med Teach*. 2012;34(1):e58–63.

35. McCauley J, Kern DE, Kolodner K, et al. The "battering syndrome": prevalence and clinical characteristics of domestic violence in primary care internal medicine practices. *Ann Intern Med*. 1995;123:737–46.

36. McCauley J, Kern DE, Kolodner K, et al. Clinical characteristics of adult female primary care patients with a history of childhood abuse: unhealed wounds. *JAMA*. 1997;277:1362–68.

37. McCauley J, Kern DE, Kolodner K, Bass EB. Relation of low severity violence to women's health. *J Gen Intern Med*. 1998;13:687–91.

CHAPTER NINE

Dissemination

. . . making it count twice

David E. Kern, MD, MPH, and Eric B. Bass, MD, MPH

DEFINITION

Dissemination refers to efforts to promote consideration or use of a curriculum or related products (e.g., needs assessment or evaluation results) by others. It also refers to the delivery of the curriculum or segments of the curriculum to new groups of learners.

WHY BOTHER?

The dissemination of a curriculum or related work can be important for several reasons. Dissemination can do the following:

- *Help address a health care problem:* As indicated in Chapter 2, the ultimate purpose of a curriculum in medical education is to address a problem that affects the health of the public or a given population. To maximize the positive impact of a curriculum, it is necessary to share the curriculum or related work with others who are dealing with the same problem.
- *Stimulate change:* Innovative curricular work can create excitement and stimulate change in educational programs and medical institutions (1). Innovations have particular impact when they are disruptive, essentially changing the nature or venue of educational activities (2, 3). Many opportunities exist for disruptive innovation with evolving learning technologies, changing practice environments, and new educational guidelines. Examples include use of the electronic medical record (4), increasingly sophisticated simulators, online educational capabilities, the patient-centered medical home, and competency-based education. New learning technology should make it easier to extend curricula beyond single institutions or countries, as in the development of massive open online courses (MOOCs) (2). Shared, innovative curricula can contribute to a continuously *learning* health care system as proposed by the Institute of Medicine in its 2013 report (5), by demonstrating methods to use health care data, build decision support, coach health care professionals and leaders, integrate patient and community perspectives, and improve coordination and communication within and across organizations.
- *Provide feedback to curriculum developers:* By disseminating curriculum-related work, curriculum developers can obtain valuable feedback from others who may have unique perspectives. This external feedback can promote further development of one's curriculum and curriculum-related work (see Chapter 8).
- *Increase collaboration:* Dissemination efforts may lead to increased exchange of ideas between people within an institution or in different institutions who are interested in the same issues. Such interchange may lead to active collaboration. The resulting teamwork is likely to lead to development of an even better curriculum or to other products that would not have been developed by individuals working separately.
- *Prevent redundant work:* Others may be struggling with the same issues that require curriculum development and evaluation. By disseminating a curriculum, curriculum developers can minimize the extent to which different people expend time and energy repeating work that has been done elsewhere. Instead, they can devote their time and energy to building on what has already been accomplished.

EXAMPLE: *Prevention of Redundancy.* All internal medicine residency programs must provide training in ambulatory medicine. When a web-based curriculum in ambulatory care medicine was developed for internal medicine residency programs, more than 80 residency programs subscribed to it, and the number has grown over time to approximately 200. By subscribing to the curriculum, residency program directors were able to build on an existing resource without each one having to create the same core set of learning materials. In addition, the income from subscriptions has permitted the curriculum developers to regularly update the curriculum's topic-based modules, thereby continuing to save time for all users of the curriculum (6–8).

- *Help curriculum developers achieve recognition and academic advancement:* Medical school faculty may devote a substantial amount of time to the development of curricula but have difficulties achieving academic advancement if this portion of their overall work is not recognized as representing significant scholarship. Properly performed, curriculum development is a recognized form of scholarship (9, 10). Promotion committees and department chairs report that they value clinician-educators' accomplishments in curriculum development (11–13). Educational portfolios detailing these accomplishments are increasingly being used to support applications for promotion (14, 15). One important criterion for judging the significance of scholarly work is the degree to which the work has been disseminated and has had an impact at a local, regional, national, or international level.

EXAMPLE: *Benefits of Dissemination.* Faculty developed innovative curricula for internal medicine residents and primary care practitioners on interviewing skills and the psychosocial domain of medical practice, starting in 1979. Dissemination of this and related curricula occurred in workshops and in published articles (16–18). This dissemination was of value to faculty at other institutions who were independently working on ways to enhance clinical training in this area. It generated feedback and promoted interactions and discussions that led to improvements in the original curriculum. It also led to collaborative work that resulted in additional publications (19–22). As a result of the successful dissemination of this curriculum-related work, the curriculum developers gained national recognition for their work. The medical school's promotion and tenure committee cited this recognition as an important achievement when the scholarly activities of responsible faculty members were reviewed. The curriculum developers were approved for promotion.

Are dissemination efforts worth the time and effort required? In many cases, the answer is yes, even for individuals who do not need academic advancement. If the curriculum developer performed an appropriate problem identification and general needs assessment, as discussed in Chapter 2, the curriculum will probably address an important problem that has not been adequately addressed previously. If this is the case, the curriculum is likely to be of value to others. The challenge is to decide how the curriculum should be disseminated and how much time and effort the curriculum developer can realistically devote to dissemination efforts. The final decision involves a trade-off between the degree of dissemination desired and the amount of time that the curriculum developer can afford to spend on dissemination.

PLANNING FOR DISSEMINATION

Curriculum developers who wish to disseminate work related to their curriculum should start planning for dissemination when they start planning their curriculum (i.e., *before* implementation) (23). To ensure a product worthy of dissemination, curriculum developers will find it helpful to follow rigorously the principles of curriculum development described in this book, particularly with respect to those steps related to the part of their work they wish to disseminate. They may also find it useful to think in advance of the characteristics of an innovation that contribute to its diffusion or dissemination. It is important to develop a coherent strategy for dissemination that clarifies the purposes of one's dissemination efforts (see above), addresses ethical and legal issues related to the protection of participants and intellectual property, identifies what is to be disseminated, delineates the target audience, and determines venues for dissemination. A realistic assessment of the time and resources available for dissemination is necessary to ensure that the dissemination strategy is feasible. These topics are discussed in the following sections of this chapter.

DIFFUSION OF INNOVATIONS

If the curriculum developer wants to disseminate all or parts of an actual curriculum, it is worthwhile to review what is known about the diffusion of innovations. Factors identified by Rogers (24) that promote the likelihood and rapidity of adoption of an innovation include the following:

- *Relative advantage*—the degree to which an innovation is perceived as superior to existing practice.
- *Compatibility*—the degree to which an innovation is perceived by the adopter as similar to previous experience, beliefs, and values.
- *Simplicity*—the degree to which a new idea is perceived as relatively easy to understand and implement.
- *Trialability*—the degree to which an innovation can be divided into steps and tried out by the adopter.
- *Observability*—the degree to which the innovation can be seen and appreciated by others.

Additional factors include impact on existing social relations, modifiability, reversibility, time investment, risk/uncertainty, and commitment (25).

> **EXAMPLE:** *Diffusion of Team-Based Learning.* Team-based learning (TBL) is an adaptation of small group and problem-based learning (PBL) that also engages small groups of students in the analysis and solving of problems but permits one or a few faculty facilitators to manage multiple small groups. It involves seven core design elements: team formation, readiness assurance (learners must prepare in advance and are tested on arrival), sequencing, in-class problem solving, four S's (significant problem, same problem by all groups, specific choices, and simultaneous reporting), incentive structure, and peer review (see Chapter 4). Developed more than 20 years ago for use in business schools, TBL has been adopted by medical schools in multiple countries. While guidelines related to efficacy of TBL have been established, the problem-based exercises can be adapted by different faculty, for different purposes, and for different subject matter (26). TBL also has an advantage over small group and PBL because it requires fewer faculty resources.

According to the conceptual model described by Rogers (24), individuals pass through *several stages* when deciding whether to adopt an innovative idea. These stages include: 1) acquisition of *knowledge* about an innovation, 2) *persuasion* that the innovation is worth considering, 3) a *decision* to adopt the innovation, 4) *implementation* of the innovation, and 5) *confirmation* that the innovation is worth continuing.

One of the main implications of diffusion theory and research is that efforts to disseminate an innovative curriculum should involve more than just communication of knowledge about the curriculum. The dissemination strategy should include efforts to *persuade* individuals of the need to consider the curricular innovation. Efforts at persuasion are best directed at individuals who are most likely to make decisions about implementation of a curriculum or who are most likely to influence other individuals' attitudes or behavior regarding implementation of a curricular innovation. The dissemination strategy also should include efforts to identify barriers to curricular transfer and to *support* those individuals who decide to implement the curriculum. The emerging field of implementation science adds a perspective in this realm by emphasizing the need to assess readiness, supply coaching, and engage necessary systems support for implementation (27, 28). Such efforts usually require direct interpersonal communication. Regardless of the mode of communication, it usually is best to identify a specific individual or leadership group who will direct the effort to transfer an innovative curriculum to the targeted institution.

Ideally, a collaborative relationship will develop between the original curriculum developer and the adopting group. A collaborative approach is ideal because most curricula require modifications when transferred to other settings. Moreover, the establishment of an ongoing collaborative relationship generally strengthens the curriculum for all users and stimulates further innovation and products.

PROTECTION OF PARTICIPANTS

If publication of curriculum-related work is anticipated, the work is likely to be considered educational research. While federal regulations governing research in the United States categorize many educational research projects as exempt from the regulations if the research involves the study of normal educational practices or records information about learners in such a way that they cannot be identified, institutional review boards (IRBs) often differ in their interpretation of what is exempt. Also, with the rise of practice-based improvement, comparative effectiveness research, and the use of existing ("big") data to assess and improve performance, the traditional distinctions between research and practice are becoming blurred (29). It is wise for curriculum developers to check in advance with their IRBs. IRBs will be concerned about whether participating learners, faculty, patients, or others could incur harm as a result of participation. Issues such as informed consent, confidentiality, the use of incentives to encourage participation in a curriculum, and funding sources may need to be considered (30). Failure to consult one's IRB before implementation of the curriculum can have adverse consequences for the curriculum developer who later tries to publish research about the curriculum (31). (See Chapter 6, Implementation, "Scholarship," and Chapter 7, Evaluation and Feedback, "Task VII: Address Ethical Concerns," for additional details.)

INTELLECTUAL PROPERTY AND COPYRIGHT ISSUES

When considering dissemination of curriculum-related work, curriculum developers need to address intellectual property issues, with respect to both copyrighted content in the curriculum and protecting their own intellectual property. A curriculum that is used locally for one's own learners generally falls under the exceptions contained in the Copyright Act, often referred to as fair use privilege provided by Section 107 of U.S. copyright law (Title 17 of the U.S. Code) (32). "Fair use" provides for use of material without the author's permission if it is being used for teaching, scholarship, or research, and it generally implies no commercial use of the material (33). In recent times, with the increasing ease of online dissemination, the law is being interpreted more narrowly by universities. Once work—such as a syllabus, a presentation, or a multimedia site with images—is disseminated, it may no longer fall under fair use guidelines. Careful attention to the proper use of copyrighted materials may require additional citations and/

or written permissions from publishers for the use of graphs and images. A curriculum developer who is a member of a university should be familiar with the university's copyright policy and seek expertise *before* disseminating the work.

The use of online learning management systems has created some additional concerns. Online material is covered by the same copyright rules as printed materials. A helpful guideline and best practices document is available from the Copyright Clearance Center (34).

Curriculum developers may wish to protect their disseminated products from unlawful use, alteration, or dissemination beyond their control. One approach is to license the material, and most universities have expertise to assist with this process as well. More recently there has been growing interest in using the Internet to increase the availability of educational and research materials to all. *Open access* refers to free sharing of content on the Internet. Several universities are involved in free sharing of educational materials online. *Creative Commons* is a nonprofit organization that has designed several copyright licenses to allow creators of content to publish that content with a range of copyright privileges. More information about publishing under a Creative Commons license is available at its website (35).

Most universities have multiple resources to assist faculty in understanding these issues. Additional resources include the U.S. Copyright Office, the Association of Research Libraries (36), the American Libraries Association Office of Intellectual Freedom (37), and resources maintained by the University of Texas (38), including a "Copyright Crash Course"(39).

WHAT SHOULD BE DISSEMINATED?

One of the first decisions to make when developing plans for disseminating curriculum work is to *determine whether the entire curriculum, parts of the curriculum, or curriculum-related work should be disseminated.* The curriculum developer can refer to the problem identification and general needs assessment to determine the extent of the need for the curriculum and to determine whether the curriculum truly represents a new contribution to the field. The results of the evaluation of a curriculum will also help determine whether any aspect of the curriculum is worth disseminating.

In some cases, dissemination efforts will focus on promoting adoption of a *complete curriculum* or *curriculum guide* by other sites. Often this requires some allowance for modifications to meet the unique needs of the learners at these sites.

EXAMPLE: *Complete Curriculum.* The Healer's Art is a 15-hour, quarter-long elective that has been taught annually at the University of California, San Francisco, since 1993 and has been disseminated to more than 70 medical schools. The course's educational strategy is based on a discovery model that uses principles of adult education, contemplative studies, humanistic and transpersonal psychology, cognitive psychology, formation education, creative arts, and storytelling. The course addresses professionalism, meaning, and the human dimensions of medical practice. Faculty development workshops, guidebooks, and curricular materials prepare faculty to plan and implement the course at their institutions (40–42).

EXAMPLE: *Curriculum Guide.* Members of the Society of General Internal Medicine and the Clerkship Directors in Internal Medicine, under a contract from the federal Health Resources and Services Administration (HRSA), designed a curriculum guide for improving existing core clerkships in internal medicine. The guide described the need for the curriculum, specific learner objectives, proposed educational strategies, and methods of evaluation. This guide was published by HRSA in 1995 and distributed to internal medicine clerkship directors in all U.S. medical schools (43). The work also was disseminated through presentations at meetings of the Association of American Medical Colleges, the Clerkship Directors in Internal Medicine, and the Society of General Internal Medicine. A follow-up survey demonstrated that, by 1998, clerkship directors in 80 of the 125 medical schools in the United States had used the guide (44). The objectives were subsequently updated in the framework of Accreditation Council for Graduate Medical Education (ACGME) competencies (45).

In other cases, it is appropriate to limit dissemination efforts to *specific products of the curriculum development process* that are likely to be of value to others. We provide examples below of products of the curriculum development process that have been disseminated through publication in peer-reviewed journals, although curricular work can also be disseminated through presentations, workshops, and courses delivered at other institutions and at professional meetings, as well as through books (see the Healer's Art example, above, and Longitudinal Program in Curriculum Development in Appendix A).

The *problem identification and general needs assessment* (Step 1) may yield new insights about a problem that warrant dissemination. This may occur when a comprehensive review of the literature on a topic has been performed, or when a systematic survey on the extent of a problem has been conducted.

> **EXAMPLE:** *Step 1, Systematic Review.* A team working on an innovative medical student curriculum that used social media to promote humanism and professionalism performed systematic reviews on social media use in medical education and on the teaching of empathy to medical students (46, 47). The reviews helped to identify a wide range of methods used, their efficacies, and associated challenges.

> **EXAMPLE:** *Step 1, Systematic Survey.* A colorectal surgeon and a pediatric urologist surveyed fellowship directors and program graduates in their fields as part of their work in developing a model for surgical subspecialty fellowship curricula. Questions addressed the educational and assessment methods used, how the methods were valued, and the perceived achievement of competencies. The findings were published in three articles (48–50).

The *targeted needs assessment* (Step 2) may yield unique insights about the need for a curriculum that merit dissemination because the targeted learners are reasonably representative of other potential learners. When this occurs, the methods employed in the needs assessment will need to be carefully described so that other groups can determine whether the results of the needs assessment are valid and applicable to them.

> **EXAMPLE:** *Step 2.* A survey of targeted learners in internal medicine, neurology, and family practice residency programs at three teaching hospitals found that residents rated most principles of professionalism highly important to medical practice but difficult to incorporate into daily practice. Duty-hour requirements created special challenges (51).

In some cases, the formulation of learning *objectives* for a topic (Step 3) may, by itself, represent an important contribution to a field, thereby calling for some degree of dissemination.

> **EXAMPLE:** *Step 3.* A team of educators used a systematic, evidence-based consensus-building process to establish agreement about educational competencies and learning objectives in disaster preparedness for hospital-based health care workers (52).

In other cases, it may be worthwhile to focus the dissemination efforts on specific *educational methods* (Step 4) and/or on *implementation* strategies (Step 5).

EXAMPLE: *Step 4.* Faculty developed a three-year longitudinal, intensive, theory- and evidence-based curriculum to teach medical residents to become as competent in dealing with common psychosocial and mental health problems as in dealing with medical problems. Because it addressed an important societal need and was so methodical in its development, the curriculum was published even though it had not yet undergone evaluation (53).

EXAMPLE: *Steps 4 and 5.* The Harvard Medical School–Cambridge integrated clerkship was piloted in 2004–5 with eight volunteer medical students. The objective of the innovation was to restructure clinical education to address the inadequacies of hospital-based experiences as effective learning opportunities for chronic care, continuity of care, and humanism. A dedicated group of faculty from the medical school collaborated with clinicians to design this unique approach to the clinical year. A variety of obstacles needed to be overcome, including fiscal, cultural, political, and operational ones (54). This curriculum became the model for Longitudinal Integrated Clerkships nationwide (55).

Frequently, the *measurement instruments* that have been developed for a curriculum and validated in its implementation can be disseminated. An example is the development of an observational checklist for clinical skills, such as the Objective Structured Assessment of Technical Skills for surgery residents (56). Most often, however, it is the results of the *evaluation* of a curriculum (Step 6) that are the focus of dissemination efforts, because people are more likely to adopt an innovative approach, or abandon a traditional approach, when there is evidence regarding the efficacy of each approach.

EXAMPLE: *Step 6.* Curriculum developers implemented a resident handoff bundle that included standardized handoff training, a verbal mnemonic, a new team handoff structure, and, on one of two units, a computerized handoff tool that was integrated into the medical record. Compared with performance before implementation, both medical errors and preventable adverse events decreased. More improvements in written documentation were seen on the unit that used the computerized handoff tool than on the one that did not (57).

EXAMPLE: *Step 6.* Surgical residents were videotaped while performing a laparoscopic cholecystectomy. In a randomized controlled design, experimental (deliberative practice) group residents were required to complete practice on a virtual reality simulator for each task performed below a predetermined cutoff level. The control group received informal feedback from the supervising staff surgeon. The deliberative practice group performed better than the control group on a subsequent videotaped laparoscopic cholecystectomy (58).

WHO IS THE TARGET AUDIENCE?

Dissemination efforts may be targeted at individuals within one's institution, individuals at other institutions, or individuals who are not affiliated with any particular institution. The ideal target audience for dissemination of a curriculum depends on the nature of the curricular work being disseminated.

EXAMPLE: *Determination of Target Audience.* The ideal audience for disseminating a curriculum for medical students on delivering primary care to a culturally diverse, inner-city, indigent population might be the faculty and deans of medical schools located in major cities. In contrast, a curriculum on ethical issues in genetic testing may be worth disseminating more widely because the targeted learners include health care providers in practice as well as those in training.

HOW SHOULD CURRICULUM WORK BE DISSEMINATED?

Once the purpose and content of the dissemination and the target audience have been defined and available resources identified, the curriculum developer must choose the most appropriate modes of dissemination (see Table 9.1 and text below). Ideally, the curriculum developer will use a variety of dissemination modes to maximize impact.

Presentations

Usually, the first mode of dissemination involves *written or oral* presentations to key people *within the setting where the curriculum was developed*. These presentations may be targeted at potential learners or at faculty who will need to be involved in the curriculum. The presentations may also be directed at leaders who can provide important support or resources for the curriculum.

Sometimes it may be appropriate to disseminate curriculum-related work, such as a timely needs assessment, before implementation of the curriculum at the curriculum developer's own institution. Once a curriculum has been established within the setting of its origin, dissemination to *other sites* is appropriate. An efficient way to disseminate curriculum-related work to other sites is to present it at regional, national, or international *meetings of professional societies*. A workshop or mini-course that engages the participants as learners is an appropriate format for presenting the content or methods of a curriculum. A presentation that follows a research abstract format is appropriate for presenting results of a needs assessment or a curriculum evaluation. General guidelines have been published for research presentations (59–61), and specific guidelines are provided by many professional organizations. As illustrated in Table 9.2, information from the six-step curriculum development cycle can fit nicely into the format for an abstract presentation. Although it may be necessary to follow a research-oriented format for abstracts submitted to a professional meeting, many organizations have developed formats that are tailored more specifically to innovative curriculum work.

Table 9.1.   Modes of Disseminating Curriculum Work

- Presentations of abstracts, workshops, or courses to individuals and groups within specific institutions
- Presentations of abstracts, workshops, or courses at regional, national, and international professional meetings
- Creation of a multi-institutional interest group
- Use of electronic communication systems
    Submission of curricular materials to a web-based educational clearinghouse
    Preparation and distribution of instructional audiovisual recordings
    Preparation and distribution of online educational modules
- Publication of an article in a professional journal
- Publication of a manual, book, or book chapter
- Preparation of a press release

Table 9.2.   Format for a Curriculum Development Abstract Presentation or Manuscript

---

I. Introduction
  A. Rationale
    1. Problem identification
    2. General needs assessment
    3. Targeted needs assessment
  B. Purpose
    1. Goals of curriculum
    2. Goals of evaluation: evaluation questions

II. Materials and Methods
  A. Setting
  B. Subjects/power analysis if any
  C. Educational intervention
    1. Relevant specific measurable objectives
    2. Relevant educational strategies
    3. Resources: faculty, other personnel, equipment/facilities, costs*
    4. Implementation strategy*
    5. Display or offer of educational materials*
  D. Evaluation methods
    1. Evaluation design
    2. Evaluation instruments
        a. Reliability measures if any
        b. Validity measures if any
        c. Display (or offer) of evaluation instruments
    3. Data collection methods
    4. Data analysis methods

III. Results
  A. Data: including tables, figures, graphs, etc.
  B. Statistical analysis

IV. Conclusions and Discussion
  A. Summary and discussion of findings
  B. Contribution to existing body of knowledge, comparison with work of others*
  C. Strengths and limitations of work
  D. Conclusions/implications
  E. Future directions*

---

* These items are usually omitted from presentations.

Multi-institutional Interest Groups

In some cases, presentation of curriculum work may occur within multi-institutional interest group meetings of professional societies. Once an interest group is created, back-and-forth dissemination among members of the group may occur in a number of ways, such as in-person meetings or asynchronous electronic mailing lists, and so forth.

EXAMPLE: *Multi-institutional Interest Groups.* The American Society for Bioethics and Humanities (ASBH) has an ongoing affinity group devoted to education: Ethics and Humanities Educators in the

Health Professions. This affinity group meets every year at the ASBH annual meeting. The agenda for the affinity group can include presentation and discussion of curricular projects created and implemented by group members. ASBH also manages electronic mailings for each affinity group, which allows sharing of information and related discussion throughout the year (62).

Electronic Communication Systems

The emergence of electronic communication systems provides a tremendous opportunity for curriculum developers to share curricular materials with anyone having Internet access. Written curricular materials, instructional visual and audio recordings, interactive instructional software, and measurement instruments used for needs assessment and/or curriculum evaluation can be shared widely using digital media. Online modules and courses, including MOOCs, are becoming increasingly available (2). Interpersonal educational methods used for achieving affective and psychomotor objectives are less amenable to such transfer, although there are exceptions.

EXAMPLE: *Online Curriculum on Communication Skills.* The American Academy on Communication in Healthcare and Drexel University College of Medicine cosponsor a curriculum on communication skills that includes the demonstration of key skills in 42 different learning modules. The curriculum involves video encounters with standardized patients and provides text commentary on the interviews, key principles, evidence-based recommendations, communication skills checklists, assessment/evaluation tools, and faculty resources, including facilitator guides and sample curriculum plans (63).

Educational clearinghouses, such as MedEdPORTAL (64), which publish peer-reviewed curricular materials, provide the opportunity to disseminate one's work widely. Information about the existence of an educational clearinghouse for a particular clinical domain generally can be obtained from the professional societies that have a vested interest in educational activities in that domain. (See Appendix B for additional clearinghouse information.)

Publications

One of the most traditional, but still underused, modes of disseminating medical education work is publication in a print or electronic *medical journal or textbook*. When a curriculum developer seeks to disseminate a comprehensive curriculum, it may be wise to consider preparation of a book or manual. On the other hand, the format for original research articles can be used to present results of a needs assessment or a curriculum evaluation (see Table 9.2). The format for review articles or meta-analyses can be used to present results of a problem identification and general needs assessment. An editorial or special article format sometimes can be used for other types of work, such as discussion of the most appropriate learning objectives or methods for a needed curriculum.

Many journals will consider articles derived from curriculum work. A useful bibliography of journals for educational scholarship has been compiled by the Association of American Medical Colleges (AAMC) Group on Educational Affairs (see General References). Curriculum developers who wish to publish work related to their curriculum should prepare their manuscript using principles of good scientific writing (23). Their manuscript will have an increased chance of being accepted by a journal if the results of the curriculum work are relevant to the majority of the readers of that journal and if that journal has a track record of publishing medical education articles (Table 9.3). Manuscripts should follow the Instructions for Authors provided by the journal to which they are to be submitted and, for instructions not specified, by the Uniform Requirements for Manuscripts Submitted to Biomedical Journals, published by the International Committee of Medical Journal Editors (ICMJE) (65). Curriculum evaluations will most likely be accepted for publication by peer-reviewed journals if they satisfy common standards of methodological rigor (66–68). Table 9.4 displays criteria that may be considered by reviewers of an original article on a curriculum. Several of the criteria listed in Table 9.4 have been combined into a *medical education research study quality instrument*, or *MERSQI*, score (66), which has been shown in one study to predict the likelihood of acceptance for publication (67). Seldom do even published curricular articles satisfy all of these criteria. Nevertheless, the criteria can serve as a guide to curriculum developers interested in publishing their work. Methodological criteria for controlled trials (69), systematic review articles and meta-analyses (70–73), and reports of nonrandomized educational, behavioral, and public health interventions (74) have been published elsewhere.

Table 9.3.   Peer-Reviewed Journals and Sites That Are Likely to Publish Curriculum-Related Work

Journal	N*	%†	2-yr IF‡	5-yr IF§	SJR‖	MEDLINE#
Medical education journals and sites						
Academic Medicine	291	26.2	3.5	3.7	1.7	Yes
Advances in Health Sciences Education	58	23.8	2.7	3.0	1.3	Yes
Advances in Medical Education and Practice	58	23.9	NA	NA	NA	No
Advances in Physiology Education	63	30.0	1.2	1.4	0.4	Yes
American Journal of Pharmaceutical Education	198	26.3	1.2	1.5	0.4	Yes
Anatomical Sciences Education	130	51.6	3.0††	3.0††	0.5	Yes
Best Evidence Medical and Health Professional Education (BEME)**	NA	NA	NA	NA	NA	No‡‡
Biochemistry and Molecular Biology Education	58	19.0	0.6	0.6	0.4	Yes
BMC Medical Education	254	34.3	1.4	1.7	0.7	Yes
Canadian Medical Education Journal**	NA	NA	NA	NA	NA	No
CBE Life Sciences Education	60	22.1	1.9	1.8	0.9	Yes
The Clinical Teacher	163	34.1	NA	NA	0.3	Yes
Education for Health**	NA	NA	NA	NA	0.2	Yes
Education for Primary Care**	NA	NA	NA	NA	0.3	Yes
European Journal of Dental Education	104	40.9	1.4	1.6	0.4	Yes
Focus on Health Professions Education**	NA	NA	NA	NA	NA	No
International Journal of Clinical Skills**	NA	NA	NA	NA	0.1	No
International Journal of Nursing Education Scholarship	60	44.8	NA	NA	0.4	Yes
The Internet and Higher Education	0	0.0	2.0	3.6	2.5	No
Journal of Biomedical Education	NA	NA	NA	NA	NA	No
Journal of Cancer Education	49	9.0	1.1	1.0	0.5	Yes
Journal of Continuing Education in the Health Professions	21	11.4	1.2	1.7	0.7	Yes

Table 9.3.   *(continued)*

Journal	N*	%†	2-yr IF‡	5-yr IF§	SJR‖	MEDLINE#
Journal of Dental Education	229	34.4	1.0	1.3	0.4	Yes
Journal of Graduate Medical Education	118	16.0	NA	NA	NA	Yes
*Journal of the International Association of Medical Science Educators / Medical Science Educator***	NA	NA	NA	NA	NA	No
Journal of Microbiology and Biology Education	17	6.6	NA	NA	NA	No
Journal of Nursing Education	112	20.3	0.8	1.2	0.7	Yes
Journal of Nutrition Education and Behavior	22	5.3	1.5	2.1	0.9	Yes
Journal of Surgical Education	127	25.5	1.4	1.6	0.7	Yes
Journal of Veterinary Medical Education	88	37.0	0.8	0.8	0.4	Yes
*MedEdPORTAL***	NA	NA	NA	NA	NA	No
Medical Education	128	23.2	3.6	4.0	1.8	Yes
*Medical Education Development***	NA	NA	NA	NA	NA	No
Medical Education Online	56	40.9	1.3	NA	0.4	Yes
Medical Teacher	329	32.4	2.0	2.2	1.2	Yes
Nurse Education in Practice	43	18.9	NA	NA	0.6	Yes
Nurse Education Today	179	19.0	1.5	1.6	0.7	Yes
*The Open Medical Education Journal***	NA	NA	NA	NA	NA	No
Perspectives on Medical Education	25§§	19.1§§	NA	NA	0.1	No
*Pharmacy Education***	NA	NA	NA	NA	0.1	No
Science Education	100	12.7	2.9	3.6	4.7	No
Simulation in Healthcare / Journal of the Society for Simulation in Healthcare	49	17.6§§	1.6	2.0	0.9	Yes
Studies in Science Education	11	35.5	2.4	3.1	3.6	No
Teaching and Learning in Medicine	94	31.6	1.1	1.2	0.7	Yes
Selected general and specialty health professional journals‖‖						
Academic Emergency Medicine	49	5.1	2.2	2.5	1.3	Yes
Academic Pediatrics	31	8.7	2.2	2.7	1.0	Yes
Academic Psychiatry	103	29.2	1.2	1.5	0.4	Yes
Academic Radiology	33	3.4	2.1	2.1	0.8	Yes
American Journal of Clinical Pathology	12	1.2	3.0	3.0	1.1	Yes
American Journal of Medical Quality	18	6.1	1.8	1.8	0.6	Yes
American Journal of Medicine	6	0.6	5.3	5.4	1.7	Yes
American Journal of Preventive Medicine	40	3.3	4.3	5.1	2.6	Yes
American Journal of Roentgenology	9	0.3	2.7	3.2	1.5	Yes
American Journal of Surgery	51	3.6	2.4	2.8	1.1	Yes
Anesthesia and Analgesia	6	0.4	3.4	3.3	1.5	Yes
Annals of Emergency Medicine	5	0.8	4.4	4.4	1.5	Yes
Annals of Surgery	117	1.2	7.2	8.1	3.8	Yes
BMJ Quality & Safety (previously *Quality & Safety in Health Care*)	20	3.8	3.3	3.3	1.6	Yes
British Journal of Hospital Medicine	7	0.9	0.4	0.3	0.2	Yes
British Journal of Surgery	5	0.4	5.2	5.3	2.3	Yes

Journal	N*	%†	2-yr IF‡	5-yr IF§	SJR‖	MEDLINE#
Canadian Family Physician	12	2.2	1.4	1.6	0.3	Yes
Clinical Anatomy	15	1.7	1.2	1.5	0.4	Yes
Evaluation and the Health Professions	6	4.4	1.6	1.7	0.7	Yes
Family Medicine	83	22.6	0.9	1.3	0.6	Yes
JAMA Surgery (formerly Archives of Surgery)	10##	1.3##	4.3	3.8	1.7	Yes
Journal of the American Academy of Dermatology	8	0.6	5.0	4.7	1.7	Yes
Journal of the American College of Surgeons	25	2.1	4.5	4.6	2.3	Yes
Journal of the American Geriatrics Society	23	1.6	4.2	4.7	2.1	Yes
Journal of Clinical Anesthesia	6	1.4	1.2	1.3	0.4	Yes
Journal of General Internal Medicine	51	4.7	3.4	3.7	1.9	Yes
Journal of Hospital Medicine	17	2.9	2.1	2.0	1.1	Yes
Journal of Interprofessional Care	54	12.9	1.4	1.5	0.8	Yes
Journal of the National Medical Association	13	3.5	0.9	1.2	0.4	Yes
Journal of Palliative Medicine	42	4.9	2.1	2.4	0.9	Yes
Journal of Professional Nursing	66	24.7	0.9	1.1	0.7	Yes
Journal of Surgical Research	37	1.4	2.1	2.2	0.8	Yes
Journal of Urology	8	0.3	3.8	3.9	2.0	Yes
Laryngoscope	11	0.4	2.0	2.3	0.9	Yes
Obstetrics and Gynecology	5	0.3	4.0	3.8	2.1	Yes
Patient Education and Counseling	54	4.3	2.6	3.2	1.1	Yes
Postgraduate Medical Journal	19	3.9	1.5	1.8	0.5	Yes
Progress in Community Health Partnerships	20	8.2	0.8	NA	0.4	Yes
Surgery	39	2.9	3.1	3.5	1.4	Yes
Urology	7	0.2	2.1	2.3	1.0	Yes

Note: In addition to considering the journals listed above, curriculum developers are advised to read the instructions for authors of the journals in their subspecialty area and to review past issues of those journals to see what types of curriculum-related work, if any, they have published. Data in this table are correct as of mid-January 2015.

*N = number of curriculum-related publications (articles, reviews) listed in Thomson Reuters Web of Science Search 2010–14.

†Percentage of total publications that are curriculum-related (articles, reviews) in Thomson Reuters Web of Science Search 2010–14.

‡2-yr IF = 2-year journal impact factor as reported by Thomson Reuters Web of Science, for year 2013 unless otherwise noted.

§5-yr IF = 5-year journal impact factor as reported by Thomson Reuters Web of Science, for year 2013 unless otherwise noted.

‖SJR = SCImago Journal Rank, for 2014.

#Currently indexed for MEDLINE, as listed in Journals in NCBI Databases through PubMed.

**Not included in Thomson Reuters Web of Science.

††For 2010.

‡‡Systematic reviews from BEME Collaboration are published in appropriate journals.

§§For 2012–14.

‖‖Five or more curriculum-related articles published 2010–14.

##Became JAMA Surgery in 2013; data for JAMA Surgery (2013–14) and Archives of Surgery (2010-12) are combined.

NA = not available.

Table 9.4.   Criteria That May Be Considered in the Review of an Original Article on a Curriculum or Curriculum-Related Work

Rationale
- Is there a well-reasoned and documented need for the curriculum or curriculum-related work? (Problem Identification and General Needs Assessment)

Setting
- Is the setting clearly described?
- Is the setting sufficiently representative to make the article of interest to readers? (External validity)

Subjects
- Are the learners clearly described? (Specific profession and specialty within profession; educational level [e.g., third-year medical students, PGY-2 residents, or practitioners]; needs assessment of targeted learners; sociodemographic information)
- Are the learners sufficiently representative to make the article of interest to readers? (External validity)

Educational Intervention
- Are the relevant objectives clearly expressed?
- Are the objectives meaningful and congruent with the rationale, intervention, and evaluation?
- Are the educational content and methods described in sufficient detail to be replicated? (If written description is incomplete, are educational materials offered in an appendix or elsewhere?)
- Are the required resources adequately described (e.g., faculty, faculty development, equipment)?

Evaluation Methods
- Are the methods described in sufficient detail so that the evaluation is replicable?
- Is the evaluation question clear? Are independent and dependent variables clearly defined?
- Are the dependent variables meaningful and congruent with the rationale and objectives for the curriculum? (For example, is performance/behavior measured instead of skill, or skill instead of knowledge, when those are the desired or most meaningful effects?) Are the measurements objective (preferred) or subjective? Where in the hierarchy of outcomes are the dependent variables (patient / health care outcomes > behaviors > skills > knowledge or attitudes > satisfaction or perceptions)?
- Is the evaluation design clear and sufficiently strong to answer the evaluation question? Could the evaluation question and design have been more ambitious?
    Is the design single or multi-institutional? (Latter enhances external validity)
    Has randomization and/or a control/comparison group been used?
    Are long-term as well as short-term effects measured?
- Has a power analysis been conducted to determine the likelihood that the evaluation would detect an effect of the desired magnitude?
- Are raters blinded to the status of learners?
- Are the measurement instruments described or displayed in sufficient detail? (If incompletely described or displayed, are they offered or referenced?)
- Do the measurement instruments possess content validity (see Chapter 7)? Are they congruent with the evaluation question?
- Have inter- and intra-rater reliability and internal consistency validity been assessed? (See Chapter 7.)

- Are there other forms of validity evidence for the measurement instruments (e.g., relationship to other variables evidence, such as concurrent and predictive validity)? (Desirable, but frequently not achieved in curricular publications; see Chapter 7.)
- Are the reliability and validity measures sufficient to ensure the accuracy of the measurement instruments? Have the measurement instruments been used elsewhere? Have they attained a level of general acceptance? (Rarely are the last two criteria satisfied.)
- Are the statistical methods (parametric vs. nonparametric) appropriate for the type of data collected (nominal, ordinal, numerical; normally distributed vs. skewed; very small vs. larger sample size)? Are the specific statistical tests appropriate to answer the evaluation question? Have potentially confounding independent variables been controlled for by random allocation or the appropriate statistical methods?
- Are the evaluation methods, as a whole, sufficiently rigorous to ensure the internal validity of the evaluation and to promote the external validity of the evaluation?

Results
- Is the response rate adequate?
- Has educational significance/effect size been assessed? (See Chapter 7.)
- Are the results of sufficient interest to be worthy of publication? (The paper's Introduction and Discussion can help address this question.)

Discussion/Conclusions
- Has the contribution of the work to the literature been accurately described?
- Are the strengths and limitations of the methodology acknowledged?
- Are the conclusions justified based on the methodology of the study or report?

Media Coverage

Curriculum developers should consider whether their work would have sufficient interest for the lay public to consider issuing a press release. If so, they should contact the public affairs office in their institution to request assistance in preparing a press release. Sometimes a press release will lead to requests for interviews or publication of articles in lay publications, either of which will bring attention to the curricular work.

WHAT RESOURCES ARE REQUIRED?

To ensure a successful dissemination effort, it is important for the curriculum developer to identify the resources that are required. While the dissemination of curricular work can result in significant benefits to both curriculum developers and others, it is also necessary for the curriculum developer to ensure that the use of limited resources is appropriately balanced among competing needs.

Time and Effort

Disseminating curricular work almost always requires considerable time and effort of the *individual or individuals responsible*. Unless one is experienced in disseminating curricular work, it is wise to multiply one's initial estimates of time and effort by a factor of 2 to 4, which is likely to be closer to reality than the original estimate. Submissions of already developed curricular products to an educational clearinghouse or website require the least time and effort. However, maintaining online materials may require additional, ongoing effort. More time and effort are required for presentations of abstracts, workshops, and courses. Still more time is required for the creation of online modules, instructional interactive software, and audiovisual recordings. Peer-reviewed publications generally require the most time and effort.

Personnel

In addition to the curriculum developer, other personnel may be helpful or necessary for the dissemination effort. The creation of instructional audiovisual recordings or computer software may require the involvement of *individuals with appropriate technical expertise*. Individuals with research and/or statistical expertise can help make needs assessments and evaluation research publishable. Collaborative approaches with *colleagues* permit the sharing of workload, can help group members maintain interest and momentum, and can provide the type of creative, critical, and supportive interactions that result in a better product than would have been achieved by a single individual. The identification of a *mentor* can be helpful to individuals with little experience in disseminating curricular work.

Equipment and Facilities

Equipment needs for dissemination are generally minimal and usually consist of equipment that is already accessible to health professional faculty, such as audiovisual equipment or a personal computer. Occasionally, software programs may need to be purchased. *Facilities or space* for presentations are usually provided by the recipients. Occasionally, a studio or simulation facility may be required for the development of audiovisual recordings.

Funds

Faculty may need to have time protected from other responsibilities in order to accomplish a dissemination effort. Technical *consultants* may require support. Funds may also be required for the purchase of necessary new *equipment* or the rental of *facilities*. Sometimes a faculty member's institution is able to provide such funding. Sometimes external sources can provide such funding (see also Chapter 6 and Appendix B). Well-funded curricula are often of higher quality than those that are poorly funded, and they typically fare better when it comes to publishing work related to the curricula (66, 67).

HOW CAN DISSEMINATION AND IMPACT BE MEASURED?

To determine whether dissemination efforts have the desired impact on target audiences, curriculum developers should make an effort to measure the effectiveness of dissemination. Quantitative and qualitative measurements can be helpful in assessing the degree of dissemination and impact of one's work. Such measures can help promotion committees in academic medical centers appreciate the impact of an educator's work.

For *journal articles*, there are several available measures of the influence of the journal in which an article is published:

- *Journal impact factor*—most commonly used measure: average number of citations per article in a given year for articles published during the previous *n* years; two and five years are most frequently used (75). Impact factors vary among fields, depending on the number of people in that field citing publications; for example, impact factors will be lower for medical education journals than for most clinical journals and lower for most subspecialties than for more general clinical fields.
- *Eigenfactor score*—number of times that articles published in the past five years in a given journal are cited, with citations from highly cited journals influencing the score more than citations from less frequently cited journals. References by one article to another in the same journal are removed. Eigenfactor scores are scaled so that the sum of the Eigenfactor scores of all journals listed in Thomson's Journal Citation Reports is 100 (75).
- *Article influence score*—journal's Eigenfactor score divided by the number of articles in the journal over the same time span, normalized so that the mean score is 1.00 (75).
- *Cited half-life*—median age of articles cited (75).
- *Immediacy factor*—average number of citations per article in the year of publication (75).
- *SCImago Journal Rank (SJR) indicator*—measure of the scientific influence of a journal that accounts for both the number of citations and the prestige of the journal from which the citations come (76). It also takes into account the thematic closeness of the citing and the cited journals and limits journal self-citations. SJRs may have less variation across fields than impact factors.

Curriculum developers may want to consider such measures of journal influence when choosing a journal for submission of a manuscript. However, measures of journal impact are imperfect and should not be used without taking into consideration how the readership of a targeted journal compares with the audience one wants to reach.

Perhaps a more important measure of dissemination is the number of times one's work has been cited in other journal articles. Such information can be provided by a *citation index*, such as Thomson Reuters Web of Science (75), Scopus (77), or Google Scholar (78). These indices can also provide a measure, called an *h-index*, for authors who have had a number of publications in a field. The value of *h* is equal to the number of an author's papers (*n*) that have *n* or more citations. For example, an *h*-index of 20 means there are 20 items that have 20 citations or more. The *h*-index thus reflects both the number of publications an author has had and the number of citations per publication. The index was developed to improve on simpler measures such as the total number of citations or publications (79). It is more appropriately used for authors who have been publishing for some time than for relatively junior authors. It is best used in conjunction with a list of publications accompanied by the number of citations for each, since it does not distinguish between authors with the same *h*-index, one of whom has had several publications with many more citations than *h*, and another who has had only publications with a few more citations than *h*. In addition, the *h*-index works properly only for comparing academicians working in the same field, such as education. Desirable *h*-indices vary widely among different fields, such as medical student education, biochemistry, and clinical cardiology research.

For *curricular materials*, one can *keep track of the number of times they have been requested by others*. This is easiest for online material, where one can build in a tracking mechanism for access and completion. MedEdPORTAL, for example, provides authors with usage reports that give total download counts, educational reasons for downloads, and the downloading user's role, affiliated institution, and country (64). For other forms of dissemination, impact can be measured in a variety of ways. For *books*, one can keep track of *sales*, *book reviews*, and *communications* regarding the book. Google Scholar includes book as well as journal article citations (78). For *workshops* and *presentations*, one can keep track of the *number* and *locations* of those that are peer-reviewed and requested. Another measure of dissemination is *media coverage* of one's work, which can be assessed by running an Internet search for any news coverage of the work.

Fortunately, new software metrics are being developed to measure how often one's work (e.g., books, presentations, datasets, videos, and journal articles) are downloaded or mentioned in social media, newspapers, government documents, and reference managers, in addition to being cited in journal articles. One such approach, developed by Altmetric (80), quantifies references to an article in social media. It is included for some journal articles indexed in Scopus (77).

Most of the above measures provide quantitative information about the dissemination of one's work. Curriculum developers can elect to collect additional information, including qualitative information about how their ideas and curricular materials have been used, as well as the impact they have had, through either *informal communications* or *systematic assessment strategies*. For example, one can build evaluation strategies into the use of a disseminated electronic curriculum.

> **EXAMPLE:** *Systematic Evaluation Strategy to Assess Dissemination.* An online curriculum in ambulatory care medicine was developed for internal medicine residency programs, and approximately 200 residency programs now subscribe to this curriculum. Information on the use of modules and resident performance is routinely collected. Periodic surveys of the program directors or curriculum administrators at each site assess how the curriculum is used (6–8). The curriculum is also structured to generate reports related to each module (81–83).

CONCLUSION

The dissemination of a new or improved curriculum can be valuable to the curriculum developer and curriculum, as well as to others. To be effective in disseminating a curriculum or the products of a curriculum development process, the curriculum developer must create a coherent strategy that determines what is worth disseminating, employs appropriate modes of dissemination, and makes the best use of available time and resources. When dissemination efforts are done well, measurement of the degree and impact of the dissemination can be very rewarding.

QUESTIONS

For a curriculum that you are coordinating, planning, or would like to be planning, please answer or think about the following questions:

1. What are the *reasons* why you might want to disseminate part or all of your work?

2. *Which* steps in your curriculum development process would you expect to lead to a discrete *product* worth disseminating to other individuals and groups?

3. *Describe a dissemination strategy* (target audiences, modes of dissemination) that would fulfill your reasons for wanting to disseminate part or all of your work. Usually this requires more than one mode of dissemination (see Table 9.1).

4. *Estimate the resources, in terms of time and effort, personnel, equipment/facilities, and costs*, that would be required to implement your dissemination strategy. Is the strategy feasible? Would you need to identify mentors, consultants, or colleagues to help you develop or execute the dissemination strategy? Would your plans for dissemination need to be altered or abandoned?

5. What would be a *simple strategy for measuring the degree/impact of your dissemination efforts*? Consider your goals for dissemination and the importance of documenting the degree and impact of your dissemination.

6. Imagine the *pleasures and rewards* of a successful dissemination effort. Could you afford to abandon your goals for dissemination?

GENERAL REFERENCES

AAMC-Regional Groups on Educational Affairs (GEA): Medical Education Scholarship, Research, and Evaluation Section. Annotated Bibliography of Journals for Educational Scholarship. Available at www.aamc.org/download/184694/data/annotated_bibliography_of_journals.pdf. This annotated bibliography, compiled by medical educators in the AAMC's Group on Educational Affairs, lists 38 journals and repositories, with structured annotations, including descriptions, topics, types of manuscripts, and audience.

Garson A, Gutgesell HP, Pinsky WW, McNamara DG. The 10-minute talk: organization, slides, writing and delivery. *Am Heart J.* 1986;111(1):193–203. Classic, still useful article that provides practical instruction on giving 10-minute oral presentations before a professional audience.

Kern DE, Branch WT, Green ML, et al. Making It Count Twice: How to Get Curricular Work Published. May 14, 2005. Available by searching google.com for Making It Count Twice or from: www.sgim.org/File%20Library/SGIM/Communities/Education/Resources/WG06 -Making-it-Count-Twice.pdf. Practical tips from the editors of the first medical education issue of the *Journal of General Internal Medicine* on planning curricular work so that it is likely to be publishable, on preparing curriculum-related manuscripts for publication, and on submitting manuscripts to journals and responding to editors' letters. 33 pages.

Oldenburg B, Glanz K. Diffusion of innovations, Chapter 13. In: Glanz K, Rimer BK, Viswaneth K, eds. *Health Behavior and Health Education*, 4th ed. San Francisco: Jossey-Bass; 2008. Pp. 313–33. This chapter discusses various aspects of diffusion theory and their practical application in the development and implementation of broad-based health behavior change interventions.

Rogers EM. *Diffusion of Innovations*, 5th ed. New York: Free Press; 2003. Classic text that presents a useful framework for understanding how new ideas are communicated to members of a social system. 551 pages.

Westberg J, Jason H. *Fostering Learning in Small Groups: A Practical Guide*. New York: Springer Publishing Co.; 2004.
    Practical book, drawing on years of experience, on practical strategies for planning and facilitating small groups. Can be applied to giving workshops. 288 pages.

Westberg J, Jason H. *Making Presentations: Guidebook for Health Professions Teachers*. Boulder, Colo.: Center for Instructional Support, Johnson Printing; 1991.
    User-friendly resource for health professionals on all aspects of preparing and giving presentations, stage fright, audiovisuals, and strategies to enhance presentations. 89 pages.

SPECIFIC REFERENCES

1. Sharf BF, Freeman J, Benson J, Rogers J. Organizational rascals in medical education: mid-level innovation through faculty development. *Teach Learn Med.* 1989;1:215–20.
2. Bateman J, Davies D. The challenge of disruptive innovation in learning technology. *Med Educ.* 2014;48:225–33.
3. Srinivasan M. Disruptive and deliberate innovations in healthcare. *J Gen Intern Med.* 2013;28(9):1117–18.
4. Pageler NM, Friedman CP, Longhurst CA. Refocusing medical education in the EMR era. *JAMA.* 2013;310(21):2249–50.
5. Smith M, Saunders R, Stuckhardt L, McGinnis JM, eds., Institute of Medicine Committee on the Learning Health Care System in America. *Best Care at Lower Cost: The Path to Continuously Learning Health Care in America.* Washington, D.C.: National Academies Press; 2013. Available at www.iom.edu/Activities/Quality/LearningHealthCare.aspx.
6. Sisson SD, Hughes MT, Levine D, Brancati FL. Effect of an Internet-based curriculum on post-graduate education: a multicenter intervention. *J Gen Intern Med.* 2004;19(5 Pt 2):505–9.
7. Sisson SD, Rastegar DA, Rice TN, Hughes MT. Multicenter implementation of a shared graduate medical education resource. *Arch Intern Med.* 2007;167:2476–80.
8. Sisson SD, Kalal D. Internal medicine residency training on topics in ambulatory care: a status report. *Am J Med.* 2011;124(1):86–90.
9. Glassick CE. Boyer's expanded definitions of scholarship, the standards for assessing scholarship, and the elusiveness of the scholarship of teaching. *Acad Med.* 2000;75:877–80.
10. Simpson D, Fincher RM, Hafler JP, et al. Advancing educators and education by defining the components and evidence of educational scholarship. *Med Educ.* 2007;41:1002–9.
11. Atasoylu AA, Wright SM, Beasley BW, et al. Promotion criteria for clinician-educators. *J Gen Intern Med.* 2003;18:711–16.
12. Beasley BW, Wright SM, Cofrancesco J Jr., et al. Promotion criteria for clinician-educators in the United States and Canada: a survey of promotion committee chairpersons. *JAMA.* 1997;278:723–28.
13. Gusic ME, Baldwin CD, Chandran L, et al. Evaluating educators using a novel toolbox: applying rigorous criteria flexibly across institutions. *Acad Med.* 2014;89(7):1006–11.
14. Baldwin C, Chandran L, Gusic M. Guidelines for evaluating the educational performance of medical school faculty: priming a national conversation. *Teach Learn Med.* 2011;23(3):285–97.
15. Simpson D, Hafler J, Brown D, Wilkerson L. Documentation systems for educators seeking academic promotion in U.S. medical schools. *Acad Med.* 2004;79:783–90.
16. Kern DE, Grayson M, Barker LR, et al. Residency training in interviewing skills and the psychosocial domain of medical practice. *J Gen Intern Med.* 1989;4:421–31.
17. Roter DL, Cole KA, Kern DE, Barker LR, Grayson MA. An evaluation of residency training in interviewing skills and the psychosocial domain of medical practice. *J Gen Intern Med.* 1990;5:347–54.

18. Roter DL, Hall JA, Kern DE, et al. Improving physicians' interviewing skills and reducing patients' emotional distress: a randomized clinical trial. *Arch Intern Med.* 1995;155: 1877–84.

19. Williamson PW, Smith R, Kern DE, et al. The medical interview and psychosocial aspects of medicine: residency block curricula. *J Gen Intern Med.* 1992;7:235–42.

20. Branch WT Jr., Kern DE, Gracey K, et al. Teaching the human dimensions of care in clinical settings. *JAMA.* 2001;286:1067–74.

21. Kern DE, Branch WT Jr., Jackson JL, et al. Teaching the psychosocial aspects of care in the clinical setting: practical recommendations. *Acad Med.* 2005;80(1):8–20.

22. Gracey CF, Haidet P, Branch WT, et al. Precepting humanism: strategies for fostering the human dimensions of care in ambulatory settings. *Acad Med.* 2005;80(1):21–28.

23. Kern DE, Branch WT, Green ML. Making It Count Twice: How to Get Curricular Work Published (workshop presented at the 27th Annual Meeting of the Society of General Internal Medicine, May 14, 2005). Available at www.sgim.org/File%20Library/SGIM/Communities /Education/Resources/WG06-Making-it-Count-Twice.pdf.

24. Rogers EM. *Diffusion of Innovations*, 5th ed. New York: Free Press; 2003. Pp. 219–66.

25. Oldenburg B, Glanz K. Diffusion of innovations, Chapter 13. In: Glanz K, Rimer BK, ViswanethK, eds. *Health Behavior and Health Education*, 4th ed. San Francisco: Jossey-Bass; 2008. Pp. 313–33.

26. Burgess AW, McGregor DM, Mellis CM. Applying established guidelines to team-based learning programs in medical schools: a systematic review. *Acad Med.* 2014;89:768–88.

27. Halle T. Implementation Science and Its Applications to State-level Integrated Professional Development Systems for Early Care and Education (slide presentation). National Center of Child Care Professional Development Systems and Workforce Initiative (PDW Center). Available at www.naeyc.org/files/naeyc/ImplementationScienceWebinar_May30.pdf.

28. Fixsen DL, Naoom SF, Blase KA, Friedman RM, Wallace F. *Implementation Research: A Synthesis of the Literature.* University of South Florida. 2005. Available at http://nirn.fpg .unc.edu/resources/implementation-research-synthesis-literature.

29. Kass NE, Faden RR, Goodman SN, et al. The research-treatment distinction: a problematic approach for determining which activities should have ethical oversight. *Hastings Cent Rep.* 2013 Jan-Feb;Spec No:S4–15. doi:10.1002/hast.133.

30. Roberts LW, Geppert C, Connor R, Nguyen K, Warner TD. An invitation for medical educators to focus on ethical and policy issues in research and scholarly practice. *Acad Med.* 2001;76(9):876–85.

31. Tomkowiak JM, Gunderson AJ. To IRB or not to IRB? *Acad Med.* 2004 Jul;79(7):628–32.

32. Copyright Act of 1976, Pub. L. No. 94–553, 90 Stat. 2541 (1976).

33. U.S. Copyright Office. Fair use [Internet]. Available at www.copyright.gov/fls/fl102.html.

34. Copyright Clearance Center. Using Course Management Systems: Guidelines and Best Practices for Copyright Compliance [Internet]. Available at www.copyright.com/content /dam/cc3/marketing/documents/pdfs/Using-Course-Management-Systems.pdf.

35. CreativeCommons.org [Internet]. Available at www.creativecommons.org.

36. Association of Research Libraries. Available at www.arl.org.

37. American Libraries Association Office of Intellectual Freedom. Available at www.ala.org.

38. University of Texas Office of General Counsel Copyright. Available at www.utsystem.edu/ogc /intellectualproperty/copyrighthome.htm.

39. University of Texas. Copyright Crash Course [Internet]. Available at http://copyright.lib.utexas .edu.

40. Institute for the Study of Health and Illness. The Healer's Art. Available at www.ishiprograms .org/programs/medical-educators-students.

41. Rabow MW, Srubel J, Remen RN. Authentic community as an educational strategy for advancing professionalism: a national evaluation of the Healer's Art curriculum. *J Gen Intern Med.* 2007;22(10):1422–28.

42. Rabow MW, Newman M, Remen RN. Teaching in relationship: the impact on faculty of teaching "The Healer's Art." *Teach Learn Med.* 2014;26(2):121–28.

43. Goroll AH, Morrison G, Bass EB, Fortin AH, Mumford L. *Core Medicine Clerkship Guide.* Washington, D.C.: Health Resources and Services Administration; 1995.

44. Jablonover RS, Blackman DJ, Bass EB, Morrison G, Goroll AH. Evaluation of a national curriculum reform effort for the medicine core clerkship. *J Gen Intern Med.* 2000;15:484–91.

45. CDIM/SGIM Core Medicine Clerkship Curriculum Guide Version 3.0 Update Taskforce. *Core Medicine Clerkship Version 3.0.* Clerkship Directors in Internal Medicine/Society of General Internal Medicine Curriculum; 2006. Available at http://connect.im.org/p/cm/ld/fid=385.

46. Cheston CC, Flickinger TE, Chisolm MS. Social media use in medical education: a systematic review. *Acad Med.* 2013;88(6):893–901.

47. Batt-Rawden SA, Chisolm MS, Anton B, Flickinger TE. Teaching empathy to medical students: an updated, systematic review. *Acad Med.* 2013;88(8):1171–77.

48. Gearhart SL, Wang MH, Gilson MM, Chen BM, Kern DE. Teaching and assessing technical proficiency in surgical subspecialty fellowships. *J Surg Ed.* 2012;69(4):521–28.

49. Monn MF, Wang MH, Gilson MM, et al. ACGME Core Competency Training, Mentorship, and Research in Surgical Subspecialty Fellowship Programs. *J Surg Ed.* 2013;70(2):180–88.

50. Wang MH, Chen B, Kern DE, Gearhart S. Pediatric urology fellowship training: are we teaching what they need to learn? *J Pediatr Urol.* 2013;9(3):318–21.

51. Ratanawongsa N, Bolen S, Howell EE, et al. Residents' perceptions of professionalism in training and practice: barriers, promoters, and duty hour requirements. *J Gen Intern Med.* 2006;21(7):758–63.

52. Hsu EB, Thomas TL, Bass EB, et al. Healthcare worker competencies for disaster training. *BMC Med Educ.* 2006;6:19.

53. Smith RC, Laird-Fick H, D'Mello D, et al. Addressing mental health issues in primary care: an initial curriculum for medical residents. *Patient Educ Couns.* 2014;94(1):33–42.

54. Ogur B, Hirsh D, Krupat E, Bor D. The Harvard Medical School–Cambridge integrated clerkship: an innovative model of clinical education. *Acad Med.* 2007;82(4):397–404.

55. Thistlethwaite JE, Bartle E, Chong AAI, et al. A review of longitudinal community and hospital placements in medical education: BEME Guide No. 26. *Med Teach.* 2013;35(8):e1340–64. doi:10.3109/0142159X.2013.806981.

56. Hopmans CJ, de Hoed PT, van der Laan L, et al. Assessment of surgery residents' operating skills in the operating theater using a modified Objective Structured Assessment of Technical Skills: a prospective multicenter study. *Surgery.* 2014;156(5):1078–88.

57. Starmer AJ, Sectish TC, Simon DW, et al. Rates of medical errors and preventable adverse events among hospitalized children following implementation of a resident handoff bundle. *JAMA.* 2013;310(21):2262–70.

58. Palter VN, Grantcharov TP. Individualized deliberate practice on a virtual reality simulator improves technical performance of surgical novices in the operating room: a randomized controlled trial. *Ann Surg.* 2014;259(3):443–48.

59. Garson A, Gutgesell HP, Pinsky WW, McNamara DG. The 10-minute talk: organization, slides, writing and delivery. *Am Heart J.* 1986;111(1):193–203.

60. Kroenke K. The ten-minute talk. *Am J Med.* 1987;83:329–30.

61. Bourne PE. Ten simple rules for making good oral presentations. *PLoS Comput Biol.* 2007;3(4) e77.

62. American Society for Bioethics and Humanities [Internet]. Available at www.asbh.org/membership/content/affinity-groups.html.

63. DocCom: An Online Communication Course. Available at www.aachonline.org/dnn/DocCom.aspx.

64. Association of American Medical Colleges [Internet]. MedEdPORTAL. Available at www.mededportal.org.

65. International Committee of Medical Journal Editors (ICMJE). Recommendations for the Conduct, Reporting, Editing, and Publication of Scholarly Work in Medical Journals [Internet]. Available at www.icmje.org.
66. Reed DA, Cook DA, Beckman TJ, et al. Association between funding and quality of published medical education research. *JAMA.* 2007;298:1002–9.
67. Reed DA, Beckman TJ, Wright SM, et al. Predictive validity evidence for medical education research study quality instrument scores: quality of submissions to *JGIM*'s medical education supplement. *J Gen Intern Med.* 2008;23(7):903–7.
68. Reed D, Price EG, Windish DM, et al. Challenges in systematic reviews of educational intervention studies. *Ann Intern Med.* 2005;142:1080–89.
69. Consolidated Standards of Reporting Trials (CONSORT) Statement, Explanation and Elaboration, Checklist, and Flow Diagram [Internet]. 2010. Available at www.consort-statement.org.
70. Moher D, Liberati A, Tetzlaff J, Altman DG, PRISMA Group. Preferred reporting items for systematic reviews and meta-analyses: the PRISMA statement. *Ann Intern Med.* 2009; 151(4):264–69.
71. Liberati A, Altman DG, Tetzlaff J, et al. The PRISMA statement for reporting systematic reviews and meta-analyses of studies that evaluate health care interventions: explanation and elaboration. *Ann Intern Med.* 2009;151(4):W65–94.
72. Gordon M, Gibbs T. STORIES statement: publication standards for healthcare education evidence synthesis. *BMC Med.* 2014;12(1):143.
73. Sharma R, Gordon M, Dharamsi S, Gibbs T. Systematic reviews in medical education: a practical approach. AMEE Guide 94. *Med Teach.* 2014;14:1–17.
74. Des Jarlais DC, Lyles C, Crepaz N, TREND Group. Improving the reporting quality of nonrandomized evaluations of behavioral and public health interventions: the TREND statement. *Am J Public Health.* 2004;94:361–66. Available with checklist at www.cdc.gov/trendstatement.
75. Thomson Reuters' Web of Science [Internet]. Available at http://wokinfo.com.
76. SCImago.com. SJR—SCImago Journal and Country Rank [Internet]. Available at www.scimagojr.com.
77. Scopus.com [Internet]. Available at www.scopus.com.
78. Google Scholar.com [Internet]. Available at http://scholar.google.com.
79. Hirsch JE. An index to quantify an individual's scientific research output. *Proc Natl Acad Sci USA.* 2005;102:16569–72.
80. Altmetric. Available at www.altmetric.com.
81. Rastegar DA, Bertram A, Sisson SD. Use of an Internet-based curriculum to teach internal medicine residents about addiction. *J Addict Med.* 2010;4(4):233–35.
82. Sisson SD, Bertam A. Changes in knowledge of diabetes guidelines during internal medicine training. *Prim Care Diabetes.* 2010;4(3):193–95.
83. Estrella MM, Sisson SD, Roth J, Choi MJ. Efficacy of an internet-based tool for improving physician knowledge of chronic kidney disease: an observational study. *BMC Nephrol.* 2012;13:126.

CHAPTER 10

Curriculum Development for Larger Programs

Patricia A. Thomas, MD

INTRODUCTION

Thus far, this book has focused on the application of concepts to smaller curricular projects, often contained within larger educational programs. It is the natural history of medical educators, however, that with increasing experience and broadening of interest, they become responsible for larger educational programs—often extending over many years for an individual learner. Examples include degree-bearing programs, residency or fellowship training programs, certificate programs, and maintenance-of-certification programs.

Many of these programs are in need of significant curriculum development. The recent interest in shortening medical training has required new program structures, such as the combined baccalaureate and medical degree programs in the United States (1) and the 0–5 surgical subspecialty training programs (2, 3). The past decade has also seen a number of landmark white papers, studies, and consensus reports articulating a vision for how medical education can better address societal health care needs (4, 5). These include the Carnegie Foundation's report *Educating Physicians: A Call for Reform of Medical School and Residency* (6), the Accreditation Council for Graduate Medical Education's (ACGME) Next Accreditation System (7), the Royal College of Physicians and Surgeons of Canada's CanMeds competency framework (8), the Interprofessional Education Collaborative's Competencies for Collaborative Practice (9), and the Institute of Medicine's report on graduate medical education (10). These guidelines and reports will drive curriculum renewal across the continuum of medical education and will require the careful design of enhancements to existing curricula, if change is to be successful.

In the late twentieth century, *integrated* curricula became the norm for most U.S. medical schools. In an integrated curriculum, content is taught not by discipline but rather in an interdisciplinary model that includes basic science, clinical science, and social sciences together. Harden has described the continuum of integration from siloed, discipline-based courses to a transdisciplinary (or real-world experience) curriculum as an 11-step ladder (11). As curricular designs progress up the ladder, there is increasing need for a central curriculum organizational structure, broad participation of faculty and content experts in curriculum planning, and strong communication lines (11, 12).

This chapter discusses curriculum development and maintenance for large educational programs, using the six-step model as a framework for the discussion. In addition to the bedrock of good curriculum design that has evolved from the six-step model, there are unique aspects to the successful design and implementation of larger programs, such as external accreditation systems, curriculum integration and mapping, resource utilization, and succession planning. Management requires the assembly and maintenance of a collaborative team of educators and stakeholders and the use of modern practices of organizational management. One of these practices is active monitoring of the various elements of the program. As discussed below, *curriculum mapping*, which tracks the congruence of objectives, methods, content, and assessments, is key to effective curriculum development and management in large and long programs. *Table 10.1 highlights these elements within the six-step framework.*

Table 10.1.   Special Considerations in the Development and Maintenance of Larger Educational Programs

---

Step 1: Problem Identification and General Needs Assessment: Understanding Societal Needs, Institutional Mission, and Accreditation Requirements
- Understanding the numbers, distribution, and competencies of graduates required to meet the health care needs of the population
- Understanding the mission of the institution in which the program resides
- Understanding legal and accrediting body requirements and standards
- Anticipating new competencies that graduates will need

Step 2: Targeted Needs Assessment: Selecting Learners and Assessing the Learners and Learning Environment
- Recruiting and selecting learners likely to meet program requirements, enhance the professional learning community, and meet the needs of served populations
- Assessing the knowledge, skills, and needs of a diverse learner population
- Assessing capacity for flexibility and individualization of learning
- Assessing the degree of alignment of the following with educational program mission and goals:
  - Institutional policies and procedures
  - Clinical, research, and business mission goals and mechanisms
  - Institutional culture: e.g., hidden and informal curricula
- Assessing a wide variety of stakeholders: administrators, faculty, staff, and others who need to provide resources or other support to, need to participate in, or will otherwise affect the educational program

Step 3: Goals and Objectives: Prioritizing Objectives, Defining Level of Mastery, and Ensuring Congruence
- Aligning program mission and goals with societal needs and external standards/requirements
- Communicating program goals effectively to all stakeholders
- Reaching consensus on level of mastery expected for learners
- Emphasizing core ideas
- Writing objectives that truly direct educational content and methods
- Working in competency-based frameworks
- Monitoring congruence of objectives with educational strategies and assessments
- Using curriculum mapping and management systems

Step 4: Educational Strategies: Aligning and Integrating Content and Choosing Methods
- Aligning educational content and methods with institutional and program values, mission, and goals
- Aligning educational strategies with varying learner needs and developmental levels to achieve desired milestones, competencies, and entrustable professional activities
- Aligning educational strategies with institutional resources
- Using curriculum mapping and management systems

Step 5: Implementation: Establishing Governance, Ensuring Quality, and Allocating Resources
- Creating a learning system in the educational program
- Establishing an effective leadership team and governance structure that is participatory, transparent, and equitable
- Incorporating quality assurance into governance
- Designing distribution of responsibility
- Effectively identifying and equitably distributing required resources
- Using curriculum mapping and management systems

Step 6: Evaluation and Feedback: Using Learning Analytics and Dashboards
- Tracking competency development of multiple learners over time
- Managing multiple types of evaluation data from multiple sources
- Using evaluation data to modify and further improve the educational program

STEP 1: PROBLEM IDENTIFICATION AND GENERAL NEEDS ASSESSMENT: UNDERSTANDING SOCIETAL NEEDS, INSTITUTIONAL MISSION, AND ACCREDITATION REQUIREMENTS

The numerous calls for medical education reform in the early twenty-first century frequently cite the gaps in delivery of a properly skilled health care workforce. Even more than with smaller curricular projects, the leadership of medical education degree or certification programs needs to be aware of how well societal health needs are being met or not being met by the existing programs. For larger programs, these needs are often framed in terms of producing a workforce that matches the current and future health care needs of the population (10, 13). Are programs producing enough graduates who are appropriately trained and committed to serving the target populations? Or is there a mismatch between the competencies of graduates and societal health care needs?

If there is a mismatch between the competencies of current graduates and the current and anticipated workforce needs, program directors need to understand the root causes of that mismatch. Examples that have been named include the length and cost of medical school attendance that drives students to select high-paying subspecialty careers when there is a growing need for primary care (14–17); a health care reimbursement system that does not sufficiently compensate primary care providers (18, 19); the location of nearly all graduate medical education training in hospital-based settings even though most physicians practice in ambulatory settings (10); the competitive and hierarchical learning environments that result in graduates with less empathy and compassion than matriculates (20, 21); training in silos that leaves graduates with a poor understanding of other health professionals' contributions to quality care (22, 23); and a paucity of training in behavioral and population health that results in graduates untrained in managing population health, chronic care, or comorbidity (24). Understanding the root causes of these deficiencies enables the curriculum developer to be strategic about which of these areas might be addressed in the curriculum (24–27).

Many of the gaps between curricula and the delivery of a properly skilled health care workforce relate less to discipline-specific knowledge, attitude, and psychomotor skills and more to generalizable skills and behaviors that are relevant across many curricula in an educational program, such as adaptive problem solving, cultural competency, commitment to quality improvement, and shared interprofessional values. For an educational program to address these skills, the leadership team needs to articulate the problem and the gaps (i.e., general needs assessment), create a vision for addressing them, and begin the work of designing a consistent and developmental approach across a time-limited educational program.

As noted in Chapter 2, program leaders need to confirm that the program is supporting *the mission and the vision of the institution* within which it resides. A state-funded school or residency program may have a more defined population (e.g., a rural or underserved urban population) that is a primary mission focus. Another school or program may choose to focus on its contribution to the next generation of physician-scientists. These different missions will necessitate different approaches. Making the connection to institutional mission will facilitate the allocation of sufficient resources in Step 5 (described below).

Chapter 2 refers to the accrediting bodies and standards as *resources* for Step 1. For large programs, attention to accreditation and regulatory boards is not an option but a *requirement*, and program leaders need to have a thorough awareness of the language and intent of accreditation standards that apply to their program.

A truly visionary medical education leadership is attuned not only to today's problems but also to anticipated future problems in improving the health of the public. A changing demographic of one's population, the ease of global travel, increasing access to information, and the communication power of social media will demand mastery of new content and skills in the next generation of health providers. Leaders can remain abreast of these societal needs through journals, active membership in professional societies, and attention to accreditation and regulatory standards.

STEP 2: TARGETED NEEDS ASSESSMENT: SELECTING LEARNERS AND ASSESSING THE LEARNERS AND LEARNING ENVIRONMENT

In this step, the curriculum developer assesses the targeted learners and the targeted learning environment. Step 2 addresses Tanner and Tanner's second critical function of the curriculum paradigm: the needs of learners (28).

Selecting Learners

For many curriculum developers of smaller curricula, the learners for a given program have already been selected or are being recruited from a previously selected group. For larger programs, the selection of learners is a significant step in the design of the program. Decisions about who is an appropriate learner for a given program can have an impact far beyond the time course of the program itself. Selection of the appropriate students into medical schools has been described as a critical step in the transformation of U.S. health care into a system that achieves greater patient access, lower cost, and higher quality (29).

Medical school admission committees must consider not only the academic skills but also the interpersonal and intrapersonal competencies of applicants. While assessing individual applicants' qualifications and characteristics, the admissions committee must also have an eye toward building an optimal *learning community* that addresses the institutional mission. Most U.S. programs are striving to achieve gender, racial, and ethnic diversity that better reflects the U.S. population or the geographic area served by the medical school, recognizing that diversity in the student body generates a workforce that can better meet the needs of the population (27, 30–32). Achieving diversity in medical school matriculates has been a challenge, however (33). To ensure a diverse and qualified group of learners, a process must be created that minimizes innate biases in the selection procedure. Efforts to reduce bias may include active recruitment of groups not currently represented in the student body, education of the selection committee on nonconscious bias and the error inherent in overvaluing standardized testing, and monitoring the diversity of the selection committee itself (34).

Assessing Targeted Learners

The complexity of Step 2 for large programs is increased by the number and diversity of learners, where the challenge is to address a spectrum of learner needs so that each learner has the opportunity for success. A typical U.S. medical school entering class can have an age range from 22 to 40 years, suggesting that students arrive with a range of pre–medical school educational and life experiences. Each student in this class, however, is expected to attain competence in several domains within a narrow time-line. At the undergraduate medical education (UME) level, addressing learners' needs may mean offering enrichment programs to students with nonscience backgrounds, or coaching in new educational methods for nontraditional students, or acknowledging previously learned content with more flexible coursework. Graduate medical education (GME) programs recruit from a breadth of medical schools with differing curricula, educational methods, and assessment systems. Both UME and GME programs are accepting students with very different skills than even a decade ago, including individuals with undergraduate experiences in team learning and "flipped classrooms," international experiences, familiarity with technology, and social media expertise. Understanding that the learners are changing requires a reassessment of a program's overall philosophy and educational methods in concert with its incoming students. Is there sufficient engagement with learning, tapping into students' resources, cultural identities, and life experiences? Have expectations about the locus of responsibility for learning shifted, and, if so, have administrators clearly articulated them? Does the assessment system reflect these changes?

Step 2 is also a challenge for board certification and maintenance-of-certification programs, with participants who span decades of educational backgrounds and a variety of practice patterns.

EXAMPLE: *Participation in Maintenance of Certification.* Maintenance of Certification (MOC) was adopted by the American Board of Medical Specialties in 2000, to move board certification from a model of self-directed lifelong learning and recertification to a model of continuous quality improvement and accountability. The American Board of Family Medicine began its transition of diplomates into MOC in 2003. An analysis of participants seven years after this transition found that 91% of active, board-certified family physicians were participating in MOC. Physicians who practiced in underserved areas, worked as solo practitioners, or were international medical graduates were less likely to participate in MOC (35).

Assessing the Targeted Learning Environment

The targeted learning environment of large programs may include a variety of environments—not only classrooms, small group learning spaces, and lecture halls but also office and clinical practices, clinical sites and staff, and affiliated health systems. The educational leadership needs to understand and to strengthen lines of communication with disparate stakeholders of the program, engage representatives in curriculum design and quality control, be explicit about educational objectives, and provide resources and feedback on performance. Failure to actively or sufficiently engage with these educational partners can facilitate a hidden or "collateral" curriculum that undermines the objectives of the formal curriculum. For large programs, ongoing analysis of the learning environment may identify factors that need greater scrutiny.

EXAMPLE: *Institutional Approach to Student Mistreatment.* Research has shown that the behaviors of faculty, residents, and nurses toward medical students are frequently unprofessional and abusive, particularly during clinical experiences. To proactively address this situation, a medical school developed policies in which students received one hour of mandatory training in anticipation of these situations, and residents received a mandatory 30-minute training program during orientation. Faculty experts also provided workshops and talks at Grand Rounds and faculty meetings at the major teaching hospital and extended these to clinical affiliates. After 13 years of this approach, analysis of student questionnaires indicated that more than half of medical students continued to experience mistreatment. The lack of improvement suggested that other aspects of the environment, such as work stress for faculty, residents, and nurses or the lack of consequences for bad behaviors, were facilitating the mistreatment. Further interventions have been suggested, including tracking departmental performance and linking it to incentive systems, addressing institutional stressors for faculty and residents, and further empowering students to participate in the reporting of mistreatment (36).

Health systems are integral to medical education at the UME and GME levels, but they can be unequal partners to the medical schools. The educational program leadership needs to be aware of an affiliated health system's mission, policies, procedures, and culture. Accreditation standards require that clinical affiliation agreements stipulate a "shared responsibility for creating and maintaining an appropriate learning environment" (37). Affiliation agreements may not be sufficiently nimble, however, to respond to conflicts between educational and clinical missions, and mechanisms should be in place for the leadership to address these issues as they arise. A case in point is the introduction of the electronic medical record (EMR) into academic medical centers and GME training just as duty-hour restrictions were increased. Residents often experience a professional conflict in time management when they are told not to use the "cut and paste" function but to remain within duty-hour limits, and often experience conflict in communication when they are urged to use "billable" terms rather than more effective language. Medical student education has also been affected.

> **EXAMPLE:** *Conflict between Health System Policy and Educational Program Goals.* Medical schools have a responsibility to teach students skills in electronic documentation. Health systems' issues of provenance, integrity of information, patient privacy, and compliance with billing have frequently limited medical students' access to EMRs during clinical rotations. A 2012 national survey of clerkship directors found that two-thirds of programs allowed student *access* to the EMR, of which only two-thirds allowed students to *write notes* in the EMR (38). In addition to limiting students' training and competence in use of the EMR, these policies introduced issues of professionalism into the learning environment, as students found other ways to access the records.

In a rapidly changing health system environment, the alignment of mission and goals for education often needs assessment and renewal.

Another aspect of assessing the learning environment relates to the adequacy of facilities for learning. Accreditation standards stipulate that a medical education program must have adequate buildings and facilities to support the program. Expanding class sizes and increasing use of active learning approaches can make existing facilities obsolete. Medical schools have been cited for not having enough seats in the lecture halls or adequate lockers for students. Residency programs may need space for teaching conferences and call rooms in clinical spaces.

> **EXAMPLE:** *Duty Hours and Call Rooms for Residents.* A residency program planning its response to the 2011 ACGME Duty Hours standard realized that call rooms had not been available for PGY-2 residents and above. To provide adequate space for rest, the medical school partnered with the hospital to find new space for medical student call rooms and open call rooms for residents close to the hospital team spaces.

STEP 3: GOALS AND OBJECTIVES: PRIORITIZING OBJECTIVES, DEFINING LEVEL OF MASTERY, AND ENSURING CONGRUENCE

By virtue of their size and duration, large and/or integrated programs often have expansive, multidimensional goals. This can be problematic in writing objectives at the program level, particularly as content experts and other stakeholders petition for the inclusion of additional content. Long, unwieldy lists of learning objectives that are useful neither to learners nor to faculty can result from attempts to reflect all the content in a large program. In addition, inclusion of all the potential *measurables* may result in a loss of generalizable goals that are the core values or goals of the program (such as problem solving, critical thinking, and self-directed learning) and may unintentionally prioritize content that can be assessed (28, 39). If the program developers write specific measurable objectives intended to describe terminal objectives for the entire program, these objectives may be too advanced to inform program matriculates about what is expected.

In a long program, building a bridge between the broad expansive goals of the program—such as "to graduate physicians who are altruistic, dutiful, skillful, and knowledgeable (see the Example below) and who will best meet the needs of our state and local communities"—and the specific, measurable course or event objectives requires, in effect, several *levels of objectives*. Different levels of objectives should be written for individual educational events (such as a lecture or simulation activity); for a course, block, or rotation; for a year or milestone; and finally, for summative objectives or competencies of the program. These different levels communicate increasing specificity as one drills down to the individual events and the increasing inclusiveness and integration of content and builds toward the overall program goal, and together they create a *map* that guides faculty and learners toward achievement of the overall program goals.

> **EXAMPLE:** *Medical School Program Objectives.* In 1999, the Association of American Medical Colleges published the first report of a consensus effort to describe the knowledge, attitudes, and skills expected of medical school graduates. The report describes four attributes expected of graduates and, within each, a number of learning objectives: physicians must be *altruistic* (7 learning objectives); physicians must be *knowledgeable* (6 learning objectives); physicians must be *skillful* (11 learning objectives); and physicians must be *dutiful* (6 learning objectives). An example of the knowledge objectives is "before graduation, a student will have demonstrated, to the satisfaction of the faculty, knowledge of the various causes (genetic, developmental, metabolic, toxic, microbiologic, autoimmune, neoplastic, degenerative and traumatic) of maladies and the ways in which they operate on the body (pathogenesis)" (40). Curriculum leaders designing a second-year pathophysiology course instructed each organ system block leader to ensure that these nine etiologies of disease were addressed in their respective course block.

The *knowledge* domain has been especially problematic in this process of defining a level of specificity for level of learner. The nature of medical knowledge in the twenty-first century is undergoing rapid, sometimes described as exponential, change. Discipline-based faculty are often distressed that there is not sufficient time to teach their discipline, but this has probably always been an issue in higher education, which historically has experienced tension between subject matter specialists and those who argue for relevance (39). Rather than gauge one discipline's time against another's, it is more useful to step back and reflect on the *overall goal of the educational program*. For example, Tanner and Tanner define curriculum not as the presentation of a body of knowledge but rather as the "reconstruction of knowledge and experience that enables the learner to grow in exercising intelligent control over subsequent knowledge and experience" (28). With this overall goal, comprehensive coverage of content is not appropriate. Tyler challenges content experts in larger educational programs with the question: "What can your subject contribute to the field of young people who are *not* going to be specialists in your field?" (39).

Before objectives can be defined, then, faculty need to reach a consensus regarding *level of mastery* (i.e., the amount of content that the program can reasonably expect learners to master), which entails a balance of specificity and generalizability. This involves a process of prioritization at the program level, in view of overall program mission and goals.

> **EXAMPLE:** *Level of Mastery in a Master's Degree.* A medical school planned to offer a new Master of Science in Physician Assistant (PA) Studies. The state Board of Regents required that all courses in the degree program be at the graduate level. The existing graduate-level Pharmacology course designed for PhD students focused on topics such as drug development and was not a good match for the needs of the PA program students, who needed more practical knowledge for prescribing. The Pharmacology faculty worked with the PA program leadership to design a Pharmacology for Physician Assistants course that contained appropriate content and level of mastery.

The good news is that true expertise seems to begin with a deep understanding of big ideas and concepts (see Chapter 4) (41). Educational programs, then, should clearly articulate these big ideas in the program goals and learning objectives and provide opportunities to repeatedly apply these concepts in new contexts. This changing understanding of the nature of knowledge and learning has directed many long educational programs to emphasize *core ideas* and release students from rote memorization of minutiae.

> **EXAMPLE:** *Emphasis of Core Concepts: University of Calgary Medical School's Clinical Presentation Curriculum.* The University of Calgary Medical School developed a "clinical presentation" curriculum in the mid-1990s, which has since been adopted by at least 15 other schools. In this model, teaching is organized around 120 ± 5 clinical presentations. The clinical presentations can take the form of patient history points (e.g., chest pain), physical examination signs (e.g., hypertension), or laboratory abnormalities (e.g., elevated serum lipids). This structure subsumes more than 3,200 diagnostic entities known in medicine and organizes them within the framework of the finite (120 ± 5) ways in which patients present to their physicians. The teaching faculty have created classification systems, or *schemes*, clinical problem-solving pathways that form the framework for building a knowledge of basic and clinical sciences throughout the curriculum (42).

Because of the complexity and numbers of stakeholders, the curricula of large programs are constantly under threat of *drifting* from their intended goals and objectives. Once program objectives have been adopted, it is important to review the *congruence* between implementation of the program and its intended goals and objectives.

> **EXAMPLE:** *Review of Residency Program–Level Objectives.* In 1996, the Federated Council of Internal Medicine (FCIM) published a resource guide for a curriculum in internal medicine residency, listing content in 20 integrative disciplines (e.g., humanism, medical ethics, legal medicine) and 22 clinical areas (43). The guide defined the core knowledge and skills expected in the clinical topics required to practice adult primary care. A subsequent content analysis of three years of Morning Report conferences in one internal medicine residency program found that 60% to 86% of FCIM focus areas and topics were addressed (44).

The move to *competency-based* frameworks in medical education has facilitated articulation of an appropriate level of educational program objectives (see Chapter 4). The *competency domains* and *milestones* serve to communicate the core concepts in these systems, and the *entrustable professional activities* (*EPAs*) communicate the assessment plan. *Milestones* in a program are higher-level integrated learning objectives, defined either by time (such as year) or by level of achievement (such as novice), and describe observable behaviors expected for that milestone.

> **EXAMPLE:** *Residency Milestone.* One competency expected of pediatric residents in the domain of patient care is: "Gathers essential and accurate information about the patient." A milestone for this competence that might be expected early in PGY-1 is: "Clinical experience allows linkage of signs and symptoms of a current patient to those encountered in previous patients. Still relies primarily on analytic reasoning through basic pathophysiology to gather information, but the ability to link current findings to prior clinical encounters allows information to be filtered, prioritized, and synthesized into pertinent positives and negatives as well as broad diagnostic categories" (45).

Implementing a competency-based approach for a larger program is not a small undertaking, however. Competency-based education requires major investments in understanding the developmental nature of the competency, in designing the opportunities to achieve competence across multiple educational venues (Step 4), and in assessing the achievement of milestones for each learner (Step 6).

External influences on a program's competency framework have strengthened in recent years, with a move in American medical education toward uniformity of competency across medical schools. In 2013, the Association of American Medical Colleges (AAMC) published its *Core Entrustable Professional Activities for Entering Residency* and launched the Curriculum Inventory project, requiring each school to map to the Physician Competency Reference Set (PCRS) (46). Educational leaders need to be aware of these changes and participate in national conversations during their development. The PCRS was developed with an early twenty-first century view of physician competency; it is likely that new health care challenges will modify this view, and leadership needs to be aware of new trends. At the same time, accreditation will almost certainly depend on sufficient documentation of students' achievement of these competencies and EPAs.

Regardless of whether a program's educational objectives are framed in competencies or in other core ideas, curriculum developers will need to demonstrate that the educational strategies and assessments of each component of the curriculum are congruent with these objectives. This activity is now frequently achieved with curriculum mapping software, as described below.

STEP 4: EDUCATIONAL STRATEGIES: ALIGNING AND INTEGRATING CONTENT AND CHOOSING METHODS

Chapter 5 defines educational strategies as *content* and *methods*. Nothing conveys a stronger message regarding the core values of an educational program than the educational strategies that the program employs.

> **EXAMPLE:** *Internal Medicine Residency and Patient-Centered Care.* An internal medicine residency program introduced a unique general inpatient service rotation in which teams cared for a smaller number of patients but were asked to incorporate a number of patient-centered activities into the care of every patient. These activities included medication reconciliation, home assessments, postdischarge

phone follow-up, and participation in multidisciplinary care teams. The exposure of every resident to this model of care communicated the value of patient-centered care in the mission and goals of the program (47).

EXAMPLE: *Orthopedic Surgery Residency Training.* A residency training program assigned incoming residents to one of three groups, including two traditional residency tracks and a third, competency-based intensive surgical skills training track. The intensive surgical skills track began the residency program with a 30-day laboratory course of intensive learning and practice in technical surgical skills, prior to residents' entering the traditional program of clinical rotations. Objective assessments of technical skills found that residents in the intensive skills track achieved higher scores. The program leadership's decision to test the new model and rigorously evaluate it communicated a commitment to education over service in this training program (48).

Aligning and Integrating Educational Content

The decisions about educational *content* in large programs follow from the discussions above regarding goals and objectives. The usual approach is to decide on the "big concepts" that the program will strive to have learners master, then to develop a sequential delivery with time-limited courses, blocks, or rotations that have more specific learning goals and objectives. Within each course or block, smaller events such as lectures, small group sessions, or simulation exercises will have more specific learning objectives and, therefore, more specific content. These more specific learning objectives should support the development of the course, block, or rotation learning objectives, which in turn support the development of the overall program objectives and competencies. This relationship is referred to as *curricular mapping*.

Curricular mapping is the system that allows content to be mapped across the curriculum and adjusted to minimize gaps and unnecessary redundancies. In the past, curricular mapping was often a paper exercise, in which faculty and administration collected data about a curriculum and organized it in a calendar framework (49). These "maps" were then analyzed for gaps and repetitions of content, as well as potential areas for improved integration. Lastly, assessments were matched to program objectives and accreditation standards. Software is increasingly used for these curricular mapping functions in large, integrated medical education programs. Typically, curricular events are entered into a calendar. *Key concepts* or *keywords* may be identified within each event, and often the *instructional method* is tracked as well. The event and its objectives are linked to the next higher level of objective, such as the course objectives, which in turn are linked to the next higher level of objective, such as the year or milestone objectives, and so on. When the overall curriculum is placed into curriculum management software, the location of content can be identified and quantified across multiple courses, rotations, and years (50).

Knowing where content is taught is critical not only to the curriculum leadership but also to individual teaching faculty and students. One of the major challenges in an *integrated curriculum* that is taught by interdisciplinary faculty is presenting content with appropriate sequencing and scaffolding that facilitates learning (12).

EXAMPLE: *Use of Curriculum Mapping to Improve Quality of Teaching Palliative Care.* The new Director of Palliative Care Medicine questioned whether there was adequate teaching of palliative care medicine in a medical student curriculum. The Associate Dean for Curriculum was able to search the curriculum and find multiple events that addressed palliative care, including a dedicated session during the Pain Care course, a one-week intersession in the clinical curriculum, a case discussion in the Geriatrics Core

Clerkship, and an advanced communication exercise in the Transition to Residency course. The Associate Dean for Curriculum and the Director of Palliative Care Medicine determined that continuity and reinforcement of learning would be enhanced if each event referred to principles introduced in the previous event, and new opportunities to apply principles of palliative care medicine were added to two core clerkships.

Choosing Educational Methods

Choosing educational methods for large programs requires attention to the core values of the program, the needs of learners, the developmental nature of longer programs, the available experiences and faculty expertise, and the feasibility of resources. Decisions about *educational methods* can have more impact in large programs. Large integrated programs are known more for their educational methods than for the specific content delivered. For example, the McMaster University Michael G. DeGroote School of Medicine is known for the use of Problem-Based Learning; the University of Virginia's Next Generation "Cells to Society" curriculum and Johns Hopkins University's "Genes to Society" curriculum emphasize systems thinking; the Commonwealth Medical College in Pennsylvania uses a community-based curriculum with a longitudinal integrated clerkship year, during which students follow a panel of patients from an outpatient practice for the entire year. The choice made for each of these methods conveys a strong message to learners about the core values of the curriculum.

As discussed above and in Chapter 5, the *diversity of students* also drives a need for multiple educational methods, so that each student has the greatest likelihood of successful learning. *Flexibility* in educational methods communicates a respect for individual student preferences and needs. Since the learners are constantly changing, the curriculum leadership needs to understand the needs of the new matriculates with each new cohort.

Attention to the *developmental* nature of the curriculum is an additional issue in long-term curricula. Grow describes staged levels of self-directed learning, from the dependent learner to the interested, the involved, and, finally, the self-directed learner (51). The nature of the educational method and the work of the teacher at each of these stages similarly evolves. It is rare in short educational programs to see this development, but it is critical in longer programs to anticipate and encourage self-directedness in order to facilitate the necessary life-long learning required of health professionals. In medical education programs, this means that reliance on one method throughout the program is inappropriate. For example, curriculum developers may be excited to introduce a new form of active learning, such as practice in a virtual reality simulated experience. Incoming learners, however, may never have learned with simulation and may need appropriate preparation for this methodology to develop a sense of comfort and motivation to learn with it. With time, these same learners may tire of simulation and be eager for real-life clinical experiences. In GME, attention to increasing levels of responsibility needs to be built across the curriculum, even though rotations are occurring in the same sites throughout the calendar year.

The *feasibility* of an educational method often determines its adoption in a larger program (see Step 5, below). What may have worked in a pilot program with smaller numbers of self-selected learners and committed faculty may not work when scaled up to an entire class or cohort. Facilities such as standardized patients or simulation-center time may be constrained. There may be too few rooms for interprofessional small groups to meet. Additional faculty may need to be identified, released from other duties, and trained in the new method. The introduction of a new method may be disruptive to other components of the curriculum, and there may be a transient drop in performance during a transition. For all of these reasons, changes in methodology should incorporate robust evaluation plans to assist the leadership in understanding both positive and negative impacts on all stakeholders. (See Step 6, below.)

STEP 5: IMPLEMENTATION: ESTABLISHING GOVERNANCE, ENSURING QUALITY, AND ALLOCATING RESOURCES

Large, integrated, and longitudinal programs are often described as complex machines with many moving parts. Implementing these curricula requires attention to the many details of these moving parts, as well as appreciation of the coherent whole and its impact on and relation to even larger institutions, such as the overall university or health system or the population served by the graduates of the program. Skilled leadership of these programs requires the ability to *delegate* the implementation details to appropriate individuals and groups, while attending to the perspectives of a range of stakeholders. For example, stakeholders for a medical school curriculum may include government funders with concerns about the career selection of graduates and population health outcomes, university leadership and alumni with concerns about national rankings and reputation, faculty with concerns about academic freedom, staff with concerns about changing workflow and skill sets, and residency training program directors with concerns about preparedness for residency roles and responsibilities. Educational program leaders should also feel accountable to current learners and their patients, often seen as the most vulnerable participants of these complex systems.

Establishing Governance

No single person or leadership role can provide adequate oversight of implementation in these complex systems. These programs require effective governance structures. Governance, which is often invisible to the students, has powerful implications for curricular quality and outcomes and needs to be carefully constructed for large, integrated programs so that the governance reflects the core values of the school or program. Traditional hierarchical, bureaucratic governance centralizes decision making and authority and emphasizes standardization; a flat or networked governance structure gives faculty and students access to authority and decision making and facilitates innovation and adaptation to change. The governance structure powerfully communicates institutional values about the relationship among students, faculty, and administration.

In discipline-based medical school curricula, courses are governed within individual departments. Course names often reflect the names of the department, such as "Pharmacology" and "Pediatrics." The department chair assigns the course leadership and allocates faculty teaching effort. Departmental faculty determine course content and methods; budgets for teaching are contained within departmental budgets.

Moving to organ system–based curricula in the second half of the twentieth century was the first step toward *integrating* disciplines across a long period of time, such as a year of the curriculum. Integration is now seen across four years of the curriculum in areas such as ethics, patient safety, and clinical reasoning. With highly integrated curricula, governance and decision making no longer rest within individual departments. Blocks of curricula in integrated frameworks are designed by interdisciplinary faculty who determine appropriate levels of objectives, plan content and methods, and review evaluations. The work can be tedious and contentious but is critical to the success of the curriculum. Without true integration, students experience a disjointed and fragmented presentation of content, rather than a developmental or "scaffolded" presentation (12). Correcting this can be problematic because an unintended consequence of this integrated design can be a disengagement of departmental discipline-based leadership from an MD curriculum that no longer reflects specific departmental effort.

The lesson for integrated curricula is that governance needs to be structured as *transparent, participatory*, and *equitable*. Effective governance includes robust program evaluation and quality assurance processes that provide feedback on performance to individual faculty, their academic supervisors, the course and content leaders, and the budgetary process for teaching and evaluation (see Step 6). This flow of information supports transparency and equity. In North America, the Liaison Committee on Medical Education (LCME) mandates a centralized curriculum governance structure that has the authority and resources to implement and maintain a high-quality curriculum (52). Schools often structure the curriculum governance to reflect the "structure" of the curriculum. For instance, there may be a centralized committee with subcommittees that reflect the major content areas or competencies within the curriculum, such as Basic Science, Clinical Sciences, and the thesis requirement. These subcommittees are made up of interdisciplinary design teams, which monitor objectives, methods, and assessments for the relevant content areas. Other schools use more detailed structures with a combination of elected and appointed faculty to oversee the curriculum.

Ensuring Quality

It has been suggested that educational programs should emulate the systems and processes of *effective industrialization models*. Competitive manufacturers maintain their edge by focusing on clarity and specificity of outcomes, creating *learning systems* that immediately identify gaps and rapidly modify processes to improve outcomes (53). Learning systems not only collect timely information on performance but also ensure that the information is communicated to and acted on by those who can respond with authority and resources.

Continuous quality improvement is vital to a large curriculum, and that role often rests in another peer committee of faculty who oversee student assessments, achievement, and program evaluation. For learner assessment, promotion, and remediation, the program needs clear policies and guidelines that are broadly publicized (see Kalet and Chou in General References). Inclusion or broad representation of stakeholders in the governance structure is the first step toward *participatory leadership*, a key feature of successful curricular change (54). In GME, the role of quality oversight often falls to an associate program director, charged with ongoing monitoring of performance outcomes.

As an example of this broader view of governance, there is increasing recognition that student advising and the informal curriculum are an integral part of the overall curriculum, especially as it relates to the competency domain of personal and professional development (see Chapter 5). At a minimum, administrators in the office of student affairs need to be aware of the curriculum's flow, work demands, and milestones. Ideally, student affairs faculty would partner with the curriculum leadership to design developmental events for career advising, recognition of important milestones, and support of curriculum goals, so that there is a seamless presentation of goals to the students. To do this, those charged with student affairs and advising should be included as active members of curriculum planning and governance.

> **EXAMPLE:** *Inclusion of Student Affairs in Curriculum Planning.* The Student Rising Clinician Ceremony marks the transition of medical students from the preclerkship to the clerkship curriculum. This time can often herald a new set of professional challenges for students, such as assuming roles in clinical teams, working longer days and having less control over their time, and needing to demonstrate achievement in competitively graded clerkships. Sensitive to these challenges, the Student Affairs Deans created an annual ceremony to acknowledge this important transition and provide students with an opportunity to reflect on the core values and goals of the educational program. The ceremony includes recognition of the Arnold P. Gold Foundation Humanism and Excellence in Teaching Awards, which are given each year to six residents chosen by clinical students for this award (55). Resident award recipients are announced and asked to speak at the Student Rising Clinician Ceremony. The event concludes with the rising students' recitation of their class oath. Planning for this event includes communication with curriculum leadership to ensure optimal timing, with program directors to ask for release of residents, and with clinical students to solicit nominations and choose award recipients.

Residency programs are broadening the representation of stakeholders in their governance structures by including nursing and hospital administration staff, and board certification programs are including patients and patient advocates as members of their governance.

Allocating Resources

The issues of *personnel*, *time*, *facilities*, and *funding* are shared by new curricula, ongoing curricula, and curricula in the midst of change. *Personnel* issues include identifying appropriate faculty to lead and implement a curriculum, having an overall program of acknowledging and rewarding faculty effort in teaching (56, 57), and developing a staff workflow that maximizes available resources. Educational leaders may have to enlist and support individuals not under their supervisory control; this requires political skill.

Forward-thinking leaders will also recognize that there should be a *succession plan* for important educational roles in a complex curriculum. Planning for succession means identifying faculty or staff who could eventually assume leadership roles and providing the opportunities to develop leadership or advanced educator skills. Medical teaching faculty may not have had access to leadership development or may not have thought to use it, and it may fall to the program director to encourage it. Many universities and health systems have local leadership development skills training; if not available locally, faculty can be referred to their own professional societies for this training. (See also Appendix B for faculty development opportunities.)

Decisions about the allotment of *curricular time* include monitoring the informal as well as formal hours in a curriculum, to ensure that there is adequate time for students' self-directed learning, reflection, and other enrichment activities, and explicitly addressing the perception of many that time equals importance in a curriculum. Once again, a curricular management system can be very helpful in tracking program-level information (such as the number of formal curricular hours per week or the amount of time spent in didactic vs. active learning) and identifying conflicts when faculty or students organize "optional" events.

Facilities are critical to curriculum effectiveness and also have an impact on the learning environment, as discussed above. Educational methods, such as immersive simulation or team-based learning, can fail if the facilities are not appropriate to the task or to the number of learners. At a time when virtual space has become as important as actual space for learning, facilities must now include optimal *informational technology* access and design of virtual learning environments.

Perhaps the most important task at the program level is the *allocation of funds* in the educational program. Medical schools have three basic sources of revenue: grants and contracts, tuition, and philanthropy; some schools also receive state funding. Less grant money is available for research and development in medical education than in biomedical research; almost no external funding is available for ongoing core curriculum functions (58). State funding is increasingly at risk in a climate of conservative fiscal policy. The curriculum, then, must be funded by tuition and philanthropy. Given the average indebtedness of the U.S. medical school graduate, there is tremendous pressure to limit any further increases in tuition (15). Decisions to incur new costs in a program must be carefully balanced with the goal of delivering high-value education at the lowest cost possible.

STEP 6: EVALUATION AND FEEDBACK: USING LEARNING ANALYTICS AND DASHBOARDS

Chapter 7 addresses the evaluation of learners and curricula. Similarly, large educational programs must have an overall plan for evaluation and must monitor that evaluation in real time. If programs have moved to a competency-based framework, a program will want to track competency development by multiple learners over long time periods, often using a variety of assessments. To do this effectively, educational programs have adopted *learning portfolios* to track documentation of learner achievement (59–62) (see Chapter 5). The Next Accreditation System for GME is an example of using a portfolio of achievement at the individual and program levels (7). Electronic portfolios allow individual learners to upload "exhibits" (i.e., documentation of achievement of competence), share with faculty evaluators, and receive feedback. These software programs can also track the achievement of milestones at the aggregate or program level (*learning analytics*).

The focus in Chapter 7 was on learner and learning outcomes, but directors of larger programs are also managing other types of evaluation data, such as faculty time, budgets, utilization of rooms, simulation space, benchmarks with peer institutions and programs, candidate interest in programs, and surveys of nonattendees to a program. Educators are increasingly expected not just to implement improvements in a program but to have processes in place for ongoing quality assurance of the program. The use of *dashboards* to monitor key performance indicators of a program is a response to the quality assurance directives (63, 64). Dashboards can be populated by several supporting systems, including the student learning portfolios, the curriculum management and assessment systems, and internal student data warehouses.

EXAMPLE: *Dashboards to Monitor Program Evaluation Data.* A medical program set as one of its program objectives that every student would be certified in Basic Life Support (BLS) before starting the core clinical rotations. Students were instructed to upload their certification documents to the electronic portfolio after completion of the BLS training. A customized dashboard of educational outcomes, such as BLS certification, USMLE Step 1, Step 2, Step 3 scores, and key indicators from the AAMC Graduation Questionnaire, was developed by the Curriculum Oversight Committee and reviewed each quarter to monitor trends in important outcomes, as well as the impact of educational interventions. When it was noted that students were starting core clerkships without BLS certification, the school responded by verifying that students had access to training and reminding them of the requirement.

Even in the absence of dashboards, programs should have a nimble relationship with the information on learners' performance as they progress through the program, in order to make timely changes for each cohort.

EXAMPLE: *Use of Residency Inservice Training Examination.* Each fall, an internal medicine residency program required all three years of residents to take the Internal Medicine Inservice Training Examination (65). Results were reviewed by the Program Director and the Competency Committee for the program, who noted that the PGY-2 residents scored lower than the national average in gastroenterology. Faculty immediately revised the required rotation in gastroenterology to include a weekly session in board review preparation, and the noon conference series increased the coverage of gastroenterology.

LEADING CURRICULUM ENHANCEMENT AND RENEWAL IN LARGER EDUCATIONAL PROGRAMS

Major reform efforts, which have been widespread in American medical education over the past two decades (6), can be disruptive and resource-intensive and require even more creative engagement of stakeholders. The drivers for curriculum renewal include the changing needs of society, the changing needs of learners, and the changing nature of knowledge, all of which are appearing in medical education at an increasing pace (6, 10, 66–68). The role of the leader in curriculum reform is critical to managing the climate and expectations during the reform and in seeing a reform effort through to its successful implementation.

Understanding the factors that promote successful organizational change efforts is therefore an important attribute for the curriculum leader (54, 69–73). These factors include

- Development and communication of a shared vision and rationale
- Collaboration with and engagement of key stakeholders
- Openness to data and diverse perspectives
- Flexibility
- Formation of an effective leadership team
- Provision of necessary support/protection for others to act on the vision
- Beginning with successes, even if small, and building on them with multiple activities
- Alignment with institutional culture, policies, and procedures to the degree possible; institutionalization of changes
- Effective communication throughout the process with all stakeholders

Familiarity with the community of stakeholders and their needs is also important and is aided by the ability to appreciate one's organization through *multiple perspectives*. Bolman and Deal have termed these perspectives "frames" and describe organizational frames as: 1) structural: the formal roles and relationships; 2) human resource: the needs of the organization's people, such as development, training, and rewards;

3) political, such as the need to allocate resources; and 4) symbolic/value-based (74). When conflicts and barriers affect organizational functioning, the ability to view the situation from more than one perspective allows a deeper understanding of the root cause and creative solutions.

Numerous leadership skills are relevant to directors of larger educational programs (Table 10.2), some of which are mentioned in previous sections of the chapter. They include: being an effective change agent (see Chapter 6) (75, 76), communication (72, 77, 78), motivation (79, 80), collaboration (81, 82), working in teams (78, 83), delegation (80), feedback (78, 84), coaching (85), conflict management (86), and succession planning (87–90).

Effective leaders are also cognizant of different management styles and able to match their approach to situational needs (80). Leadership style can have an impact on the organizational climate, which can result in either an effective, adaptive, and learning organization or an organization riddled with problems and paralyzed in the face of change. Generally speaking, leaders who are visionary, inclusive, and supportive develop more positive learning climates than those who are more authoritative (91, 92).

EXAMPLE: *Using Organizational Understanding and Leadership Skills to Address Conflict in Curriculum Reform.* A medical school planned a new curriculum with a vision to enhance the systems thinking of its graduates, necessitating inclusion of more social and behavioral science. Basic science faculty who had less allotted time expressed concern that the curriculum was less rigorous and would diminish the reputation of the school—that is, would not uphold the core value of research and discovery. Recognizing that the discussions about allocation of time (a political frame) were actually value-based, the Dean responded to faculty concerns by articulating a vision for the new curriculum in symbolic and value-based terms, noting a new research requirement and plans to enhance the development of physician-scientists.

Because of the broad skill set required to effectively oversee large educational programs and organizational change efforts, it behooves those responsible to develop themselves in the areas noted above. As previously mentioned, leadership development programs are available locally at many universities and also through professional societies.

Table 10.2   Leadership Skills for Curriculum Implementation, Maintenance, Enhancement, and Renewal

- Communicating and motivating
- Understanding and exercising flexibility in management style
- Leading teams
- Delegating
- Collaborating
- Providing feedback and coaching
- Managing conflict
- Leading organizational change
- Planning succession

CONCLUSION

The size and complexity of large, longitudinal programs present challenges, so it is perhaps most useful to think of them as complex systems or organizations. Effective systems and structures are critical to ensure that a program is meeting its goals. The field of organizational development has much to offer educators in understanding the nature and functions of their curricular systems. Special considerations applied to the six-step approach can provide a foundation for developing, implementing, sustaining, and enhancing large or longitudinal programs.

ACKNOWLEDGMENTS

The author wishes to thank Dr. Sanjay Desai, Program Director for the Johns Hopkins Internal Medicine Osler Housestaff Training Program, Dr. Colleen O'Connor Grochowski, Associate Dean, Curricular Affairs, Duke University School of Medicine, and Dr. John Mahoney, Associate Dean for Medical Education, University of Pittsburgh School of Medicine, for their careful reviews and thoughtful comments on earlier versions of this chapter.

QUESTIONS

For the program you are coordinating, planning, or would like to be planning, please answer or think about the following questions:

1. Cite the evidence that the program promotes societal health care needs and the institutional mission. What do you see as future changes in health care delivery, and how can the curriculum address these?

2. Describe the trends you see in the demographics, preparedness, or motivations of learners in your program. How can you structure your selection process to recruit the best learning community for your program? What characteristics of learners do you need to monitor to address their learning needs?

3. Describe how the educational program objectives were developed for the program and how they relate to national competency frameworks.

4. What system is in place for monitoring the curriculum for congruence of objectives, methods, and assessments; sequencing and coordination of content; and vertical and horizontal integration?

5. Describe how faculty are developed, supported, and rewarded for teaching in your program. How are faculty needs and actual faculty effort monitored to ensure there is an appropriate match?

6. How is information on program outcomes used to improve the quality of the program?

7. If a curriculum renewal process is in progress, note any conflicts or barriers to its success. How can these be addressed by leadership, faculty, and students?

GENERAL REFERENCES

Bland CJ, Starnaman S, Wersal L, et al. Curricular change in medical schools: how to succeed. *Acad Med*. 2000;75:575–94.
This systematic study of the published literature on medical curricular change, although looking at twentieth-century reforms, has not been replicated, and its lessons are still timely. The authors synthesized their review into characteristics that contribute to success. These include: organization's mission and goals, history of change, politics, organizational structure, need for change, scope and complexity of the innovation, cooperative climate, participation, communication, human resource development, evaluation, performance dip, and leadership.

Bolman LG, Deal TE. *Reframing Organizations: Artistry, Choice, and Leadership*, 5th ed. San Francisco: Jossey-Bass; 2013.
An updated synthesis of the authors' framework for organization theory, with a number of modern examples. The four frames discussed are: 1) the Structural Frame, the social architecture of the organization; 2) the Human Resource Frame, the properties of people and organizations; 3) the Political Frame, the allocation of resources and struggles for power; and 4) Organizational Symbols and Culture. The book concludes with Leadership in Practice. 526 pages.

Cooke M, Irby DM, O'Brien BC. *Educating Physicians: A Call for Reform of Medical School and Residency*. Stanford, Calif.: Jossey-Bass; 2010.
A qualitative study of medical education in the United States 100 years after the 1910 Flexner Report. The authors conclude that, while much is outstanding, there is a need for reform in four key areas that incorporate a contemporary understanding of how people learn and the gaps in the current model. The four recommendations are: 1) standardization of outcomes and individualization of learning process; 2) better integration of medical knowledge and clinical experience; 3) development of habits of inquiry and innovation; and 4) a focus on personal development and professional identity formation. 304 pages.

Eden J, Berwick D, Wilensky G, eds. *Graduate Medical Education That Meets the Nation's Health Needs*. Washington, D.C.: National Academies Press; 2014.
The Institute of Medicine committee's report proposes significant revisions to rectify current shortcomings and to create a GME system with greater transparency, accountability, strategic direction, and capacity to innovate.

Hafferty FW, O'Donnell JF, eds. *The Hidden Curriculum in Health Professional Education*. Lebanon, N.H.: Dartmouth College Press; 2014.
This book examines the history, theory, methodology, and application of hidden curriculum theory in health professional education. Includes chapters devoted to professional identify formation, social media, and longitudinal integrated clerkships. 322 pages.

Interprofessional Education Collaborative Expert Panel. *Core Competencies for Interprofessional Collaborative Practice: Report of an Expert Panel*. Washington, D.C.: Interprofessional Education Collaborative; 2011.
The Interprofessional Education Collaborative consists of six health professions educational organizations, representing dental medicine, medicine (allopathic and osteopathic), nursing, pharmacy, and public health. The consensus report describes the need for development of collaborative practice and lays out four competency domains—roles and responsibilities, shared values and ethics, interprofessional communication, and teamwork—and learning objectives within each domain. The document has been a major force in the design of interprofessional education.

Kalet A, Chou CL, eds. *Remediation in Medical Education: A Mid-Course Correction*. New York: Springer Publishing Co.; 2014.
This multiauthored text collates the literature and experience to date in the context of defined competencies for physicians, the limitations of assessment, and approaches to remediation. One section, authored by a student affairs dean, looks at program-level issues such as privacy, technical standards, fitness for duty, and the official academic record. 351 pages.

Leadership

Fairholm MR. The Themes and Theory of Leadership: James MacGregor Burns and the Philosophy of Leadership (Working Paper CR01-01). George Washington University Center for Excellence in Municipal Management. 2001.
Good overview of transactional versus. transformational leadership. Transactional leaders focus on rewards and punishments to achieve performance. Transformational leaders engage with others to raise one another to higher levels of motivation and morality, and tap into values.

Goleman D. Leadership that gets results. *Harvard Business Review*, Mar–Apr 2000.
Describes different management styles (coercive, authoritative, affiliative, democratic, pacesetting, coaching — Hay Group) and the importance of being able to flex one's management style. Also discusses emotional intelligence.

Heifetz RA, Lurie DL. The work of leadership. *Harvard Business Review*, Dec 2001.
Good overview of adaptive leadership. Distinguishes between addressing technical or routine problems or situations and adaptive challenges where "business as usual" will no longer work. The latter requires special leadership traits.

Merton RK. The social nature of leadership. *Am J Nurs*. 1969;69:2614–18.
A good article on the relational aspects of leadership. Distinguishes authority from leadership. Authority involves the legitimated rights of a position that require others to obey; leadership is an interpersonal relation in which others comply because they want to, not because they have to.

Stewart J. Transformational leadership: an evolving concept examined through the works of Burns, Bass, Avolio, and Leithwood. *Can J Educ Admin Policy.* 2006 (June 26); Issue no. 54.
An in-depth article on transformational leadership.

Organizational/Culture Change

Collins J. *Good to Great: Why Some Companies Make the Leap . . . and Others Don't*. New York: Harper Collins Publishers; 2001. 300 pages.

Collins J. *Good to Great and the Social Sectors: A Monograph to Accompany Good to Great*. London: Random House Business; 2006.
The first book is a study of businesses. The second is a less formal reflection on how the principles of "Good to Great" work in the social sector, based upon observations and discussions. 35 pages.

Heath C, Heath D. *Switch: How to Change Things When Change Is Hard*. New York: Broadway Books, Random House; 2010.
Written for the lay reader but based on years of social science research on how people change. Presents the analogy of the Rider (rational self) and the Elephant (emotional self): the Rider can direct the Elephant as long as he or she concentrates on/devotes energy to the task, but eventually wears out if the Elephant wants to go elsewhere. The more choices and the more complicated the path, the harder the change. Engaging the emotional self is helpful, as is making the path easy. The book is replete with examples. 320 pages.

Kotter JP. *Leading Change.* Boston: Harvard Business Review Press; 2012.
An excellent book on leading change in today's fast-paced, global market. Although oriented toward business, it is applicable to most organizations. Based on his years of experience and study, Dr. Kotter, Professor Emeritus at Harvard Business School, discusses eight steps critical to creating enduring *major change in organizations*. 208 pages.

Westley F, Zimmerman B, Patton MQ. *Getting to Maybe: How the World Is Changed*. Toronto: Random House Canada; 2006.
  This book is complementary to Kotter's work. It focuses on complex organizations and social change, and addresses change that occurs from the bottom up as well as from the top down. Richly illustrated with real-world examples, it explains an approach to complex, as distinct from simple or complicated, problems. 272 pages.

Examples of Institutional/Culture Change Efforts

Cottingham AH, Suchman AL, Litzelman DK, et al. Enhancing the informal curriculum of a medical school: a case study in organizational culture change. *J Gen Intern Med*. 2008;23:715–22.
  The Indiana University School of Medicine (IUSM) culture change initiative to improve the informal or hidden curriculum.

Krupat E, Pololi L, Schnell ER, Kern DE. Changing the culture of academic medicine: the C-Change Learning Action Network and its impact at participating medical schools. *Acad Med*. 2013;18:1252–58.

Pololi L, Krupat E, Schnell ER, Kern DE. Preparing culture change agents for academic medicine in a multi-institutional consortium: the C-Change Learning Action Network. *J Contin Educ Health Prof*. 2013;33(4):244–57.
  These two papers present a culture change project shared by five medical schools. Institutional leadership and faculty met regularly as a consortium to create a learning community that would foster a collaborative, inclusive, and relational culture in their constituent institutions.

SPECIFIC REFERENCES

1. Cosgrove EM, Harrison GL, Kalishman S, et al. Addressing physician shortages in New Mexico through a combined BA/MD program. *Acad Med*. 2007;82:1152–57.
2. Schanzer A, Nahmias J, Korenda K, et al. An increasing demand for integrated vascular residency training far outweighs the limited supply of positions. *J Vasc Surg*. 2009;50:1513–18.
3. Lee JT, Teshome M, de Virgilio C, et al. A survey of demographics, motivations, and backgrounds among applicants to the integrated 0–5 vascular surgery residency. *J Vasc Surg*. 2010;51:496–503.
4. Ludmerer K. The history of calls for reform in graduate medical education and why we are still waiting for the right kind of change. *Acad Med*. 2012;87:34–40.
5. Skochelak SE. A decade of reports calling for change in medical education: what do they say? *Acad Med*. 2010;85:S26–33.
6. Cooke M, Irby DM, O'Brien BC. *Educating Physicians: A Call for Reform of Medical School and Residency*. Stanford, Calif.: Jossey-Bass; 2010.
7. Nasca TJ, Philibert I, Brigham T, Flynn TC. The Next GME Accreditation System—rationale and benefits. *N Engl J Med*. 2012;366:1051–56.
8. Royal College of Physicians and Surgeons of Canada. CanMeds2015 [Internet]. Available at www.royalcollege.ca/portal/page/portal/rc/canmeds/canmeds2015.
9. Interprofessional Education Collaborative Expert Panel. *Core Competencies for Interprofessional Collaborative Practice: Report of an Expert Panel*. Washington, D.C.: Interprofessional Education Collaborative; 2011.
10. Eden J, Berwick D, Wilensky G, eds. *Graduate Medical Education That Meets the Nation's Health Needs*. Washington, D.C.: National Academies Press; 2014.
11. Harden R. The integration ladder: a tool for curriculum planning and evaluation. *Med Educ*. 2000;34:551–57.

12. Muller JH, Jain S, Loeser H, Irby DM. Lessons learned about integrating a medical school curriculum: perceptions of students, faculty and curriculum leaders. *Med Educ*. 2008; 42:778–85.

13. Association of American Medical Colleges. AAMC Workforce Policy Recommendations: Fixing the Doctor Shortage Initiatives [Internet]. September 13, 2012. Available at www .aamc.org/download/304026/data/2012aamcworkforcepolicyrecommendations.pdf.

14. Robert Graham Center. Specialty and Geographic Distribution of the Physician Workforce: What Influences Medical Student & Resident Choices? [Internet]. Available at www.graham center.org/dam/rgc/documents/publications-reports/monographs-books/Specialty-geo graphy-compressed.pdf.

15. Greysen SR, Chen C, Mullan F. A history of medical student debt: observations and implications for the future of medical education. *Acad Med*. 2011;86:840–45.

16. Youngclaus JA, Koehler PA, Kotlikoff LJ, Wiecha JM. Can medical students afford to choose primary care? An economic analysis of physician education repayment. *Acad Med*. 2013;88:16–25.

17. Phillips JP, Petterson SM, Bazemore SW, Phillips RL. A retrospective analysis of the relationship between medical school debt and primary care practice in the US. *Ann Fam Med*. 2014;12(6):542–49.

18. Macinko J, Starfield B, Shi L. Quantifying the benefits of primary care physician supply in the United States. *Int J Health Serv*. 2007;37:111–26.

19. Vaughn BT, DeVrieze SR, Reed SD, Schulman KA. Can we close the income and wealth gap between specialists and primary care physicians? *Health Aff (Millwood)*. 2010;29(5):933–40.

20. Hafferty FW, Franks R. The hidden curriculum, ethics teaching and the structure of medical education. *Acad Med*. 1994;69:861–71.

21. Neumann M, Edelhauser F, Tauschel D, et al. Empathy decline and its reasons: a systematic review of studies with medical students and residents. *Acad Med*. 2011;86:996–1009.

22. Hall P. Interprofessional teamwork: professional cultures as barriers. *J Interprof Care*. 2005;Suppl 1:188–96.

23. Lawlis TR, Anson J, Greenfield D. Barriers and enablers that influence sustainable interprofessional education: a literature review. *J Interprof Care*. 2014;28:305–10.

24. Cuff PA, Vanselow NA, eds. *Improving Medical Education: Enhancing the Behavioral and Social Science Content of Medical School Curricula*. Washington, D.C.: National Academies Press; 2004.

25. Boscardin CK, Grbic D, Grumbach K, O'Sullivan P. Educational and individual factors associated with positive change in and reaffirmation of medical students' intention to practice in underserved areas. *Acad Med*. 2014;89:1490–96.

26. Stepien KA, Baernstein A. Educating for empathy: a review. *J Gen Intern Med*. 2006;21: 524–30.

27. Ko M, Edelstein RA, Heslin KC, et al. Impact of the University of California, Los Angeles / Charles R. Drew University Medical Education Program on medical students' intentions to practice in underserved areas. *Acad Med*. 2005;80:803–8.

28. Tanner D, Tanner L. *Curriculum Development Theory into Practice*, 4th ed. Columbus, Ohio: Pearson Prentice-Hall; 2007.

29. Mahon KE, Henderson MK, Kirch DG. Selecting tomorrow's physicians: the key to the future healthcare workforce. *Acad Med*. 2013:88:1806–11.

30. Pamies RJ, Lawrence LE, Helm EG, Strayhorn G. The effects of certain student and institutional characteristics on minority medical student specialty choice. *J Natl Med Assoc*. 1994;86:136–40.

31. Saha S, Guilton G, Wimmers PF, Wilkerson L. Student body racial and ethnic composition and diversity-related outcomes in US medical schools. *JAMA*. 2008;300(10):1135–45.

32. Sullivan LW, Suez Mittman I. The state of diversity in the health professions a century after Flexner. *Acad Med*. 2010;85(2):246–53.

33. Iglehart JK. Diversity dynamics—challenges to a representative U.S. medical workforce. *N Engl J Med.* 2014;371:1471–74.

34. Association of American Medical Colleges. *Roadmap to Diversity: Key Legal and Educational Policy Foundations for Medical Schools.* Washington, D.C.: Association of American Medical Colleges; 2008.

35. Xierali IM, Rinaldo JC, Green LA, et al. Family physician participation in maintenance of certification. *Ann Fam Med.* 2011;9(3):203–10.

36. Fried JM, Vermillion M, Parker NH, Uijtdehaage S. Eradicating medical student mistreatment: a longitudinal study of one institution's efforts. *Acad Med.* 2012;87:1191–98.

37. Liaison Committee on Medical Education. Functions and Structure of a Medical School: Standards for Accreditation for Programs Leading to the M.D. Degree [Internet]. March 2014. P. 1 (Standard 1.4). Available at www.lcme.org/publications.htm.

38. Hammond MY, Margo K, Christner JG, et al. Opportunities and challenges in integrating electronic health records into undergraduate medical education: a national survey of clerkship directors. *Teach Learn Med.* 2012;24:219–24.

39. Tyler RW. *Basic Principles of Curriculum and Instruction.* Chicago: University of Chicago Press; 2013.

40. Medical School Objectives Writing Group. Learning objectives for medical school education—guidelines for medical schools: report I of the Medical School Objectives Project. *Acad Med.* 1999;74:13–18.

41. Bransford JD, Brown AL, Cocking RR, eds. *How People Learn: Brain, Mind, Experience, and School.* Washington, D.C.: National Academies Press; 2000.

42. University of Calgary Medical School. Introduction to the Curriculum [Internet]. Available at www.ucalgary.ca/mdprogram/current-student/introduction-curriculum.

43. Ende J, Kelley M, Sox H. The Federated Council of Internal Medicine's resource guide for residency education: an instrument for curricular change. *Ann Intern Med.* 1997;127(6):454–57.

44. Durning SJ, Sweet JM, Cation LJ. Morning report: an analysis of curricular content and comparison to national guidelines. *Teach Learn Med.* 2003;15:40–44.

45. Pediatrics Milestone Project: A Joint Initiative of the Accreditation Council for Graduate Medical Education and the American Board of Pediatrics [Internet]. 2015. Available at https://www.acgme.org/acgmeweb/Portals/0/PDFs/Milestones/PediatricsMilestones.pdf.

46. Association of American Medical Colleges. Core Entrustable Professional Activities for Entering Residency (CEPAER) [Internet]. Washington, D.C. March 2014. Available at www.mededportal.org/icollaborative/resource/887.

47. Ratanawongsa N, Rand CS, Magill CF, et al. Teaching residents to know their patients as individuals: the Aliki Initiative at Johns Hopkins Bayview Medical Center. *Pharos Alpha Omega Alpha Honor Med Sci.* 2009;72:4–11.

48. Sonnadara RR, Van Vliet A, Safir O, et al. Orthopedic boot camp: examining the effectiveness of an intensive surgical skills course. *Surgery.* 2011;149:745–49.

49. Jacobs HH. *Mapping the Big Picture: Integrating Curriculum and Assessment K-12.* Alexandria, Va.: Association for Supervision and Curriculum Development; 1997.

50. Lee MY, Albright SA, Alkasab T, et al. Tufts Health Sciences database: lessons, issues, opportunities. *Acad Med.* 2003;78:254–64.

51. Grow G. Teaching learners to be self-directed: a stage approach. *Adult Educ Q.* 1991;41:125–49.

52. Liaison Committee on Medical Education. Functions and Structure of a Medical School: Standards for Accreditation for Programs Leading to the M.D. Degree [Internet]. March 2014. P. 14 (Standard 8.1). Available at www.lcme.org/publications.htm.

53. Armstrong EG, Mackey M, Spear SJ. Medical education as a process management problem. *Acad Med.* 2004;79:721–28.

54. Bland CJ, Starnaman S, Wersal L, et al. Curricular change in medical schools: how to succeed. *Acad Med.* 2000;75:575–94.

55. Arnold P. Gold Foundation. Humanism in Medicine; Humanism and Excellence in Teaching Award [Internet]. Available at http://humanism-in-medicine.org/programs/awards/humanism-and-excellence-in-teaching-award.

56. Nutter DO, Bond JS, Coller BS. Measuring faculty effort and contributions in medical education. *Acad Med.* 2000;75:199–207.

57. Stites S, Vansaghi L, Pingleton S, Cox G, Paolo A. Aligning compensation with education: design and implementation of the educational value unit (EVU) system in an academic internal medicine department. *Acad Med.* 2005;80(12):1100–1106.

58. Geraci SA, Devine DR, Babbott SF, et al. AAIM Report on Master Teachers and Clinician Educators Part 3: finances and resourcing. *Am J Med.* 2010; 23(10):963–67.

59. Friedman Ben David M, Davis MH, Harden RM, et al. AMEE Medical Education Guide No. 24: portfolios as a method of student assessment. *Med Teach.* 2001;23(6):535–51.

60. Webb C, Endacott R, Gray M, et al. Evaluating portfolio assessment systems: what are the appropriate criteria? *Nurs Educ Today.* 2003;23:600–609.

61. McCready T. Portfolios and the assessment of competence in nursing. *Int J Nurs Stud.* 2007;44:143–51.

62. Tochel C, Haig A, Hesketh A, et al. The effectiveness of portfolios for postgraduate assessment and education: BEME Guide No. 12. *Med Teach.* 2009;12:299–318.

63. Gorniak RJ, Flanders AE, Sharpe RE. Trainee report dashboard: tool for enhancing feedback to radiology trainees about their reports. *Radiographics.* 2013;33(7):2105–13.

64. Hoekzema G, Abercrombie S, Carr S, et al. Residency "dashboard": family medicine GME's step toward transparency and accountability? *Ann Fam Med.* 2010;8(5):470.

65. American College of Physicians. ACP Internal Medicine Inservice Training Exam (IM-ITE) [Internet]. Available at www.acponline.org/education_recertification/education/in_training.

66. Lawley TJ, Saxton JF, Johns MM. Medical education: time for reform. *Trans Am Clin Clim Assoc.* 2005;116:311–20.

67. Seifer SD. Recent and emerging trends in undergraduate medical education—curricular responses to a rapidly changing health care systems. *West J Med.* 1998;168:400–411.

68. Childs B, Wiener C, Valle D. A science of the individual: implications for a medical school curriculum. *Annu Rev Genomics Hum Genet.* 2005;6:313–30.

69. Collins J. *Good to Great: Why Some Companies Make the Leap . . . and Others Don't.* New York: Harper Collins Publishers; 2001.

70. Collins J. *Good to Great and the Social Sectors: A Monograph to Accompany Good to Great.* London: Random House Business; 2006.

71. Heath C, Heath D. *Switch: How to Change Things When Change is Hard.* New York: Broadway Books, Random House; 2010.

72. Kotter J. Leading change: why transformation efforts fail. *Harvard Business Review,* Mar–Apr 1995.

73. Westley F, Zimmerman B, Patton MQ. *Getting to Maybe: How the World Is Changed.* Toronto: Random House Canada; 2006.

74. Bolman LG, Deal TE. *Reframing Organizations,* 5th ed. San Francisco: Jossey-Bass; 2013.

75. Meyerson DE, Scully MA. Tempered radicalism and the politics of ambivalence and change. *Organ Sci.* 1995;6:585–600.

76. Shepard, HA. Rules of thumb for change agents. In: French WL, Bell C, Zawacki RA, eds. *Organization Development and Transformation,* 6th ed. New York: McGraw-Hill/Irwin; 2005. Pp. 336–41.

77. Kim WC, Mauborgne R. Fair process: managing in the knowledge economy. *Harvard Business Review,* Jan 2003.

78. Blanchard K, Carew D, Carew EP. *The One Minute Manager Builds High Performing Teams.* New York: Harper Collins Publisher; 2009.

79. Fairholm MR. The Themes and Theory of Leadership: James MacGregor Burns and the

Philosophy of Leadership (Working Paper CR01-01). George Washington University Center for Excellence in Municipal Management. 2001.
80. Bass BM. From transactional to transformational leadership: learning to share the vision. *Organ Dyn*. 1990;18(3):19–31.
81. Palmer P. Leading from Within [Internet]. 1990. Available at www.couragerenewal.org/PDFs/Parker-Palmer_leading-from-within.pdf.
82. Raelin J. Does action learning promote collaborative leadership? *Acad Manag Learn Educ*. 2006;5(2):152–68.
83. Baker DP, Day R, Salas E. Teamwork as an essential component of high-reliability organizations. *Health Serv Res*. 2006;41(4 Pt 2):1576–98.
84. Ende J. Feedback in clinical medical education. *JAMA*. 1983;250(6):777–81.
85. Witherspoon R, White RP. Executive coaching: a continuum of roles. *J Consult Psychol*. 1996;48(2)124–33.
86. Thomas KW. *Introduction to Conflict Management: Improving Performance Using the TKI*. Mountain View, Calif.: CPP; 2002.
87. Bolton J, Roy W. Succession planning: securing the future. *J Nurs Admin*. 2004;34(12): 589–93.
88. Collins SK, Collins KS. Succession planning and leadership development: critical business strategies for healthcare organizations. *Radiol Manag*. 2007;291:16–21.
89. Collins SK, Collins KS. Changing workforce demographics necessitates succession planning in health care. *Health Care Manager*. 2007;26(4):318–25.
90. McConnell C. Succession planning: valuable exercise or pointless exercise? *Health Care Manager*. 2006;25(1):91–98.
91. Goleman D, Boyatzis R, McKee A. *Primal Leadership: Unleashing the Power of Emotional Intelligence*. Boston: Harvard Business Review Press; 2013. P. 306.
92. Goleman D. Leadership that gets results. *Harvard Business Review*, Mar–Apr 2000.

Example Curricula

This appendix provides three examples of curricula that have progressed through all six steps of curriculum development. The curricula were chosen to demonstrate differences in learner level and longevity. One focuses on medical students (Essential Resuscitation Skills for Medical Students), one on residents (Teaching Internal Medicine Residents to Incorporate Prognosis in the Care of Older Patients with Multimorbidity), and one on faculty (Longitudinal Program in Curriculum Development). The reader may want to review one or more of these examples to see how the various steps of the curriculum development process can relate to one another and be integrated into a whole.

ESSENTIAL RESUSCITATION SKILLS FOR MEDICAL STUDENTS

Julianna Jung, MD, and Nicole A. Shilkofski, MD, MEd

This curriculum was developed in 2010 as part of the Transition to the Wards (TTW) course at Johns Hopkins University School of Medicine (JHUSOM). The development team was led by Dr. Julianna Jung of the Department of Emergency Medicine and Dr. Nicole Shilkofski of the Department of Anesthesiology and Critical Care Medicine. In the process of a major curriculum reform, the medical school curriculum committee recognized the lack of formal preparation provided for medical students entering the clinical years and developed the TTW course to provide students with essential knowledge and skills needed to function effectively as integral members of health care teams. Systematic assessment and initial stabilization of acutely ill patients is one of the core content areas addressed by this course. While this is a complex skill set and many aspects of acute care were covered in the curriculum, management of cardiac arrest was particularly emphasized for both teaching and assessment. This is because spontaneous cardiac arrest is a sudden and randomly timed event that could potentially occur when a medical student is alone at the bedside. Furthermore, after receiving Basic Life Support (BLS) training, students are presumed to genuinely possess the knowledge and skills to initiate appropriate resuscitation for a patient in cardiac arrest, which is less true for other pathologies for which management is less protocolized. This confers a greater degree of responsibility for students confronted with cardiac arrest, as well as a greater opportunity to personally influence the outcome of the patient.

Step 1: Problem Identification and General Needs Assessment

The authors conducted a literature search in preparing this step.

Problem Identification	In-hospital cardiac arrest outcomes are highly variable both between and within hospitals (1, 2). While the reasons for this are certainly multifactorial, provider training and performance is likely to be a contributor. The importance of this issue is highlighted by the ever-increasing body of literature demonstrating the link between resuscitation quality and cardiac arrest survival rates. Survival following cardiac arrest has been linked to chest compression continuity (3, 4), rate (5), and depth (6), and animal studies suggest the potential for significant harm from hyperventilation (7). All of these variables are dependent on individual human performance, and, in addition to psychomotor skill, they require correct prioritization and effective leadership of the resuscitation team. The impact of these factors on survival outcomes underscores the critical importance of education to facilitate the best possible performance on the part of health care workers managing cardiac arrest patients.
Current Approach	Certification courses such as Basic and Advanced Cardiovascular Life Support (BLS and ACLS), while essential, have not been shown to be sufficient to produce competence among trainees. Several studies demonstrate poor baseline resuscitation performance

by ACLS-certified medical trainees tested using high-fidelity simulation, with checklist scores ranging from 44% to 75% (8–10). These findings demonstrate the need for additional training to ensure competence, particularly among future physicians who will be expected not only to provide lifesaving care for patients but also to serve as leaders of resuscitation teams.

Ideal Approach	Simulation has been shown to be superior to traditional teaching methods for improving resuscitation performance in the simulation lab (8, 9, 11, 12) as well as in clinical practice (10, 12, 13) and has been associated with better patient outcomes (14, 15). Simulation was therefore a natural choice as the core instructional method for this curriculum. Additionally, expert consensus has identified specific approaches within simulation that are particularly associated with effective learning. Deliberate practice (DP), a concept originally developed to explain how elite athletes master complex skills, is one such approach (16, 17). In the DP paradigm, learners strive to attain a well-defined goal through focused practice followed by specific feedback. This feedback informs further practice, which in turn leads to additional feedback, and the cycle continues in perpetuity until learners achieve mastery. The authors felt that DP was particularly well suited to the goal of enabling the learners to achieve mastery-level performance of key resuscitation skills, and they therefore emphasized this approach in the curriculum.

Step 2: Targeted Needs Assessment

For this step, the authors were particularly interested in the baseline resuscitation performance of students within the existing JHUSOM curriculum. While the literature suggests that certification courses alone do not guarantee adequate performance, it was unclear whether routine clinical education filled the "gap" and provided students with the additional knowledge and skills needed for resuscitation competence.

Targeted Learners	The authors polled the students informally and found that they had very little confidence in their emergency management skills and rated resuscitation as a major area of need within their curriculum. To quantify students' resuscitation performance, the authors recruited a volunteer cohort of 24 BLS-trained senior medical students to participate in formal simulation-based assessment. Each student participated individually in a standardized high-fidelity simulation scenario depicting a case of acute myocardial infarction complicated by ventricular fibrillation arrest.

Resuscitation performance in this group was far from optimal, with only 45% of students initiating chest compressions within one minute of arrest, 58% placing a cardiac monitor, and 25% initiating ventilation. Seventy-five percent of students defibrillated within three minutes of arrest, but many did so inappropriately, |

either without apparent knowledge of the cardiac rhythm or without adhering to accepted protocols for shock frequency. These findings confirmed the authors' belief that additional resuscitation education was necessary to ensure medical graduates' competence to provide basic lifesaving care during residency and beyond.

As noted above, the authors recognized that students could potentially encounter cardiac arrest during their clinical rotations in medical school and that they had both the obligation and the opportunity to provide lifesaving care for patients in cardiac arrest while waiting for help to arrive. For this reason, the authors targeted second-year medical students in the TTW course as learners for this curriculum. All students were formally certified in BLS prior to participating.

Targeted Environment	The resuscitation curriculum was implemented as part of the Transition to the Wards course, as described above, and was part of a larger module on acute care skills covering common in-hospital emergencies such as respiratory distress, shock, and altered mental status. The hospitals in which students complete their clerkships have rapid response teams that are available within several minutes.

The curriculum was conducted in a 10,000-square-foot state-of-the-art simulation center featuring high-fidelity human patient simulators and advanced audiovisual technology. Simulations were conducted using Laerdal SimMan 3G and were recorded digitally using SimCapture software. All instructors were board-certified specialists in Emergency Medicine or Anesthesiology/Critical Care Medicine, with specific expertise in resuscitation education.

Step 3: Goals and Objectives

Goals	Based on the authors' findings from Steps 1 and 2, the fundamental goal of the curriculum was to transmit the necessary knowledge, skills, and attitudes to allow all students to initiate high-quality resuscitation for patients in cardiac arrest, in strict accordance with current guidelines and protocols.
Specific Objectives	The authors further operationalized this goal into specific learning objectives.

- By the end of the resuscitation curriculum, all students will be able to:
- Demonstrate an appropriate initial assessment for patients in cardiac arrest, including prioritization of circulation over respiration and limitation of time devoted to assessment

- Demonstrate an appropriate call for help when confronted with any life-threatening emergency in any clinical or nonclinical setting

- Demonstrate correct chest compression technique, including use of quality adjuncts for in-hospital resuscitation

- Identify shockable cardiac rhythms and differentiate these from nonshockable cardiac rhythms

- Demonstrate correct use of both automated and manual defibrillators, including appropriate rhythm check, delivery of shock if indicated, and correct shock interval

- Demonstrate effective bag-valve-mask ventilation with correct coordination between compressions and breaths

- Demonstrate effective teamwork and communication practices to optimize resuscitation performance

Step 4: Educational Strategies

As discussed above, simulation was the foundation for teaching resuscitation skills in this curriculum. Simulation sessions were supplemented with didactic instruction and hands-on skills demonstration. In accordance with deliberate practice principles, the authors repeatedly reinforced essential core skills such as systematic assessment and recommended interventions throughout the entire acute care curriculum, though there was only one session specifically devoted to cardiac arrest management. While the basic approach remained constant, certain elements of the curriculum were refined over the years in response to assessment data (see Step 6: Evaluation and Assessment, and Curriculum Maintenance and Enhancement, below). The emphasis on deliberate practice was increased over time.

Step 5: Implementation

Resources	- Johns Hopkins Medicine Simulation Center
	- Human patient simulators
	- Durable medical equipment (defibrillator, crash cart, etc.)
	- Consumable supplies (defibrillator pads, bag-valve masks, etc.)
	- Expert faculty educators to precept sessions (4 faculty preceptors, 8 hours/day, for 1 week each year)
	- Technicians to operate simulators and assist with sessions (though, in many cases, faculty operated their own simulators)
Support	- Salary support for curriculum developers and educators

	■ Institutional support for the TTW course in general and for resuscitation content specifically
Administration	■ A single faculty member as director of the resuscitation skills curriculum
	■ Administrative staff from the Office of Curriculum for scheduling and communications
	■ Simulation staff from the Simulation Center
Barriers	■ Large class size (sessions had to be run repeatedly over several days, with larger group sizes than ideal)
	■ Significant time required for implementation and assessment (would have been prohibitive without salary support for faculty)
Introduction	■ No formal pilot of curriculum itself was conducted
	■ Targeted needs assessment served as pilot for the assessment tool as well as providing valuable insight for curriculum development.

The curriculum was initially implemented as part of the required TTW course in 2010 and has been repeated annually since that time. The four-hour resuscitation curriculum is delivered repeatedly to small groups of students over one week to ensure that 120 students are accommodated. The curriculum occupies the entire Simulation Center for its duration.

Step 6: Evaluation and Assessment

Users	■ Learners themselves use the evaluation data to understand and improve their own performance.
	■ Faculty and curriculum developers use the data to understand the strengths and weaknesses of the curriculum and to optimize instructional strategies, in order to maximize educational outcomes and learner satisfaction.
	■ Institutional leadership uses the data to document students' attainment of an essential clinical competency and to assess the job performance of the curriculum developers.
	■ The data have allowed curriculum developers to present at national meetings and have promoted professional development.
	■ Educators from other institutions have used the data, which have been presented in several national meetings, as the data provide evidentiary support for an educational technique that they may find useful in their own settings.

Uses	
	▪ Formative feedback to learners gives them insight into their strengths and weaknesses and helps them to develop learning plans to facilitate future performance improvement.
	▪ Summative assessment data can be used to determine whether learners achieved the stated learning objectives.
	▪ Aggregated summative data have allowed faculty to assess the effectiveness of the curriculum and to target improvements appropriately.
	▪ Aggregated formative data have allowed faculty and curriculum developers to understand learners' perceptions of the educational experience.
	▪ Both types of program-level data have been used to justify allocation of resources to the course, to support applications for promotion and other types of recognition for the curriculum developers, and for dissemination to other educators.
Resources	▪ The authors were granted institutional support that provided protected time for curriculum development, implementation, and collection of assessment data.
	▪ Administrative support for collation and analysis of the data was not readily available, which could have been problematic. However, the authors were fortunate to recruit three residents who were interested in the curriculum as an academic project and assisted with data entry and analysis. Equipment, facilities, and personnel with technical expertise in simulation were available through the institution's Simulation Center.
Evaluation Questions	▪ By the end of the curriculum, what percentage of learners demonstrated correct and timely performance of essential assessment techniques and therapeutic interventions in the setting of a simulated resuscitation scenario?
	▪ When learners did not correctly perform needed assessments and interventions, what were their common errors or misconceptions?
	▪ What was the perceived effectiveness of the curriculum on the part of learners? What were the strengths and weaknesses of the curriculum?
	▪ "Correct and timely performance" was operationally defined for each "essential assessment technique" and "therapeutic intervention" prior to implementation of the curriculum. Where possible, these definitions were based on accepted national standards (e.g., American Heart Association guidelines).
Evaluation Design	X - - - O design. This approach allowed documentation of learners' proficiency following the intervention. It did not permit ex-

clusion of preexisting proficiency or natural maturation over the course of the observation period. However, as the curriculum was implemented over a very short period and was targeted to novice learners, these were not thought to be major concerns.

Evaluation Methods and Instruments	*Direct observation* of individual performance in a simulated resuscitation scenario was the principal measurement method. This method had the advantage of allowing the authors to provide specific, direct, formative feedback to each learner. Use of *performance checklists* that were based on observable behavior allowed a high degree of precision and objectivity in data collection. The main disadvantage of this approach is that it is highly labor-intensive. It is also possible that simulation performance may not be predictive of future "real-life" performance. Development of an appropriate data collection instrument was simplified by the existence of well-documented and universally accepted protocols for resuscitation in cardiac arrest. Content validity was ensured by basing all checklist items on these established protocols, and reliability was aided by linking each item to a predefined observable behavior.
Ethical Concerns	The authors took steps to ensure confidentiality for participants, both in the curriculum itself and in assessment. Prior to participating in the curriculum, all learners were oriented to the importance of confidentiality for the maintenance of a safe learning environment. Access to assessment data was restricted to curriculum developers and course leaders, and all data were stored in password-protected devices. Learners were informed in advance of how their individual assessment data would be used in computing their final score and determining pass/fail status.
	Informed consent was not required by the Institutional Review Board for the research aspects of this program, as all data were deidentified and analyzed only in the aggregate on a post-hoc basis. The X - - - O evaluation design was selected to minimize resource consumption, and the lifesaving nature of the content was deemed sufficiently important to merit the resources expended in assessment. The authors felt that the potential impact of the assessment data was minimal. The small subset of learners with inadequate performance received remediation to enhance their skills. No failing grades were recorded on transcripts or records, and no academic consequences were associated with the need for remediation.
Data Collection	The authors collected assessment data as an end-of-course Objective Structured Clinical Examination (OSCE). Participation in the OSCE was required for all learners, ensuring a response rate of 100%. A faculty member personally observed all learners during the resuscitation portion of this exam and collected data on a standardized behavioral checklist, using pen and paper. All

sessions were videotaped to ensure the accuracy of data and to permit post-hoc assessment of interobserver reliability. Data were entered into a spreadsheet, and missing or illegible values were determined through video review.

Data Analysis	Data were analyzed using simple descriptive statistics to determine the proportion of students completing necessary assessment and treatment maneuvers in a timely fashion. Descriptive statistics could then be used to ascertain that 98.4% of learners initiated CPR, but only 81.2% did so within the 30-second timeframe recommended by American Heart Association guidelines. When curricular improvements were made, data were aggregated and comparisons made between pre-improvement and post-improvement groups, using Fisher's exact test for categorical variables and unpaired t-tests for interval variables such as time.
Reporting of Results	Formative feedback was provided immediately to individual learners. Summative results, including group averages for comparison, were made available within four weeks after the end of the course. These aggregate data were also provided to faculty so that curricular needs could be discussed and improvements planned.

Curriculum Maintenance and Enhancement

Student evaluations of the curriculum have been uniformly positive, with 96% to 99% of students each year giving the Acute Care curriculum the highest rating on the TTW course evaluation. While the authors found this pleasing, they must emphasize that the fundamental goal of the curriculum was not to satisfy the students but to improve their resuscitation performance. To that end, assessment data from the OSCE were analyzed each year and used to evaluate the strengths and weaknesses of the curriculum. The curriculum was then revised accordingly, with the goal of optimizing student performance.

In the first year of the curriculum, the authors were frankly disappointed with students' performance on the OSCE. Only 58% of students initiated chest compressions within one minute, and only 47% defibrillated within three minutes, both of which are essential interventions that would be expected to influence cardiac arrest survival in clinical practice. In response to these poor outcomes, the authors analyzed the OSCE data to identify common patterns of error. They then adjusted the didactic portion of the curriculum to clarify areas of apparent confusion for the students and reorganized the simulation component to emphasize the deliberate practice paradigm, with the goal of ensuring that learners spent more time actually *performing* the desired skills instead of *discussing* how they should perform them. Following this adjustment in the second year, the percentage of students initiating timely CPR rose to 75%, which the authors did not deem adequate. Timely defibrillation rates also did not improve.

Analysis of the second year's OSCE data revealed that students appeared to have difficulty prioritizing the myriad tasks that must be performed in the initial stages of resuscitation, leading to unacceptable delays in the most critical tasks. The authors therefore further adjusted the curriculum in the third year of implementation to emphasize and reinforce appropriate prioritization of tasks within the resuscitation. The conceptual basis for task prioritization was addressed in the didactic curriculum, and learners were forced to sequence tasks in the simulation rather than performing them simultaneously. Following these adjustments in the third year, 98% of students initiated CPR within one minute, and 83% defibrillated within three minutes.

It should be emphasized that learner satisfaction was uniformly high throughout these three years although the educational outcomes were very different, indicating that learners will value a curriculum that they enjoy even if it is not optimally effective. This finding underscores the importance of using objective educational outcome data to measure curricular impact, rather than simply relying on more readily accessible learner satisfaction data. It should also be emphasized that assessment provides valuable insight into the strengths and weaknesses of a curriculum, and educators can use this insight to improve the curriculum and optimize educational outcomes.

Dissemination

Educational outcome data from this curriculum have been presented at institutional educational leadership and research meetings as well as at national professional meetings, in both poster and oral forms. The original version of the curriculum itself has been published on MedEdPORTAL. The data have not yet been published in a peer-reviewed journal, but the authors are currently working on a manuscript describing the iterative cycles of assessment, analysis, and curricular improvement that have led to substantial increases in the quality of learners' resuscitation performance over time.

REFERENCES

1. Merchant RM, Berg RA, Yang L, et al. Hospital variation in survival after in-hospital cardiac arrest. *J Am Heart Assoc.* 2014;3(1):e000400. doi:10.1161/JAHA.113.000400.
2. Perberdy MA, Ornato JP, Larking GL, et al. Survival from in-hospital cardiac arrest during nights and weekends. *JAMA.* 2008;299(7):785–92.
3. Christenson J, Andrusiek D, Everson-Stewart S, et al. Chest compression fraction determines survival in patients with out-of-hospital ventricular fibrillation. *Circulation.* 2009;120(13):1241–47.
4. Vaillancourt C, Everson-Stewart S, Christenson J, et al. The impact of increased chest compression fraction on return of spontaneous circulation for out-of-hospital cardiac arrest patients not in ventricular fibrillation. *Resuscitation.* 2011;82(12):1501–7.
5. Idris AH, Guffey D, Aufderheide TP, et al. Relationship between chest compression rates and outcomes from cardiac arrest. *Circulation.* 2012;125(24):3004–12.
6. Stiell IG, Brown SP, Christenson J, et al. What is the role of chest compression depth during out-of-hospital cardiac arrest resuscitation? *Crit Care Med.* 2012;40(4):1192–98.
7. Aufderheide TP, Sigurdsson G, Pirrallo RG, et al. Hyperventilation-induced hypotension during cardiopulmonary resuscitation. *Circulation.* 2004;109(16):1960–65.
8. Wayne DB, Butter J, Siddall V, et al. Mastery learning of advanced cardiac life support skills by internal medicine residents using simulation technology and deliberate practice. *J Gen Intern Med.* 2006;21(3):251–56.
9. Wayne DB, Butter J, Siddall VJ, et al. Simulation-based training of internal medicine residents

in advanced cardiac life support protocols: a randomized trial. *Teach Learn Med*. 2005; 17(3):210–16.

10. Wayne DB, Didwania A, Feinglass J, et al. Simulation-based education improves quality of care during cardiac arrest team responses at an academic teaching hospital: a case-control study. *Chest*. 2008;133(1):56–61. Epub 2007 Jun 15.

11. Oermann MH, Kardong-Edgren S, Odom-Maryon T, et al. Deliberate practice of motor skills in nursing education: CPR as exemplar. *Nurs Educ Perspect*. 2011;32:311–15.

12. Sawyer T, Sierocka-Castaneda A, Chan D, et al. Deliberate practice using simulation improves neonatal resuscitation performance. *Simul Healthc*. 2011;6:327–36.

13. Steinemann S, Berg B, Skinner A, et al. In situ, multidisciplinary, simulation-based teamwork training improves early trauma care. *J Surg Educ*. 2011;68:472–77.

14. Draycott TJ, Crofts JF, Ash JP, et al. Improving neonatal outcome through practical shoulder dystocia training. *Obstet Gynecol*. 2008;112:14–20.

15. Phipps MG, Lindquist DG, McConaughey E, et al. Outcomes from a labor and delivery team training program with simulation component. *Am J Obstet Gynecol*. 2012;206:3–9.

16. Issenberg SB, McGaghie WC, Petrusa ER, et al. Features and uses of high-fidelity medical simulations that lead to effective learning: a BEME systematic review. *Med Teach*. 2005;27:10–28.

17. McGaghie WC, Issenberg SB, Cohen ER, et al. Medical education featuring mastery learning with deliberate practice can lead to better health for individuals and populations. *Acad Med*. 2011;86:e8–9.

TEACHING INTERNAL MEDICINE RESIDENTS TO INCORPORATE PROGNOSIS IN THE CARE OF OLDER PATIENTS WITH MULTIMORBIDITY

Nancy L. Schoenborn, MD, and Matthew K. McNabney, MD

This curriculum was developed in 2012–13 by Dr. Nancy Schoenborn and Dr. Matthew McNabney as part of the Longitudinal Curriculum Development Course in the Johns Hopkins University Faculty Development Program. The curriculum development coincided with the publication of a landmark consensus document by the American Geriatrics Society (AGS), "Guiding Principles for the Care of Older Adults with Multimorbidity" (1). This document and an accompanying pocket card urged physicians caring for older adults with multiple chronic medical conditions to implement five guiding principles, with the goal of improving health care and outcomes for these complex patients who were largely excluded from the patient populations used to develop individual disease treatment guidelines. Guiding Principle III is the "Prognosis Domain," which encourages clinicians to frame clinical management decisions within the context of risk, burdens, benefits, and prognosis (remaining life expectancy, functional status, quality of life).

Dr. McNabney and Dr. Cynthia Boyd (who served as a consultant to this project) were co-chairs of the expert panel that authored the consensus document. Though a pocket card was created to help to disseminate these principles, they understood that changing behavior would require more targeted and intensive educational intervention. Thus, this curriculum was designed as a resource for programs aiming to train physicians to implement these principles in their practice.

Step 1: Problem Identification and General Needs Assessment

The authors, with the help of a medical informationist, conducted literature searches in PubMed. A table of relevant search terms related to the Prognosis Domain is given in the AGS Guiding Principles (1). They also searched in educational portals such as the Portal of Geriatric Online Education and MedEdPORTAL to help prepare for this step (2, 3). The goal was to look not only for full available curricula but also for related curricula in calculating and communicating prognosis and incorporating prognosis into clinical discussions.

Problem Identification	Multimorbidity, defined as the coexistence of two or more chronic conditions, is a common problem that affects more than half of older adults (1, 4). Multimorbidity is associated with higher mortality, disability, institutionalization, decreased quality of life, and higher rates of adverse effects of treatment or interventions (5). A significant portion of older adults with multimorbidity have limited prognosis, especially when multimorbidity is also associated with functional limitations (1). Central to the challenge of caring for older adults with multimorbidity is the lack of provider training specific to caring for this population. Medical training has traditionally focused on single disease entities. Similarly, clinical practice guidelines also address single disease entities (6). Caring for older adults with multimorbidity, however, is much more

than simply combining the care plans for each of the individual conditions. In fact, combining guidelines often leads to contradictory recommendations, a higher likelihood of adverse effects, and higher cost (6). Failure to consider prognosis in the context of clinical decision making can lead to poor care, which is particularly relevant for older adults with multimorbidity. There are suggestions that assessment and incorporation of prognosis in clinical decision making are currently suboptimal. For example, there are numerous reports on underutilization of hospice, inadequate screening of healthy older adults, and excess screening of older adults with poor prognosis (7–10). Physicians tend to underestimate patients' need for information and overestimate patients' understanding and awareness of their prognosis (11–13). Yet, patients consider it very important to know their prognosis and to discuss it with their physicians (14–18).

Furthermore, patient preferences for specific treatment options change significantly when the predicted treatment outcomes are different (19, 20). Since the likelihood of a patient experiencing benefit from a test or treatment is predicated on the patient living long enough to experience the benefit, prognostic information is necessary to inform patients' decisions. Indeed, it is impossible to effectively elicit and respect patient preferences without incorporating prognostic information to provide the context within which patients' values can be framed.

Current Approach

Some existing curricula teach about caring for patients with chronic diseases in general (21–24), but they typically focus on single diseases (25–29), and none address the unique challenges when older adults have multiple coexisting chronic diseases. The AGS convened a consensus panel to review the literature and draft guiding principles for the care of older adults with multimorbidity. The recommendations and the references were published in journals, and a pocket card was circulated.

Despite its importance, physicians find prognosis difficult and stressful and report inadequate training (30). Current teaching regarding prognosis exists only as part of curricula on palliative care or oncologic care (31–33). Even in those contexts, the focus is often on how to assess and communicate a prognosis based on a terminal illness, not how to assess prognosis for older adults with multimorbidity who may not necessarily be at the very end of life.

Ideal Approach

Ideally, a prognosis curriculum will help learners develop the knowledge, skills, and attitudes to effectively:

1) *assess* prognosis among older patients with multimorbidity,

2) *discuss* prognosis with patients, and

3) *incorporate* prognosis into clinical decision making.

Since these are complex psychomotor skills, the curriculum should provide tools to facilitate deliberate practice of each of these skills and opportunities for feedback. The curriculum should be easily adaptable to different levels of learners, such as geriatrics fellows and practicing clinicians at other institutions, and easily updateable as the body of evidence supporting best practices in this area grows.

Step 2: Targeted Needs Assessment

Targeted Learners — The authors identified targeted learners to be the internal medicine residents at their institution—the Johns Hopkins Bayview Medical Center. They chose residents because residency is one of the most formative times in clinical training. Also, most older adults are cared for by providers who are trained in internal medicine or family practice, who may not have specialty training in geriatric medicine (34). Therefore, teaching to trainees in residency, rather than geriatric fellowship, will have a broader impact. In addition, assessing and incorporating prognosis in clinical practice are part of the key competencies for residents as described by professional societies and regulatory bodies. For example, competency milestones from the Accreditation Council for Graduate Medical Education (ACGME) and the American Board of Internal Medicine (ABIM) for medicine residents include "customize care in the context of patient's preferences and overall health" (35). Key geriatrics competencies for medicine residents developed by a consensus committee from multiple professional societies also include "individualize standard recommendations . . . based on life expectancy, functional status, patient preference, and goals of care" (36). The authors did not initially target residents of a specific training year, but as described in Step 5, below, due to considerations of available curricular time, number of residents in specific rotations, and the related teaching time required, they eventually decided to implement the curriculum for first-year residents.

Targeted Environment — The authors chose to target the outpatient clinic as the learning environment. While prognosis is critically relevant to inpatient care, the literature suggests that physicians and patients prefer to discuss prognosis in the context of established, trusting relationships and to have such discussions over time (37, 38). Both of these preferences are characteristics of an outpatient continuity practice setting.

Needs Assessment/Targeted Learners — The authors assessed the needs of the targeted learners through several means: they reviewed their existing curricula, met with key stakeholders, surveyed a subset of the residents at a teaching conference, and informally interviewed the resident clinic preceptors.

Using an innovative hybrid method of in-person surveying, the authors presented a case discussion at the resident morning teaching conference to illustrate the importance of incorporating prognosis in patient care and how doing so affects clinical decision making. They embedded survey questions in the presentation and used an audience response system to gather anonymous responses from the residents in real time. As they were able to immediately see the pooled responses to each question, the authors then invited voluntary comments from the audience to clarify and elaborate on their answers.

Among the 24 attendees at the teaching conference, 14 were residents in the three-year internal medicine training program with continuity clinics and were therefore included in the survey; the other 10 were medical students or residents in a one-year preliminary program without continuity clinics. Two-thirds (9 of 14 targeted learners) responded that they did not regularly assess prognosis in their clinics, citing lack of knowledge as the biggest barrier, followed by competing demands in clinic. None of the respondents regularly discussed prognosis with patients, citing lack of knowledge, competing demands, and patient-related factors as top barriers. Although 87% responded that they regularly incorporated prognosis in clinical decision making, further discussion with the audience suggested that those who responded in this way meant that they considered patients' multiple comorbidities in clinical decision making, but no one volunteered any examples of actually incorporating prognosis. Lack of knowledge, insufficient skills, and competing demands were top barriers.

Needs Assessment Targeted Learning Environment	Within the several existent outpatient curricula for the residents, there was limited teaching on goals of care and advance directives; the only specific teaching on prognosis was a small component within the oncology curriculum. There was no specific teaching about multimorbidity or prognosis for patients with multimorbidity.

The authors met with and obtained support from the residency program director, the resident ambulatory care faculty leader, and the resident clinic preceptors. They all confirmed the lack of any existing curriculum on multimorbidity or prognosis. The clinic preceptors mentioned that they themselves did not regularly or systematically consider prognosis in the care of patients who have multimorbidity. They requested a short online module to teach them key concepts about prognosis for patients with multimorbidity; they also suggested easily accessible resources and tools such as pocket cards for reference during preceptor sessions.

Step 3: Goals and Objectives

Based on the information obtained in Step 2, the authors wrote specific learning objectives, with attention to congruence among objectives, educational strategies, and learner evaluation.

Goals	The curricular goal was to help internal medicine residents develop the knowledge, skills, and attitudes to regularly and appropriately assess, communicate, and incorporate prognosis in the care of older adults with multimorbidity in the outpatient continuity clinic. The authors expected that incorporating prognosis would then lead to improved care and patient outcomes for older adults with multimorbidity.
Objectives	Objectives were divided into domains related to attitude, knowledge, skills, and behavior, as follows: *Attitude:* ▪ Identify rationale for incorporating prognosis ▪ Rank incorporating prognosis as important *Knowledge:* ▪ Demonstrate assessing prognosis using available tools ▪ Demonstrate applying prognostic information to inform clinical decisions *Skill:* ▪ Demonstrate incorporating prognosis in discussion of risks and benefits ▪ Demonstrate communication about prognosis *Behavior:* ▪ Routinely assess, communicate, and incorporate prognosis in clinical care of older adults with multimorbidity

Step 4: Educational Strategies

The curriculum consisted of three sessions (120, 150, 60 minutes, respectively) over the course of 4 weeks, to include the following elements:

Small Group Didactics/ Discussions	There were two didactics: the first addressed the objectives on attitude and knowledge; the second addressed the objective on communication skill. These sessions took place in small groups of six to eight learners due to the logistics of existing rotation structure, but should be transferrable to larger or smaller groups.
Case-Based Learning	In addition to having illustrative cases during the didactic sessions, learners were asked to bring their own patient cases for practicing assessment and application of prognosis information. This process was guided by a structured worksheet and was

done in two iterations: first, in a group setting following the didactic on this topic, where the faculty facilitator was available for troubleshooting and residents could also learn from one another; second, the same exercise repeated individually as part of an assignment to prepare for a real-life clinic visit discussion.

Role Play	Standardized patients were used for the learners to practice the skills related to communicating prognosis. A teaching case was developed with specific instructions for the learners, as well as for the standardized patients. The exercise was conducted in groups of two or three learners. A faculty facilitator led debriefing after each encounter and provided feedback; the observing learners also provided peer feedback, followed by reflection at the end of all encounters.
Clinical Experience and Reflection	After the didactics, case-based exercise, and role-play exercises, the learners were given the assignment to assess, incorporate, and communicate prognosis with one of their own continuity clinic patients. They were asked to reflect on the experience and share the reflection with the group. The rotation structure includes an interim of several weeks between the first teaching sessions and the final reflection session, allowing time to complete the assignment. During the session, after each learner shared her or his experience and reflection, the faculty facilitator solicited group feedback and comments. At the end of the session, learners were asked to complete a survey that included questions about how they expected to change their behavior in the area of incorporating prognosis in clinical care.

Step 5: Implementation

The authors obtained support from the Internal Medicine Residency Director, the faculty leader of the resident clinic, and the course director of the outpatient rotation Evidence-Based Medicine, where this curriculum was given its curricular time. The authors also met with all the faculty members who precept in the resident clinic for a needs assessment, as well as to obtain support. They were able to obtain external grant funding to support evaluation strategies and the cost of standardized patients.

Resources	*Personnel:* In the initial curriculum development stage: one geriatrics fellow and one geriatrics faculty met for 4 hours per week for the 9 months of the Longitudinal Curriculum Development Course to develop the curriculum. Subsequently, to implement the curriculum, the Evidence-Based Medicine rotation runs three times a year for the 20 first-year internal medicine residents, which translates to repeating the curriculum three times with one faculty member committing 5 hours per rotation, totaling 15 hours in direct teaching time per year. One to two additional faculty spent up to 4 or 5 hours each as facilitators in the standardized patient exercises.

	Facilities and Equipment:
	• Conference room for didactics/discussion and standardized patient exercises
	• Standardized patients
	• Computer with projected screen
	Funding: The authors applied for and received funding from the Picker/Gold Graduate Medical Education Challenge Grant.
Support	The residency program director and the resident clinic faculty all welcomed the program. The geriatrics faculty were deeply invested in the program and donated their time.
Administration	The Evidence-Based Medicine rotation has existing support staff who scheduled the lectures and reserved the conference rooms, so no additional coordination was needed.
Barriers	The external funding was for one year, and there was no continuing funding source for standardized patient expenses or for faculty time. Dr. Schoenborn transitioned from fellow to faculty and plans to continue teaching the curriculum on a volunteer basis. The authors are exploring the development of video materials to teach the communication skills with a faculty facilitator to replace the standardized patient exercises and thus help minimize long-term costs.
Introduction	The curriculum was developed during 2012–13 and implemented in January 2014, with plans to continue in the coming years.

Step 6: Evaluation

The evaluation was based on congruence with the learning objectives and the different levels of educational outcomes. A Johns Hopkins Institutional Review Board approved the study, which includes all the evaluation plans, and informed consent was obtained from all participants.

Users	• Internal medicine residents
	• Resident clinic faculty
	• Funding agency
Uses	• Formative information to help residents achieve learning objectives
	• Summative information for the funding agency on the program's effectiveness

Resources	• Funding as mentioned above, which covered a part-time re-search assistant

Evaluation Questions	
	1) Is the curriculum acceptable to the participants?
	2) Does the curriculum improve the participants' attitude with regard to incorporating prognosis in the care of older patients with multimorbidity, as compared with nonparticipants?
	3) Does the curriculum improve the participants' knowledge on how to use available prognostic assessment tools and incorporate the information in specific clinical decisions, as compared with nonparticipants?
	4) Does the curriculum improve the participants' self-rated skills on communicating prognosis, as compared with nonparticipants?
	5) Does the curriculum improve the rate of incorporating prognosis in clinical practice, as documented in clinical visit charts, among participants compared with nonparticipants?
	6) How are participants incorporating prognosis in their real-life clinical communication when prompted to do so after the curriculum?
	7) How do patients perceive the clinical communication and clinical care?

Evaluation Design	
	1) X - - - O
	2–4) E O_1 - - - X - - - O_2
	C O_1 - - - - - - - O_2
	5) E O_1 - - - X - - - O_2
	C O_1 - - - - - - - O_2
	6, 7) X - - - O
	The control group was the first-year internal medicine residents at a separate residency training program.

Evaluation Methods	
	1–4) Questionnaires
	5) Chart review
	6) Audio recording of clinic visits, with subsequent qualitative analysis of the transcript
	7) Patient surveys

Data Collection	Questionnaire for 1) was administered in person; questionnaires for 2) to 4) were administered online through Surveymonkey.com. Chart review was conducted by Dr. Schoenborn and research assistants. A research assistant also conducted the audio recording and administered the patient surveys.
Data Analysis	Quantitative data were analyzed using descriptive statistics and paired t-tests. Audio recordings were analyzed using qualitative methods.
Reporting of Results	The results are currently being collected and analyzed with a plan for submission to peer-reviewed journals for publication.

Curriculum Maintenance and Enhancement

The major anticipated challenge is to support faculty time and to reinforce the curricular concepts among learners over time. The authors have enlisted the help of the faculty who precept in the resident clinic to reinforce these concepts, but this may be challenging because the faculty themselves are not familiar with these concepts and have many other competing demands.

The preliminary feedback and evaluation data from the first year of implementation were reviewed with the Curriculum Development team. The curriculum was well-received, and no changes were planned immediately. However, the authors plan to develop videos related to the prognosis communication aspect of the curriculum to improve the long-term sustainability of the curriculum and its ability to disseminate to other programs.

Actions toward sustaining the curriculum team and related activities that strengthen the curriculum:

- The curriculum and its related evaluation results are being submitted for publication.
- There is a plan to adapt the curriculum to other levels of learners—specifically, practicing clinicians.
- There is ongoing collaboration to develop videos related to the prognosis communication aspect of the curriculum with other geriatrics researchers in the area of prognostication.

Dissemination

Target Audience(s)	- Generalist practitioners in training - Geriatricians in training - Practicing primary care physicians
Reasons for Dissemination:	To improve the incorporation of prognosis to inform clinical decision making in the care of older adults with multimorbidity
Content:	Curricular material and evaluation results

Method(s):	Curriculum needs assessment was presented in abstract form at the national AGS meeting and the national Society of General Internal Medicine (SGIM) meeting (39, 40). Curricular materials were shared at an Educational Innovations forum at a national AGS meeting.

REFERENCES

1. American Geriatrics Society Expert Panel on the Care of Older Adults with Multimorbidity. Guiding principles for the care of older adults with multimorbidity: an approach for clinicians. *J Am Geriatr Soc*. 2012;60(10):E1–25.

2. Portal of Geriatric Online Education. www.pogoe.org.

3. MedEdPORTAL. www.mededportal.org.

4. Fortin M, Hudon C, Haggerty J, et al. Prevalence estimates of multimorbidity: a comparative study of two sources. *BMC Health Serv Res*. 2010;10:111.

5. Boyd CM, Fortin M. Future of multimorbidity research: how should understanding of multimorbidity inform health system design? *Public Health Rev*. 2010;32:451–74.

6. Boyd CM, Darer J, Boult C, et al. Clinical practice guidelines and quality of care for older patients with multiple comorbid diseases: implications for pay for performance. *JAMA*. 2005;294:716–24.

7. Casarett D, Karlawish J, Morales K, et al. Improving the use of hospice services in nursing homes: a randomized controlled trial. *JAMA*. 2005;294:211–17.

8. Walter LC, Covinsky KE. Cancer screening in elderly patients: a framework for individualized decision making. *JAMA*. 2001;285:2750–56.

9. Mehta KM, Fung KZ, Kistler CE, et al. Impact of cognitive impairment on screening mammography use in older US women. *Am J Public Health*. 2010;100:1917–23.

10. Sima CS, Panageas KS, Schrag D. Cancer screening among patients with advanced cancer. *JAMA*. 2010;304:1584–91.

11. Hamel MB, Teno JM, Goldman L, et al. Patient age and decisions to withhold life-sustaining treatments from seriously ill, hospitalized adults. SUPPORT investigators: Study to Understand Prognoses and Preferences for Outcomes and Risks of Treatment. *Ann Intern Med*. 1999;130:116–25.

12. Hancock K, Clayton JM, Parker SM, et al. Discrepant perceptions about end-of-life communication: a systematic review. *J Pain Symptom Manage*. 2007;34:190–200.

13. Wilson IB, Green ML, Goldman L, et al. Is experience a good teacher? How interns and attending physicians understand patients' choices for end-of-life care. SUPPORT investigators: Study to Understand Prognoses and Preferences for Outcomes and Risks of Treatments. *Med Decis Making*. 1997;17:217–27.

14. Ahalt C, Walter LC, Yourman L, et al. "Knowing is better": preferences of diverse older adults for discussing prognosis. *J Gen Intern Med*. 2012;27:568–75.

15. Greisinger AJ, Lorimor RJ, Aday LA, et al. Terminally ill cancer patients: their most important concerns. *Cancer Pract*. 1997;5:147–54.

16. Hagerty RG, Butow PN, Ellis PA, et al. Cancer patient preferences for communication of prognosis in the metastatic setting. *J Clin Oncol*. 2004;22:1721–30.

17. Fried TR, Bradley EH, O'Leary J. Prognosis communication in serious illness: perceptions of older patients, caregivers, and clinicians. *J Am Geriatr Soc*. 2003;51:1398–1403.

18. Parker SM, Clayton JM, Hancock K, et al. A systematic review of prognostic/end-of-life communication with adults in the advanced stages of a life-limiting illness: patient/caregiver

preferences for the content, style, and timing of information. *J Pain Symptom Manage*. 2007;34:81–93.

19. Weeks JC, Cook EF, O'Day SJ, et al. Relationship between cancer patients' predictions of prognosis and their treatment preferences. *JAMA*. 1998;279:1709–14.

20. Fried TR, Bradley EH, Towle VR, et al. Understanding the treatment preferences of seriously ill patients. *N Engl J Med*. 2002;346:1061–66.

21. Ritchie L. Integration of chronic illness care into a primary healthcare focused nursing curriculum. *Nurse Educ*. 2012;37:23–24.

22. Dent MM, Mathis MW, Outland M, et al. Chronic disease management: teaching medical students to incorporate community. *Fam Med*. 2010;42:736–40.

23. Nieman LZ, Cheng L. Chronic illness needs educated doctors: an innovative primary care training program for chronic illness education. *Med Teach*. 2011;33:e340–48.

24. Mayer RS, Shah A, DeLateur BJ, et al. Proposal for a required advanced clerkship in chronic disease and disability for medical students. *Am J Phys Med Rehabil*. 2008;87:162–67.

25. Nieman LZ. Chronic condition self-management and two teaching models for chronic conditions. *Chronic Illn*. 2009;5:15–17.

26. Bricker PL, Baron RJ, Scheirer JJ, et al. Collaboration in Pennsylvania: rapidly spreading improved chronic care for patients to practices. *J Contin Educ Health Prof*. 2010;30:114–25.

27. Newton W, Baxley E, Reid A, et al. Improving chronic illness care in teaching practices: learnings from the I(3) collaborative. *Fam Med*. 2011;43:495–502.

28. Stevens DP, Bowen JL, Johnson JK, et al. A multi-institutional quality improvement initiative to transform education for chronic illness care in resident continuity practices. *J Gen Intern Med*. 2010;25(Suppl 4):S574–80.

29. Yu GC, Beresford R. Implementation of a chronic illness model for diabetes care in a family medicine residency program. *J Gen Intern Med*. 2010;25(Suppl 4):S615–19.

30. Christakis NA, Iwashyna TJ. Attitude and self-reported practice regarding prognostication in a national sample of internists. *Arch Intern Med*. 1998;158:2389–95.

31. Kissane DW, Byland CL, Banerjee SC, et al. Communication skills training for oncology professionals. *J Clin Oncol*. 2012; 30:1242–47.

32. Montagnini M, Varkey B, Duthie E Jr. Palliative care education integrated into a geriatrics rotation for resident physicians. *J Palliat Med*. 2004;7:652–59.

33. Lim LS, Kandavelou K, Khan N. Palliative care teaching in medical residency: a review of two POGO-e teaching products. *J Am Geriatr Soc*. 2012;60:1141–44.

34. Reuben DB, Zwanziger J, Bradley TB, et al. How many physicians will be needed to provide medical care for older persons? Physician manpower needs for the twenty-first century. *J Am Geriatr Soc*. 1993;41:444–53.

35. Green ML, Aagaard EM, Caverzagie KJ, et al. Charting the road to competence: developmental milestones for internal medicine residency training. *J Grad Med Educ*. 2009;1:5–20.

36. Williams BC, Warshaw G, Fabiny AR, et al. Medicine in the 21st century: recommended essential geriatrics competencies for internal medicine and family medicine residents. *J Grad Med Educ*. 2010;2:373–83.

37. Butow PN, Dowsett S, Hagerty R, et al. Communicating prognosis to patients with metastatic disease: what do they really want to know? *Support Care Cancer*. 2002;10:161–68.

38. Wittenberg-Lyles EM, Goldsmith J, Sanchez-Reilly S, et al. Communicating a terminal prognosis in a palliative care setting: deficiencies in current communication training protocols. *Soc Sci Med*. 2008;66:2356–65.

39. Schoenborn NL, McNabney M, Cayea D, Boyd C. Developing a curriculum for medicine residents on incorporating prognosis in the care of older adults with multimorbidity. *J Gen Intern Med*. 2013;8(S1):S59–60.

40. Schoenborn NL, McNabney M, Cayea D, Boyd C. Developing a curriculum for medicine residents on incorporating prognosis in the care of older adults with multimorbidity. *J Am Geriatr Soc*. 2013;61(S1):S45.

LONGITUDINAL PROGRAM IN CURRICULUM DEVELOPMENT

David E. Kern, MD, MPH, and Belinda Y. Chen, MD

This curriculum was originally developed as part of a faculty development grant proposal to the Bureau of Health Professions, Health Resources and Services Administration, U.S. Public Health Service, in 1986 and was implemented as part of the Johns Hopkins Faculty Development Program for Clinician-Educators in 1987–88. Faculty involved in its initial development included David E. Kern, MD, MPH, Donna H. Howard, RN, DrPH, L. Randol Barker, MD, ScM, Penelope R. Williamson, ScD, and Laura M. Mumford, MD. Additional faculty involved in its subsequent maintenance and enhancement include Eric B. Bass, MD, Belinda Y. Chen, MD, Karan A. Cole, ScD, Mark T. Hughes, MD, Najlla Nassery, MD, MPH, Stephen D. Sisson, MD, Henry G. Taylor, MD, MPH, Patricia A. Thomas, MD, and Leah Wolfe, MD.

Step 1: Problem Identification and General Needs Assessment

This needs assessment has evolved since the original application, based on faculty needs and an evolving literature.

Problem Identification	• Deficiencies have been demonstrated in the knowledge, skills, and behaviors of practicing physicians and graduating students and residents, as well as in related health care outcomes (1–8).
	• The Liaison Committee on Medical Education, the Accreditation Council for Graduate Medical Education (ACGME), the Accreditation Council for Continuing Medical Education, and other organizations have called for curricular changes to enhance the ability of physicians to fulfill their societal contract of providing high-quality medical care (9–18).
	• Medical education requires ongoing curriculum development (CD) to disseminate new knowledge, incorporate revised competencies (19–20), and enable learners to achieve competencies with increased efficiency and effectiveness (16, 20).
Current Approach	• Medical schools and residency and continuing education programs are required to define learning objectives and methods for their learners (9–11).
	• These programs are expected to demonstrate the attainment of program objectives and trainee competencies (9–11).
	• Despite demands for curricular change and the recognition of CD as a faculty development need (21, 22), most faculty have no formal instruction in education or CD (23).
	• Curricula produced are often suboptimal and do not follow CD principles (24, 25).

- Although better funding results in better research and development, funding for medical education is limited (26–28).

- At the time of the inception of the program, a few faculty development programs existed but tended not to focus on CD or had not published their programs' results. Since then, several publications have described faculty training programs that include training in CD (29–40).

- Master of Education in the Health Professions (MEHP) programs have proliferated and address CD as a skill (41). However, most faculty tasked with CD do not have these credentials.

Ideal Approach	- Curriculum developers should be trained in knowledge and skills to produce high-quality curricula.

- Curriculum developers should be trained in knowledge and skills to produce high-quality curricula.

- Generic approaches to CD have been articulated by Taba, Tyler, Yura, and others (42–45) and should be adapted for the unique requirements/goals of medical professional training.

- McGaghie et al. and Golden, more than 30 years ago, articulated the importance of linking curricula in medical education to health care needs (46, 47). Cooke et al. reinforced the importance of such grounding in their 2010 call for medical school and residency education reform (16).

- A six-step approach was developed from the educational literature and adapted for a specifically medical focus and has been articulated in a standard, widely used book on the subject (25).

- Training in CD should include generally recommended methods for developing research and educational scholarship skills: skills training sessions, involvement in projects, protected time, and regular meetings with and feedback from mentors and/or peers (31, 39, 48–52). To help with time management, provide additional support, and stimulate progress, the authors added to their curriculum periodic deadlines, work-in-progress presentations, and the oral and written presentation of a final project. Several of these methods were subsequently used by other faculty development programs (30–35, 37–39).

- Involving trainees in a community of peers and role models who are successfully applying and reflecting on CD principles should help support desired attitudes about CD as an important academic skill and scholarly activity. (See Chapter 5, Educational Strategies, "Methods for Achieving Affective Objectives.")

Step 2: Targeted Needs Assessment

Targeted Learners	▪ Initially, General Internal Medicine (GIM) faculty and fellows from Johns Hopkins Medical Institutions and the geographic region
	▪ Subsequently expanded to faculty and fellows from all divisions and departments
Needs Assessment/ Targeted Learners	▪ Based on the curriculum developers' knowledge and informal information gathering, no faculty training in CD existed at Johns Hopkins at the time of the program's inception. No survey was done.
	▪ Later, a survey of all medical schools was performed as part of a national project (23).
Needs Assessment/ Targeted Learning Environment	▪ There were no related curricula available to faculty.
	▪ There were no funds available to support such a program.
	▪ There was little demand or awareness of need by institutional leaders.
	▪ However, the department chair and other institutional leaders were pleased by the opportunity for external funding.
	▪ As the program was successfully implemented, it came to be viewed as an important resource for improving educational programs.
	▪ As the approach taught in the program gained wide recognition, such an approach has come to be expected as part of institution-wide curricular reform.

Step 3: Goals and Objectives

Goals	The overarching goal of the program is for participants to develop the knowledge, attitudes, and skills required to design, implement, evaluate, and disseminate effective medical curricula.
Objectives	By the end of the program, participants will achieve the following:

1. Rate themselves as skilled in the six steps of curriculum development:

   a. problem identification and general needs assessment
   b. targeted needs assessment
   c. goals and objectives
   d. educational strategies: content and methods

  e. implementation
  f. evaluation and feedback

2. Demonstrate their knowledge and skill by having designed, piloted, and formulated plans for implementation of a curriculum in medical education relevant to a documented health care need.

3. Be practiced in the skills necessary for presenting their work to the academic community. These skills include: 1) verbal presentation of one's work and 2) preparation of a paper describing one's work, for the purposes of obtaining support for funding, sharing information, or publication.

4. Agree that CD is both an essential skill for educational leaders and a scholarly activity.

By one year after completion of the program, participants will have implemented their curriculum.

Step 4: Educational Strategies

The educational strategies were based on the ideal approach as identified in Step 1: Problem Identification and General Needs Assessment. Educational methods were selected to be congruent with the type of educational objectives.

Knowledge objectives were addressed through readings and mini-lectures during workshops and reinforced through discussion and application of the knowledge. Psychomotor objectives were achieved by having participants develop, present, and write up a real curriculum, supported by ongoing mentoring, discussion, and feedback; participants were supported by having protected time and having the project broken down into component steps with associated deadlines. Affective objectives were addressed by immersing participants in a logical approach to CD supported by the existing educational literature, enabling them to have a successful experience, exposing them to other successful curricular development examples and projects, and including them in a community of medical educators. Having participants present their work to professional audiences and having them produce a final manuscript served both psychomotor and attitudinal objectives.

Content	• The six steps of curriculum development
	• Literature searching skills
	• Online approaches to asynchronous group work
	• Survey design skills
	• Use of information technology to support education
	• Use of simulation in medical education

- Obtaining institutional review board (IRB) approval for educational projects

- Finding and applying for funding support for curriculum-related work

- Presenting, writing up, and submitting for publication curriculum-related work

Methods	The one half-day per week, 10-month longitudinal program includes the following:

- Workshops on each of the CD steps and related topics

- Readings (handouts, CD text (25), and selected articles on the above topics)

- A mentored project, with participants organized into curriculum teams focused on the development of a predetermined curriculum (participants apply and are organized into curricular teams before acceptance into the program). The process includes:

  - protected time for independent work

  - deadlines for outlines and written drafts of each CD step

  - meetings with experienced facilitators for 1 hour every 4 to 6 weeks to discuss progress and receive written feedback on their work

  - end-of-year paper on their curriculum

  - end-of-year presentation before a professional audience

- Work-in-progress sessions where participants present their needs assessment instruments, curricular segments, evaluation instruments, and other aspects of their work to facilitators and other course participants

Step 5: Implementation

Implementation of a program that resembled an ideal approach was greatly helped by sufficient external funding.

Resources	*Personnel:*

- Faculty administrator (6% FTE)

- Faculty facilitators (1.5% FTE for each mentored curriculum, 6% FTE for facilitating and presenting at total group sessions)

- Guest speakers for special topics

- Administrative coordinator (35% FTE)

Facilities, Equipment, Materials:

- Space: large conference room with one or two breakout rooms for workshops; small conference room for meetings of the project team with the facilitator

- Other: LCD projector, whiteboards/flip charts, learning management software for posting curricular materials, textbook, videoconferencing/recording equipment for distant/asynchronous learning and for review

Funding: The Bureau of Health Professions, Health Resources and Services Administration, U.S. Public Health Service, provided grant support in all but one year from 1987 to 2006. In 1993, the program introduced tuition to partly cover expenses, incorporating the existing tuition/CME benefit for full-time faculty. The program became financially independent as of 2006.

Support	- Initially, a competitively awarded external grant for primary care faculty development garnered critical institutional and departmental support. - Subsequently, the program built a reputation as the faculty development home for educators. - With increasing financial independence, the program became a resource for training faculty and fellows from all divisions and departments.
Administration	- Faculty administrator: constructs a yearly budget for the program, coordinates an annual application for CME accreditation, interviews applicants, screens proposed projects to promote the likelihood of successful implementation, and oversees all operations. - Faculty Planning Committee: reviews the yearly evaluation of the program and proposes curricular updates for the ensuing year. - Office of CME: handles tuition payments and CME credit and, along with the Office of Faculty Development, assists with marketing the program to potential applicants. - Administrative coordinator: provides general administrative, communications, evaluations, scheduling, and secretarial support.
Barriers	- Funding barriers: initially overcome by external funding; subsequently decreased by options for tuition support. Tuition is a barrier for participants from other institutions without tuition benefit. - Single participant projects are less likely to be successful and pose financial challenges to the program in terms of facilitator support.

- Emphasis on group project learning and facilitation may be a barrier to enrollment for participants unable to find a team.

- Protecting time: a specific half-day per week for 10 months.

- Faculty development: a sufficient number of faculty have now been trained to facilitate individual projects during years when a relatively large number of projects are enrolled.

- Alternative training programs: there are now more opportunities for faculty to get varying levels of training in CD, both within and beyond this institution. (See the sections "Curriculum Maintenance and Enhancement" and "Dissemination," below.)

| Introduction | The program was fully implemented in 1987 with external funding to faculty and fellows in the funded division who were interested and had their time protected for participation. Subsequently, the funding was made available to faculty from all departments and divisions (see above). |

Step 6: Evaluation

Early planning for the evaluation permitted the identification of desired outcomes and evaluation questions, construction of useful questionnaire instruments, and inclusion of a comparison group for cohorts 2 through 9 of the program. External funding was helpful but resources were limited, so the program had to rely primarily on participant self-report for assessment of skill attainment and subsequent behaviors. However, low-cost objective measures such as implementation of curricular projects and publications were included. To reduce data collection effort and boost response rates, questionnaires were administered as part of the program whenever possible. Participants and controls received a popular clinical textbook, produced by the department and available to the program at much reduced cost, as an incentive to boost response rates for the long-term follow-up study. GIM medical education fellows, supported by division grants, used evaluation of the program as mentored research projects that resulted in first-authored publications (53, 54).

Users	Predominantly curriculum faculty, but also the funding agency, CME office, and prospective participants.
Uses	Formative information to guide improvement of the curriculum for the faculty administrator and faculty facilitators; summative information for the external funding agency, for the CME office on program effectiveness/worthiness of continued support, and for dissemination.
Resources	External grant support in all but one year from 1987 to 2006 funded questionnaire development, administration, and collation. Tuition now covers the costs of ongoing evaluations, as described below. Divisional grants supported research projects to study long-term outcomes.

Evaluation Questions	A. Ongoing evaluation for formative and summative program evaluation (internal uses):

A. Ongoing evaluation for formative and summative program evaluation (internal uses):

1) Do participants in the program improve their self-assessed skills in CD?

2) Do participants produce and implement curricula as a result of participation?

3) How are the program components and facilitators rated by participants?

4) What are the program's strengths and weaknesses as perceived by the participants?

B. Additional evaluation for external funding agency and dissemination:

1) Do participants in the program improve their self-assessed skills in CD compared with nonparticipants?

2) What type of curricula are produced? Is work related to their curricula published?

3) Do participants continue to rate their skills, and their improvement in skills, more highly than nonparticipants years after completion of the program?

4) Are participants more active in CD than nonparticipants years after completion of the program?

5) What is the perceived impact of the program on its participants years after completion of the program?

Evaluation Design

A1) O_1 - - - - X - - - - O_2

A2–4)   X - - - - O_2

B1) E O_1 - - - - X - - - - O_2

   C O_1 - - - - - - - - - O_2

B2)   X - - - - O_2

B3) E O_1 - - - - X - - - - O_2 - O_3

   C O_1 - - - - - - - - - O_2 - O_3

B4) E   X - O_3

   C   - O_3

B5)   X - O_3

Evaluation Methods and Instruments   A1–4)

O_1: Survey of previous training and self-rated skills in CD.

O_2: Self-rated skills in CD, Likert-scale ratings of course components and facilitators, open-response feedback on course components and facilitators, documentation of final presentation and paper.

B1–5)

O_1: Same as O_1 above but also included matched controls who did not participate in this program.

O_2: Same as O_2 above plus facilitator and participant documentation of curricular implementation, classification of curricula produced by learner type and topic, and count of number of publications related to curricula produced.

O_3: Long-term follow-up survey of selected cohorts and matched controls inquiring about self-rated CD skills, reported CD behaviors, recent CD activities, and educational career path/achievements. Perceived impact of program for participants only.

Ethical Concerns	A Johns Hopkins IRB determined that immediate pre-post evaluation qualified for exemption from review under guidelines regarding educational program evaluation. The IRB also approved the long-term follow-up study. Responses were kept confidential, and findings were presented only in aggregate in a manner that maintains respondents' confidentiality.
Data Collection	A brief survey was sent electronically at the end of each class. More detailed surveys were sent at midterm and the end of the course. The administrative coordinator reminded participants weekly to complete the scheduled evaluations. Completion of the final survey is a requirement of the course, but responses are deidentified once the survey results are received. For the long-term outcome study, the principal investigator followed up until a response rate of >75% was obtained. Respondents received a free clinical textbook as an incentive.
Data Analysis	The administrative coordinator collated and performed descriptive statistical analysis on the immediate pre-post data for local formative and summative evaluation. For the additional studies for dissemination, the study principal investigators performed data entry and analysis with assistance from a statistical consultant.
Reporting of Results	Collated weekly evaluation results, with simple descriptive statistics, were distributed to the faculty for formative feedback. Shortly after completion of the program, the final course evaluation and summative evaluation results were shared with the Faculty Planning Committee for use in planning the following year's program.

Analysis and preparation of manuscripts for dissemination of mul-
tiyear evaluations were conducted over many months by a study
team of fellows who were graduates of the program and program
faculty. The manuscripts were submitted to peer-reviewed journals for publication (53, 54).

Curriculum Maintenance and Enhancement

Curriculum maintenance and enhancement are supported by ongoing faculty development, an experienced and committed faculty, affirmation through strong evaluations and program successes, periodic meetings, faculty interactions with educational
leaders beyond the institution, dissemination and scholarly work, and development of
ongoing funding for the program.

Understanding the Curriculum	The faculty administrator maintains a good understanding of the curriculum through presence at all total group meetings, periodic review of the progress of each curriculum project team with other facilitators, review of all evaluation results, informal discussions with participants and other facilitators, and yearly formal planning meetings.
Management of Change	Changes during the course of the year are made by the faculty administrator in response to formative feedback from participants and facilitators and in consultation with the other facilitators. At the annual evaluation and planning meeting each summer, the Faculty Planning Committee discusses and decides upon larger changes.

Examples of changes based on yearly evaluations:

- Sessions added over the years include: 1) writing for publication, Internet resources for curriculum development, and finding and applying for funding in 2002; 2) searching educational
databases and obtaining IRB approval in 2004; 3) survey
design in 2007; 4) use of simulation in medical education in
2008; 5) use of information technology to support education in
2011; 6) online approaches to asynchronous group work
in 2012; and 7) incorporation of the flipped classroom in 2013.

- As the years have passed, facilitators have focused increasingly on the implementation step of curriculum development.
For the first 16 cohorts, 84% of the curricula developed were
fully or partly implemented (53).

- In 2003, the faculty initiated a process for interviewing prospective participants and having them form project groups
before day 1 of the course. This process increased support
within the participants' departments, allowed groups to start
doing meaningful work at the first class session, increased the

likelihood of successful implementation, and provided insight into the needs of participants.

- Feedback from prospective and former participants led the faculty to tailor alternative programs to meet the CD training needs of faculty who cannot commit to the full longitudinal program. These alternative programs currently include half-day and two-day workshops, a CD mentoring program, customized CD workshops tailored to specific departments or schools, and an online course for the Johns Hopkins MEHP program.

Faculty Development Development of an expert faculty has been crucial to curriculum maintenance and enhancement.

- All of the facilitators in the program were trained in or involved in developing the program.

- A facilitator-in-training program was developed so that program graduates can work alongside an experienced facilitator during their first year as faculty.

- The development of alternative CD courses has increased faculty involvement with ongoing curriculum development. For example, in 2013–14, there were six participants and three projects in the full longitudinal program. However, the expanded faculty development program offerings reached an additional 39 participants and 20 projects and provided opportunity for seven faculty to remain involved in CD facilitation. An additional 26 participants (26 projects) were reached through the online MEHP curriculum development course.

Sustaining the Curriculum Team Several methods are used:

- CD facilitators receive salary support for their contributions to the program; the tuition charged ensures this support.

- Facilitators are involved not only in implementing the curriculum but also in the ongoing curriculum maintenance and enhancement processes, as described above.

- Review of collated evaluation results, final papers, and abstract presentations provides feedback about facilitator and team success.

- Project teams have sometimes acknowledged the significant contribution of a facilitator by including him or her on a relevant publication or on a grant.

Networking, Innovation, and Scholarly Activity CD facilitators have achieved the following:

- Presented workshops, courses, and abstracts on CD and interacted with educational leaders at other institutions, nationally and internationally

- Presented workshops on disseminating curricular work and edited a medical education issue of a major journal that included curriculum-related publications with colleagues from other institutions

- Authored several publications related to or stimulated by this curriculum (see below)

Dissemination

Dissemination has occurred in the form of both CME activities and publications.

Target Audience	- Educational program directors and other medical faculty who plan educational experiences, often without having received training or acquired experience in such endeavors and often in the presence of limited resources and significant institutional constraints.
Reasons for Dissemination	- Improve the quality of medical education - Help curriculum developers (in the authors' team and others) achieve recognition and academic advancement for curriculum-related work
Content	- National survey on status of faculty development (23) - CD principles and communication of a practical, theoretically sound approach to developing, implementing, evaluating, and constantly improving educational experiences in medicine (25) - Description and evaluations of the Longitudinal Program in Curriculum Development (53, 54) - Publications related to curricula developed by participants in the Longitudinal Program (see Chapter 9, Dissemination, "Specific References," references 6–8, 48–51, 81–83)
Methods	- Development of half-day and two-day workshops at Johns Hopkins (55) - Development of a longitudinal mentoring program at Johns Hopkins for individuals already trained in CD (55) - Development of a 12-week online asynchronous CD course as part of the Johns Hopkins MEHP program (56) - Workshops and courses on CD at other institutions in the United States and other countries

- Book publication (25)
- Peer-reviewed journal articles (23, 53, 54)

Resources	• Faculty expertise developed through review of existing literature, interaction with colleagues from other institutions, years of experience teaching in the Longitudinal Program in CD and in workshops/courses, and publishing work on the subject
	• Semi-protected academic time of some faculty and reimbursement for travel, supported by a Division of General Internal Medicine fund and external grant support
	• Funding for a statistical consultant from external grant support and a Division of General Internal Medicine fund
	• External grant support until 2006 (see above)

REFERENCES

1. Beckman HB, Frankel RM. The effect of physician behavior on the collection of data. *Ann Intern Med.* 1984;101:692–96.
2. Feinstein RE, Blumenfield M, Orlowski B, Frishman WH, Ovanessian S. A national survey of cardiovascular physicians' beliefs and clinical care practices when diagnosing and treating depression in patients with cardiovascular disease. *Cardiol Rev.* 2006;14:164–69.
3. Hanlon JT, Schmader KE, Ruby CM, Weinberger M. Suboptimal prescribing in older inpatients and outpatients. *J Am Geriatr Soc.* 2001;49:200–209.
4. Hannon EL, Racz MJ, Gold J, et al. Adherence of catheterization laboratory cardiologists to American College of Cardiology/American Heart Association guidelines for percutaneous coronary interventions and coronary artery bypass graft surgery: what happens in actual practice? *Circulation.* 2010;121:267–75.
5. Moore C, Wisnivesky J, Williams S, McGinn T. Medical errors related to discontinuity of care from an inpatient to an outpatient setting. *J Gen Intern Med.* 2003;18:646–51.
6. Roberts NK, Dorsey JK, Wold B. Unprofessional behavior by specialty: a qualitative analysis of six years of student perceptions of medical school faculty. *Med Teach.* 2014;36(7):621–25.
7. Shah BR, Hux JE, Laupacis A, Zinman B, Zwarenstein M. Deficiencies in the quality of diabetes care: comparing specialist with generalist care misses the point. *J Gen Intern Med.* 2007;22:275–79.
8. von Muhlen M, Ohno-Machado L. Reviewing social media use by clinicians. *J Am Med Inform Assoc.* 2012;19:777–81.
9. Liaison Committee on Medical Education. Functions and Structure of a Medical School: Standards for Accreditation of Medical Education Programs Leading to an M.D. Degree. [Internet]. March 2014. Available at www.lcme.org.
10. Accreditation Council on Graduate Medical Education. Common Program Requirements [Internet]. Available at www.acgme.org.
11. Accreditation Council for Continuing Medical Education. Accreditation Requirements and Descriptions of the Accreditation Council for Continuing Medical Education (ACCME) [Internet]. Updated June 2014. Available at www.accme.org.
12. Institute of Medicine. *Health Professions Education: A Bridge to Quality.* Washington, D.C.: National Academies Press; 2003.

13. Blue Ridge Academic Health Group. *Reforming Medical Education: Urgent Priority for Academic Health Centers in the New Century.* Atlanta: Robert W. Woodruff Health Sciences Center; 2003.
14. Institute of Medicine. *Academic Health Centers: Leading Change in the 21st Century.* Washington, D.C.: National Academies Press; 2004.
15. Institute of Medicine. *Improving Medical Education: Enhancing the Behavioral and Social Science Content of Medical School Curricula.* Washington, D.C.: National Academies Press; 2004.
16. Cooke M, Irby DM, O'Brien BC, Carnegie Foundation for the Advancement of Teaching. *Educating Physicians: A Call for Reform of Medical School and Residency.* San Francisco: Jossey-Bass; 2010.
17. Blue Ridge Academic Health Group. *Health Professions Education: Accelerating Innovation through Technology.* Atlanta: Robert W. Woodruff Health Sciences Center; 2013.
18. Institute of Medicine. *Graduate Medical Education That Meets the Nation's Health Needs.* Washington, D.C.: National Academies Press; 2014.
19. Epstein R, Hundert E. Defining and assessing professional competence. *JAMA.* 2002; 287(2):226–35.
20. Weinberger SE, Pereira AG, Iobst WF, Mechaber AJ, Bronze MS, Alliance for Academic Internal Medicine Education Redesign Task Force II. Competency-based education and training in internal medicine. *Ann Intern Med.* 2010;153:751–56.
21. Sherbino J, Frank JR, Snell L. Defining roles and competencies of the clinician-educator of the 21st century: a national mixed-methods study. *Acad Med.* 2014;89:783–89.
22. Harris DL, Krause KC, Parish DC, Smith MU. Academic competencies for medical faculty. *Fam Med.* 2007;39:343–50.
23. Clark JM, Houston TK, Kolodner K, et al. Teaching the teachers: national survey of faculty development in departments of medicine of U.S. teaching hospitals. *J Gen Intern Med.* 2004;19(3):205–14.
24. Sheets KJ, Anderson WA. The reporting of curriculum development activities in the health professions. *Teach Learn Med.* 1991;3(4):221–26.
25. Kern DE, Thomas PA, Hughes MT, eds. *Curriculum Development for Medical Education: A Six-Step Approach*, 2nd ed. Baltimore: Johns Hopkins University Press; 2009.
26. Kern DE. Achievements and challenges in medical education. *SGIM Forum.* 2003;26(8):1, 6–7.
27. Reed D, Kern DE, Levine RB, Wright SM. Costs and funding for published medical education research. *JAMA.* 2005;294:1052–57.
28. Reed DA, Cook DA, Beckman TJ, et al. Association between funding and quality of published medical education research. *JAMA.* 2007;298:1002–9.
29. Anderson WA, Stritter FT, Mygdal WK, Arndt JE, Reid A. Outcomes of three part-time faculty development programs. *Fam Med.* 1997;29(3):204–8.
30. Armstrong EG, Doyle J, Bennett NL. Transformative professional development of physicians as educators: assessment of a model. *Acad Med.* 2003;78(7):702–8.
31. Bland CJ, VanLoy W, Wersal L. Lessons learned from a distance-based consulting program to assist faculty development projects. *Acad Med.* 2001;76:776–90.
32. Daley S, Wingard W, Reznik V. Improving the retention of underrepresented minority faculty in academic medicine. *J Natl Med Assoc.* 2006;98:1435–40.
33. Frohna AZ, Hamstra SJ, Mullan PB, Gruppen LD. Teaching medical education principles and methods to faculty using an active learning approach: the University of Michigan Education Scholars Program. *Acad Med.* 2006;81:975–78.
34. Gruppen LD, Frohna AZ, Anderson RM, Lowe KD. Faculty development for educational leadership and scholarship. *Acad Med.* 2003;78(2):137–41.
35. Hunt J, Stubbe DE, Hanson M, et al. A 2-year progress report of the AACAP-Harvard Macy Teaching Scholars Program. *Acad Psychiatry.* 2008;32:414–19.

36. Leslie K, Baker L, Egan-Lee E, Esdaile M, Reeves S. Advancing faculty development in medical education: a systematic review. *Acad Med.* 2013;88:1038–45.
37. Rosenbaum ME, Lenoch S, Ferguson KJ. Outcomes of a teaching scholars program to promote leadership in faculty development. *Teach Learn Med.* 2005;17(3):247–52.
38. Snyder S. A program to teach curriculum development to junior faculty. *Fam Med.* 2001; 33(5):382–87.
39. Steinert Y, Nasmith L, McLeod PJ, Conochie L. A teaching scholars program to develop leaders in medical education. *Acad Med.* 2003;78(2):142–49.
40. Yudkowsky R, Tekain A. A model workshop in curriculum development for international medical audiences. *Med Teach.* 1998;20:258–60.
41. Tekian A, Harris I. Preparing health professions education leaders worldwide: a description of masters-level programs. *Med Teach.* 2012;34;52–58.
42. Taba H. *Curriculum Development: Theory and Practice.* New York: Harcourt, Brace, & World; 1962. Pp. 1–515.
43. Tyler RW. *Basic Principles of Curriculum and Instruction.* Chicago: University of Chicago Press; 1950. Pp. 1–83.
44. Yura H, Torres GJ, eds. *Faculty-Curriculum Development: Curriculum Design by Nursing Faculty.* New York: National League for Nursing; 1986. Publication No. 15-2164. Pp. 1-371.
45. Sheets KJ, Anderson WA, Alguire PC. Curriculum development and evaluation in medical education: annotated bibliography. *J Gen Intern Med* 1992;7(5):538–43.
46. McGaghie WC, Miller GE, Sajid AW, Telder TV. *Competency Based Curriculum Development in Medical Education: An Introduction.* Geneva: World Health Organization; 1978. Pp. 1–99.
47. Golden AS. A model for curriculum development linking curriculum with health needs. In: Golden AS, Carlson DG, Hogan JL, eds. *The Art of Teaching Primary Care.* New York: Springer Publishing Co.; 1982. Pp. 9–25.
48. Saha S, Christakis DA, Saint S, Whooley MA, Simon SR. A survival guide for generalist physicians in academic fellowships. Part 1: getting started. *J Gen Intern Med.* 1999;14(12): 745–49.
49. Loscalzo J, Tomaselli GF, Vaughan DE, Walsh RA. Task force 7: training in cardiovascular research. *J Am Coll Cardiol.* 2008:51:380–83.
50. Yager J, Greden J, Abrams M, Riba M. The Institute of Medicine's report on Research Training in Psychiatry Residency: Strategies for Reform—background, results, and follow up. *Acad Psychiatry.* 2004;28:267–74.
51. Sambunjak D, Straus SE, Marusic A. Mentoring in academic medicine: a systematic review. *JAMA.* 2006;296:1103–15.
52. Sambunjak D, Straus SE, Marusic A. A systematic review of qualitative research on the meaning and characteristics of mentoring in academic medicine. *J Gen Intern Med.* 2010 Jan;25(1):72–78.
53. Windish DM, Gozu A, Bass EB, et al. A ten-month program in curriculum development for medical educators: 16 years of experience. *J Gen Intern Med.* 2007;22:655–61.
54. Gozu A, Windish DM, Knight AM, et al. Long-term follow-up of a ten-month program in curriculum development for medical educators: a cohort study. *Med Educ.* 2008;42:684–92.
55. Johns Hopkins Faculty Development Program [Internet]. Available at www.hopkinsmedicine .org/jhbmc/fdp.
56. Johns Hopkins Master of Education in the Health Professions [Internet]. Available at http: //education.jhu.edu/Academics/masters/MEHP.

APPENDIX B

Curricular, Faculty Development, and Funding Resources

Patricia A. Thomas, MD, and David E. Kern, MD, MPH

Lists of specific and annotated general references appear at the end of each chapter. These lists provide the reader with access to predominantly published resources on curriculum development and evaluation. Recognizing that most people begin searches for information by looking at *online resources*, this appendix focuses mainly on online information resources for curriculum development. The appendix is organized by providing a selected list of resources for the steps of curriculum development, such as general needs assessment, learning objectives, educational strategies, and evaluation, including already developed curricula. It also provides a selected list of resources for faculty development and funding. Not meant to be all-inclusive, the lists include resources that have been relatively stable over time and useful to the authors. All websites were reviewed in March 2015 and accessed again in August 2015.

CURRICULAR RESOURCES

When searching for additional resources related to medical education curricula, we recommend the following approach (1):

a. Review websites and publications of the major accrediting bodies for medical accreditation standards that might apply to the curriculum once implemented and for other resources.

b.   Review resources and organizations devoted to particular topics or fields.

c.   Review general educational resources within medicine.

d.   Review general educational resources beyond medicine.

Many of these organizations sponsor meetings and peer-reviewed publications, a potential resource for the dissemination of the curriculum or its evaluation.

Oversight and Accreditation Organizations

- *Association of American Medical Colleges (AAMC):* The AAMC represents 141 U.S. and 17 Canadian medical schools and hundreds of teaching hospitals and health systems, as well as professional societies. The AAMC collects data and surveys and publishes annual reports on a number of topics related to Step 1: workforce, applicant, student, and resident surveys, as well as faculty and teaching hospital statistics. The Group on Educational Affairs (GEA) sponsors meetings and scholarship related to medical education. The AAMC publishes *Academic Medicine* and other publications helpful as general needs assessment resources. Available at www.aamc.org.

- *Accreditation Council for Continuing Medical Education (ACCME):* The ACCME is a voluntary accreditation body for CME-related activities and sets the standards for qualifying educational programs. Its website contains faculty development materials for those attempting to meet standards. Available at www.accme.org.

- *Accreditation Council for Graduate Medical Education (ACGME):* The ACGME is charged with accreditation of clinical residency training programs and is made up of five sponsoring organizations: the American Hospital Association, the American Medical Association (AMA), the AAMC, the American Board of Medical Specialties, and the Council of Medical Specialty Societies. The website lists specific program requirements for each specialty. ACGME sponsors an annual Education Retreat and the online *Journal of Graduate Medical Education*. Available at www.acgme.org.

- *American Medical Association (AMA):* The largest professional organization of physicians in the United States, the AMA has particular interest in professionalism and ethics (publication *Virtual Mentor*). Its Council on Medical Education formulates educational policy and makes recommendations to the AMA. FREIDA Online is a resource for medical students to research and track residency programs. There is an annual edition of the journal *JAMA* devoted to medical education. Professional resources and information are available at www.ama-assn.org.

- *American Osteopathic Association (AOA):* This organization is charged with accreditation of predoctoral DO degrees in the United States. Accreditation standards can be found on the website. As of 2015, the DO residency accreditation system begins a transition to ACGME accreditation. The AOA website is www.osteopathic.org.

- *General Medical Council (GMC):* The GMC registers and provides oversight for all practicing physicians in the United Kingdom. The GMC has published its standards for undergraduate medical education, *Tomorrow's Doctors*, as well as supplementary materials on assessment, faculty development, and clinical placements for students (available at www.gmc-uk.org/Tomorrow_s_Doctors_1214.pdf_48905759.pdf. The GMC also conducts training surveys and reports on its findings, most recently on topics of patient safety and undermining (bullying) in the learning environment. Home page is www.gmc-uk.org.

- *Liaison Committee on Medical Education (LCME):* This is a joint committee of the AMA and the AAMC (above) that has been recognized by the U.S. Department of Education as the official accreditation body for the MD degree. The LCME has developed curricular standards for the undergraduate program that are available in the document *Functions and Structure of a Medical School*, available at www.lcme .org; click on "Standards."

- *Society for Simulation in Health Care (SSIH):* This accrediting organization for simulation centers publishes accreditation standards as well as guides for accreditation self-study. A number of resources and webinars are available on the website; the organization sponsors an annual meeting of simulation educators. Available at www.ssih.org.

Topic-related Resources and Organizations

Basic Science

- *International Association of Medical Science Educators (IAMSE):* IAMSE is an international organization concerned with basic science medical education. It sponsors a peer-reviewed journal, *Medical Science Educator*, and an annual meeting and hosts faculty development resources. The website is an excellent source of content related to basic science education and a potential resource for dissemination. Available at www.iamse.org.

Clinical Sciences

- *Alliance for Clinical Education (ACE):* This is an umbrella organization for seven specialty medical student clerkship organizations. Its website contains links to all of these organizations, as well as a faculty development resource, the *Guidebook for Clerkship Directors, The Handbook on Medical Student Evaluation and Assessment*, and panel presentations from AAMC meetings, such as "Portfolios in Clinical Medical Education." Available at www.allianceforclinicaleducation.org.

- Curriculum developers working in a particular clerkship should review that specialty's website (see below) for developed core curricula that have been nationally peer-reviewed. Examples are the *Clerkship Directors in Internal Medicine Core Curriculum Guide v.3.0* (available at www.im.org under "Publications for Faculty") and the *Educational Clearinghouse* for the Association for Surgical Education (available at www.surgicaleducation.com).

Bioethics

- *American Society of Bioethics and Humanities (ASBH):* This organization includes multidisciplinary and interdisciplinary professionals in academic and clinical bioethics and medical humanities. Publications include *Core Competencies for Health Care Ethics Consultation* and a companion *Education Guide*, available from the website. In 2009, the ASBH published the *Report on Ethics and Humanities in Undergraduate Medical Education Programs* (appropriate for "Current Approach" in Step 1). Available at www.asbh.org.

Communication, Behavioral and Psychosocial Medicine

- *American Academy on Communication in Healthcare (AACH):* AACH is dedicated to advocating patient-centered health care communication (see Faculty Development resources, below). It hosts an interactive online curriculum to teach communication skills (DocCom), a newsletter, *Medical Encounter,* and numerous other resources. Available at www.aachonline.org.
- *Association for the Behavioral Sciences and Medical Education (ABSAME):* This is an interdisciplinary professional society dedicated to strengthening behavioral science teaching in medical schools, in residency programs, and in continuing medical education. ABSAME publishes *Annals of Behavioral Science and Medical Education* and provides access to publications, reports, and a curricular guide in this content area. Available at www.absame.org.

Emergency Medicine

- *American College of Emergency Physicians (ACEP):* This organization sponsors an annual meeting, a teaching fellowship, and Simulation Immersive Training Course. Available at www.acep.org.

Family Medicine

- *Society of Teachers in Family Medicine (STFM):* Curricula are available in sports medicine, substance abuse, clinical nutrition, innovative primary care for first- and second-year medical students, third-year family medicine clerkship, and other areas. Available at www.stfm.org.

Geriatrics

- *Portal of Geriatrics Online Education (POGOe):* This online clearinghouse for educators is sponsored by the Association of Directors of Geriatric Academic Programs. It includes a list of minimum geriatrics competencies for medical students, faculty development materials, and links to other geriatrics educational resources. Available at www.pogoe.org.

Informatics

- *American Medical Informatics Association (AMIA):* The AMIA is concerned with advancement of informatics professionals. It sponsors a peer-reviewed publication, *Journal of the American Medical Informatics Association* (*JAMIA*), and annual meetings related to the use of informatics in health care and for educational purposes. The organization has also developed informatics standards for educational programs. Available at www.amia.org.

Internal Medicine

- *Alliance for Academic Internal Medicine (AAIM):* This is a consortium of five academically focused specialty organizations representing departments of internal medicine at medical schools and teaching hospitals in the United States and Canada: Association of Professors of Medicine (APM), Association of Program Directors in Internal Medicine (APDIM), Clerkship Directors in Internal Medicine (CDIM), Association of Subspecialty Professors (ASP), and Administrators in Internal Medicine (AIM). AAIM provides links to constituent organizations and access to educational materials under "Educational Tools," such as an *Internal Medicine Subinternship Curriculum* and the most recent edition of the *Guidebook for Clerkship Directors.* Available at www.im.org.

- *American College of Physicians (ACP):* The ACP is the largest professional organization for internists maintains active educational resources for all levels of learners. By clicking on "Education and Recertification," then "Medical Educator Resources," one can access resources such as residency curricula in high-value care and teaching tools from the *Annals of Internal Medicine.* Available at www.acponline.org.
- *Society of General Internal Medicine:* This society offers annual meeting precourses, workshops, task force groups, and a monthly journal, the *Journal of General Internal Medicine*, which also publishes an annual medical education issue. There are numerous topic-oriented interest groups (see Chapter 9) open to interested members. Available at www.sgim.org.

Neurology

- *Consortium of Neurology Clerkship Directors / American Academy of Neurology (CNCD):* The consortium's website contains several clerkship curricular resources. There is also a one-year Medical Education Research Fellowship program. Available at www.aan.com/residents-and-fellows/clerkship-and-course-director-resources/consortium-of-neurology-clerkship-directors.

Palliative/End-of-Life Care

- *Center to Advance Palliative Care:* The website contains resources for providers with an interest in palliative care, including background documents on a number of topics. Available at www.capc.org.

Pediatrics

- *Academic Pediatric Association (APA):* Curricular materials are available in areas such as substance abuse, training of residents to serve the underserved, guidelines for residency training, a general pediatric clerkship curriculum and resource manual, and so forth. (Not a member of the Alliance for Clinical Education.) APA publishes *Academic Pediatrics.* There is also a professional development Educational Scholars Program open to members. Available at www.academicpeds.org.
- *Council on Medical Student Education in Pediatrics (COMSEP):* The "Educational Resources" tab provides access to the third- and fourth-year clerkship curricula, faculty development, and other teaching resources. Available at www.comsep.org.

Preventive Medicine

- *Association for Prevention Teaching and Research (APTR):* The organization publishes the *American Journal of Preventive Medicine.* The website also includes a wealth of curricular materials, particularly relevant for population health and interprofessional education, under the "Resources" tab. Available at www.aptrweb.org.

Public Health

- *American Public Health Association (APHA):* APHA publishes the *American Journal of Public Health*, an online newsletter entitled *The Nation's Health*, and reports and issue briefs that may be a source of content for the general needs assessment. Available at www.apha.org.

- *The Centers for Disease Control and Prevention (CDC):* The CDC has data and public health statistics (GNA) on numerous disease conditions and has set standards for public health (an example of ideal approach). Available at www.cdc.gov.

Surgery

- *Association for Surgical Education:* The website contains an educational clearinghouse in areas of the surgical clerkship, educational research, evaluation, and faculty development, including a *Manual of Surgical Objectives* and a case-based, self-directed study guide for medical students. The organization sponsors a grants program, research fellowship, and educational awards. Available at www.surgical education.com.

Women's Health

- *Association of Professors of Gynecology and Obstetrics (APGO):* This is a nonprofit, membership-based organization for women's health educators. The website has numerous educational resources, including suggested curricula, the most recent edition of the APGO *Medical Student Educational Objectives*, teaching tips, an Effective Preceptor series, and resident educational resources. Available at www .apgo.org.

  Curriculum developers should contact *professional societies in their relevant specialty/subspecialty* that are not listed above, because they may maintain curricular guidelines, curricular materials, or other resources helpful in developing specific curricula.

General Education Resources within Medicine

- *Association for Medical Education in Europe (AMEE):* AMEE is an international organization dedicated to promoting excellence in education in the health professions. It publishes the peer-reviewed journal *Medical Teacher* as well as a number of AMEE guides on topics such as teaching and learning, curriculum planning, and educational management, and it sponsors an annual conference. Available at www.amee .org.
- *Association of Standardized Patient Educators (ASPE):* This is an international organization of simulation educators promoting the advancement of standardized patient methodology for teaching, assessment, and research. The website has information on resources for best practices and webinars for training, as well as information on the annual conference. Available at www.aspeducators.org.
- *Association for the Study of Medical Education (ASME):* ASME is a British-based organization of medical educators that publishes *Medical Education* and *Clinical Teacher*, as well as a textbook, *Understanding Medical Education* (2nd ed., 2013). Available at www.asme.org.uk.
- *Best Evidence Medical Education (BEME):* This collaboration of individuals and institutions is devoted to the dissemination of high-quality information through the production and publication of systematic reviews of medical education. The website also provides links to other resources. Available at www.bemecollaboration .org.
- *MedBiquitous:* The MedBiquitous consortium creates technology standards for

health care education. It sponsors an annual meeting, MedBiquitous E-Learning Discourse (presentations available for download from the website), and workshops to train faculty in the use of SCORM (the Sharable Content Object Reference Model, a technical specification that governs how online training or "e-learning" is created and delivered to learners). The home page is at www.medbiq.org.

- *MedEdPORTAL:* Housed by the AAMC, MedEdPORTAL is designed to provide on-line access to peer-reviewed medical education curricular resources across the continuum of medical education. Content can be browsed by discipline or by key-word. Available at www.aamc.org/mededportal.
- *National Board of Medical Examiners (NBME):* The NBME administers the U.S. Medical Licensing Examinations (USMLE). Information on the annual Stemmler Medical Education Research Fund and publications related to medical education, as well as faculty development resources in assessment such as the *Item Writing Manual*, can be found on its website. Available at www.nbme.org.
- *National Guideline Clearinghouse:* This project of the Agency for Healthcare Research and Quality (AHRQ) provides a searchable clearinghouse of evidence-based practice guidelines that may serve as resources for the GNA "ideal approach." Available at www.guideline.gov.
- *The Generalists in Medical Education (TGME):* This is a relatively new organization of American medical educators who provide networking and opportunities for dissemination through their annual meeting and newsletter. Website at www.thegeneralists .org.
- *The Society for Academic Continuing Medical Education (SACME):* SACME is a North American organization that promotes research, scholarship, evaluation and development of continuing medical education (CME) and continuing professional development (CPD). SACME sponsors a biannual meeting and serves as a resource for best practices in CME/CPD education. Available at www.sacme.org.

Interprofessional Education

- *Interprofessional Education Collaborative (IPEC):* This collaborative brought to-gether six higher education health professional organizations in 2009 to develop the *Interprofessional Collaborative Practice Competencies*. Additional organizations have continued to join IPEC and participate in its efforts to advance interprofessional collaborative practice in North America. Links to 11 of these organizations are available on the IPEC website. IPEC sponsors an annual faculty development conference hosting institutional teams to design and advance interprofessional education at their home institutions and serves as a portal for a number of resources and publications in interprofessional education. Available at https://ipecollabora tive.org.

General Educational Resources beyond Medicine

- *American Education Research Association (AERA):* AERA is a national research society devoted to advancing knowledge about education, teaching, and learning. It sponsors an annual meeting for educational researchers. Available at www.aera .net.

- *The Carnegie Foundation for the Advancement of Teaching:* The foundation has sponsored a century of scholarship related to teaching and learning. Its interest in medical education dates to the 1910 Flexner Report. Its 2010 publication *Educating Physicians for the Twenty-First Century: A Call for Reform* synthesized a qualitative study of American medical education 100 years after the Flexner Report. The website houses a number of other studies and reports on general and higher education. Available at www.carnegiefoundation.org.
- *Educational Resource Information Center (ERIC):* Sponsored by the U.S. Department of Education, ERIC provides online access to a bibliography of educational publications, with links to many. It can be particularly useful when researching new educational methods or evaluation methods, such as "reflective writing," not limited to medical education. Available at www.eric.ed.gov.
- *Team-Based Learning Collaborative (TBLC):* This collaborative also sponsors an annual conference that is a great opportunity for faculty development as well as dissemination of scholarship in this educational method. The website hosts a number of resources and recommended readings for best practices. Available at www.teambasedlearning.org.

FACULTY DEVELOPMENT RESOURCES

Listed below are selected programs, courses, and written resources that address the development of clinician-educators in general and educators for specific content areas. As medical education has become increasingly professionalized, many educators are seeking advanced degrees in education, and example degree programs are also noted. Individuals should also contact *professional societies* in their field, which frequently offer workshops, courses, certificates, and fellowships, and *health professional or educational schools* in their area, which may offer faculty development programs or courses.

Faculty Development Programs/Courses

In addition to the organizations listed above, many of which sponsor faculty development courses, workshops, and fellowships, curriculum developers may want to explore the following programs:

- *Harvard Macy Institute:* Sponsors a number of programs for health professional educators, presented by multidisciplinary national and international faculty. Information at www.harvardmacy.org.
- *Johns Hopkins University Faculty Development Program:* Offers longitudinal programs in both teaching skills and curriculum development in Baltimore for physicians in the Mid-Atlantic region. Program faculty are also available to consult, develop, and present on-site programs in teaching skills and curriculum development for client institutions in any location. Information at www.hopkinsmedicine.org/johns_hopkins_bayview/education_training/continuing_education/faculty_development_program.
- *Medical Education Research Certificate (MERC) Program:* Sponsored by the AAMC and intended to provide individuals with skills to foster educational research. Par-

ticipants must complete six workshops to receive certification. Workshops are presented at the annual AAMC meeting and regionally. Information at www.aamc.org /members/gea/merc.

- *McMaster University Faculty in Health Sciences Program for Faculty Development:* Offers a series of faculty development programs in three pathways: basic educators, advanced skills, and leadership. Information at fhs.mcmaster.ca/facdev.
- *Stanford Faculty Development Center for Medical Teachers:* Offers four-week programs in Stanford, California, in clinical teaching and basic science teaching. Participants agree to return to their home institutions and disseminate what they have learned. Information at http://sfdc.stanford.edu.

Degree Programs

Degree programs in health professions education have increased dramatically in number in the past decade. A 2010 publication noted that until 1996 there were only 7 master's-level programs in health professions education and that number had grown to 76 in 2010 (2). Listed below are some of the American programs; these programs are rapidly evolving and the URLs are not stable. Interested readers are encouraged to do additional research looking for both Master's of Education and Master's of Science degrees.

- *Harvard Medical School:* Master of Medical Sciences in Medical Education. Information at http://hms.harvard.edu/masters_medical_education.
- *Johns Hopkins University:* Master of Education in the Health Professions. The Schools of Business, Education, Medicine, Nursing, and Public Health co-developed and sponsor this degree. Information at http://education.jhu.edu/Academics /masters/MEHP.
- *Loma Linda University School of Allied Health Professions:* Certificate or Master of Science in Health Professions Education. Information at www.llu.edu/central /faculty-development/currentcourses.page.
- *Southern Illinois University College of Education in partnership with the Department of Medical Education at the School of Medicine:* Master of Education, Human Resource Development, Health Profession Education Emphasis. Online 36 credit hour degree program. Information at www.siumed.edu/academy/online_masters_ descript.html.
- *University of Cincinnati College of Education and the Division of Community and General Pediatrics at Cincinnati Children's Hospital:* Master of Education (MEd). An online degree program. Information at www.cincinnatichildrens.org/ed/clinical /grad/masters.
- *University of Illinois at Chicago, Department of Medical Education:* Master of Health Professions Education (MHPE). Offered in both online and on-campus formats. Information at http://chicago.medicine.uic.edu/departments___programs/depart ments/meded/educational_programs/mhpe.
- *University of Iowa, Office of Consultation and Research in Medical Education:* Master in Medical Education (MME), a 30 credit hour degree, or a certificate program. Information at www.healthcare.uiowa.edu/ocrme/masters/programoverview.htm.
- *University of Michigan School of Education and the Medical School of the University*

of Michigan: Master of Education with a Concentration in Medical and Professional Education, a 30 credit hour degree program. Information at www.med.umich.edu /lrc/webtest/conMed/index.html.

- *University of New England College of Osteopathic Medicine and Maine Medical Center:* Master of Science (MS) in Medical Education Leadership, a 33 credit hour curriculum. Also offers certificates in program development and leadership development. Information at www.une.edu/com/mmel.
- *University of Pittsburgh, Institute for Clinical Research Education:* Master of Science in Medical Education, a 30 credit program. Also offers a 15 credit certificate program in medical education. Information at www.icre.pitt.edu/degrees/ms_meded .html.
- *University of Southern California, Keck School of Medicine in collaboration with the schools of dentistry and pharmacy:* Master of Academic Medicine. Information at http://keck.usc.edu/Education/Department_of_Medical_Education.aspx.

Other Resources for Faculty Development

- *Association of American Medical Colleges:* Maintains a listing of teaching skills resources at www.aamc.org/initiatives/cei/67772/resources_teaching.html. In addition, MedEdPORTAL (listed above) contains a number of online resources available for faculty development in teaching and assessment.
- *Center for Ambulatory Teaching Excellence (CATE):* Housed in the Department of Family and Community Medicine at the Medical College of Wisconsin, CATE hosts a number of written faculty development materials related to the Educators Portfolio, Mentoring Guidebook for Academic Physicians, precepting skills and teaching skills. Available at www.mcw.edu/Family-Medicine/Center-Ambulatory-Teaching -Excellence.htm.
- *Association of Professors of Obstetrics and Gynecology:* The website hosts a number of faculty development opportunities and teaching resources for obstetrics and gynecology educators. Available at www.apgo.org/faculty.html.
- *Te4Q:* This AAMC initiative is designed to assist clinical faculty in improving their teaching and learner assessment of patient safety and quality improvement. The website includes a listing of faculty development resources and Te4Q literature. Available at www.aamc.org/initiatives/cei/te4q.
- *Advancing Educators and Education by Defining the Components and Evidence Associated with Educational Scholarship:* This 2007 report summarizes the literature on documentation standards for educational scholarship. Available under "Publications" on the AAMC website at www.aamc.org.

FUNDING RESOURCES

Funds for most medical education programs are provided through the sponsoring institution from tuition, clinical, or other revenues or government support of the educational mission of the institution. When asked to take on curriculum development, maintenance, or evaluation activities, it is advisable to think through the resources that will be required for implementation (Chapter 6) and maintenance (Chapter 8) and to negotiate with one's institution for the support that will be required to do the job well. Institutional funding, however, is often limited. It is often desirable to obtain additional funding to protect faculty time, to hire support staff, and to enhance the quality of the educational intervention and evaluation. Unfortunately, the funding provided by external sources for direct support of the development, maintenance, and evaluation of specific educational programs is small when compared with sources that provide grant support for clinical and basic research. Some government and private entities that do provide direct support for medical education, usually in targeted areas, are listed below. Information is current at the time of writing, but websites should be checked carefully because funding priorities change over time. Additional funding can not only increase the quality of the educational intervention but also enhance the quality of related educational research (3), increase the likelihood of publication (4), and add to the academic portfolio of the curriculum developer.

General Information

- *Community of Sciences (COS) Pivot:* A database for funding opportunities. Members can set up a weekly e-mail notification based on saved searches or specified criteria. To create an account, one must be affiliated with an institution that subscribes to Pivot. Available at http://pivot.cos.com.
- *Grant Forward:* A database for searching funding opportunities. One can set up an e-mail notification based on saved searches. There are individual and institutional memberships, and a free trial. Available at www.grantforward.com.
- *Medical Center Libraries:* Libraries may subscribe to one of the above or to another service. Librarians/informationists at one's medical center can often assist in locating funding opportunities.

U.S. Government Resources

- *Agency for Healthcare Research and Quality (AHRQ):* Areas of focus include enhancing the quality (including appropriate use of data), safety, accessibility, affordability, efficiency, and cost transparency of health care. Sometimes research on the promotion of improvements in clinical practice and dissemination activities can be framed in curriculum development terms. Having had research training and having a funded mentor for the application process are very helpful. Available at www.ahrq.gov; click on "Funding & Grants."
- *Fogarty International Center:* The center is part of the *National Institutes of Health* (NIH) with a mission to support global health. The center supports research and research training focused on low- to middle-income nations. Curriculum developers with a focus on international health should look at this website. The Medical Education Partnership Initiative (MEPI) supports foreign institutions to develop or expand and enhance models of medical education. International Research Ethics Education and Curriculum Development Awards (Bioethics) support domestic and international educational and research institutions to develop or expand current graduate curricula and training opportunities in international bioethics related to performing research on acute and chronic diseases in low- and middle-income nations. There are numerous other programs, mostly related to training researchers in developing countries. Available at www.fic.nih.gov.

- *Fund for the Improvement of Postsecondary Education (FIPSE):* Nonmedical focus on precollege-, college- and graduate-level curricula and faculty development to improve quality of and access to education. Premedical or medical curricula that fit the criteria for specific programs could conceivably be funded. Probably best to inquire about a specific idea after reviewing the website and current funding opportunities. Available at www.ed.gov/about/offices/list/ope/fipse/index.html.

- *Grants.gov:* Guide to U.S. government grants. Managed by the Department of Health and Human Services (HHS), Grants.gov is an E-Government initiative operating under the governance of the Office of Management and Budget. This website provides a centralized location for information on more than 1,000 grant programs offered by 26 federal grant-making agencies. It houses a Search Grant function that can help searchers locate grant opportunities related to their area of interest. One can register to receive e-mail notifications of relevant new grant postings through a custom search profile. Available at www.grants.gov.

- *Health Resources and Services Administration (HRSA), Bureau of Health Professions (BHPr):* In the past, the Bureau of Health Professions at HRSA has funded residency training and faculty development programs under Title VII, section 747, of the Public Health Service Act, in the areas of primary care medicine and dentistry, geriatrics, nursing, public health/preventive medicine, and health administration. Grants have been substantial. For some grant programs, only applicants that satisfied a funding preference have been funded. The funding preferences were defined differently for each type of grant, but all were related to the placement of graduates in practices/settings that serve defined, underserved patient populations. The current status of these programs is uncertain. Available at http://bhpr.hrsa.gov.

- *HHS Grants Forecast:* The Department of Health and Human Services' Grants Forecast is a database of planned grant opportunities proposed by its agencies. Each Forecast record contains actual or estimated dates and funding levels for grants that the agency intends to award during the fiscal year. There is a search function. Available at www.acf.hhs.gov/hhsgrantsforecast.

- *National Institutes of Health (NIH):* Most funding is directed toward clinical, basic science, or disease-oriented research and is awarded through disease-oriented institutes. Sometimes educational research and development can be targeted toward specific disease processes and fall within the purview of one of the institutes. The NIH's increased interest in translating research into practice may create opportunities for educators to incorporate educational initiatives into grant proposals. Career development K awards can provide substantial support to individuals for periods of 3 to 5 years to develop as research scientists. R25 (Education Projects), K07 (Academic/Teacher Award), and K30 (Clinical Research Curriculum Awards) awards provide opportunity for curriculum development. NIH grants provide generous funding but are very competitive. Having had research training and having a funded mentor are very helpful. The website has a search function. One can subscribe to a weekly electronic notice of new postings by joining an NIH Guide Listserv. Available at www.nih.gov; click on "About Grants" and "Grants & Funding."

- *National Science Foundation (NSF):* The NSF funds research and education in science and engineering through grants, contracts, and cooperative agreements. The foundation accounts for about 24% of federal support to academic institutions for basic research. It might be a source for basic science curricula. The ADVANCE program focuses on increasing the participation and advancement of women in academic science and engineering careers and could support systematic faculty development efforts in basic science departments. Available at www.nsf.gov; click on "Funding."

- *Veterans Administration:* Faculty at VA hospitals in the United States should explore VA career development awards, as well as funding opportunities for individual projects. Available at www.research.va.gov/funding.

Applying for government grants in the United States is, in general, a very competitive process. Having a mentor who has served on a review board or been funded by the type of grant being applied for is strongly recommended. It is advisable for readers from other countries to acquaint themselves with the government funding resources within their countries.

Private Foundations

- *Arthur Vining Davis Foundations:* The foundations have identified health care as one of their numerous foci. In the past they have funded programs to meet the emotional, spiritual, and psychological needs of patients and families, to enhance the skills, compassion, and empathy of health care professionals, and to improve patient support through an integrated approach, but this "caring attitudes in health care" program has ended. There will be no funding in 2015 or 2016 while the trustees rethink priorities. Past applications could come from institutions and organizations that educate health care professionals and/or provide direct patient care and required a cover letter signed by the chief executive officer of the institution. Grants normally ranged from $100,000 to $200,000. Available at www.avdf.org.
- *Commonwealth Fund:* The fund is a private foundation that aims to promote a high-performing health care system that achieves better access, improved quality, greater efficiency, and improved patient education, particularly for society's most vulnerable, including low-income people, the uninsured, minority Americans, young children, and elderly adults. The fund predominantly supports health services research, but some needs assessment, educational intervention studies, and conferences might be supported. Available at www.commonwealthfund.org/grants-and -fellowships/grants.
- *Dekker Foundation:* Provides small grants to promote educational programs, raise awareness of social issues, and foster a larger sense of community among people of different backgrounds and beliefs. The foundation awards grants only to tax-exempt, nonprofit organizations. Available at www.dekkerfoundation.org.
- *The Foundation Center:* A guide to private foundations. Searching for specific foundations is free. There is a subscription fee for more advanced searches. Available at https://fdo.foundationcenter.org.
- *Arnold P. Gold Foundation for Humanism in Medicine:* The foundation funds curriculum development projects related to humanism, ethics and compassion, and research focused on an aspect of humanism in medicine, at up to $30,000 per year, for 1 to occasionally 3 years. It also provides funding in the Gold Professorship program at $50,000 per year for 3 years for assistant and associate professors to protect time for teaching, program development, and research related to the humanistic practice of medicine. Available at www.humanism-in-medicine.org.
- *John A. Hartford Foundation:* The Hartford Foundation funds numerous programs

related to geriatric education and health services. Support for unsolicited individual projects is limited and by invitation only, after submission of a one- to two-page letter of inquiry. Available at www.jhartfound.org.

- *William Randolph Hearst Foundations:* The foundations fund programs in the areas of education, health, social service, and culture and the arts. In terms of education, the goal is to prepare students to succeed in a global society. The foundations' focus is largely on higher education and includes professional and faculty development. In terms of health, the foundations fund programs designed to enhance skills and increase the number of practitioners and educators in health care. Available at www.hearstfdn.org.
- *Josiah Macy, Jr. Foundation:* The foundation's mission is to improve the health of the public by advancing the education and training of health professionals. Through its programs, it strives to foster innovation in health professional education and to align the education of health professionals with contemporary health needs and a changing health care system. The foundation's grant making is focused on projects that:
  - demonstrate or encourage *interprofessional education and teamwork* among health care professionals;
  - provide *new curriculum content* for health professional education, including patient safety, quality improvement, systems performance, and professionalism;
  - develop new models for clinical education, including graduate medical education reform;
  - improve *education for the care of underserved populations*, with an emphasis on primary care; and
  - increase faculty skills in health professions education, with a special emphasis on the *career development* of underrepresented minorities.

  The foundation has two grant programs: board grants (generally 1 to 3 years of funding, starts with a letter of inquiry) and discretionary President's grants (generally ≤1 year duration, ≤$35,000) in priority areas. It also has a Macy Faculty Scholar program ($100,000 per year for 2 years). Candidates must be nominated by the dean, give 50% of their time to pursuing an education reform project, and have ≥5 years' experience as a faculty member. Available at www.macyfoundation.org.
- *The McDonnell Foundation:* The James S. McDonnell Foundation (JSMF) was founded in 1950 by the aerospace pioneer to improve quality of life by contributing to the generation of new knowledge through its support of research and scholarship. The foundation awards grants in three program areas: *Studying Complex Systems, Brain Cancer Research*, and *Understanding Human Cognition*. JSMF reviews proposals submitted in response to foundation-initiated programs and calls for proposals. Funding is not for educational programs but could include research on learning. Investigator-initiated research awards provide up to $600,000 for up to 6 years. Available at www.jsmf.org.
- *National Board of Medical Examiners (NBME)/Edward J. Stemmler, M.D. Medical Education Research Fund:* The NBME accepts proposals from LCME- or AOA-accredited medical schools. The goal of the Stemmler Fund is to provide support for research or development of innovative assessment/evaluation approaches. Expected outcomes include advances in the theory, knowledge, or practice of assessment at any point along the continuum of medical education, from undergraduate and graduate education and training through practice. Pilot and more compre-

hensive projects are both of interest. Collaborative investigations within or among institutions are eligible, particularly as they strengthen the likelihood of the project's contribution and success. Awards are for up to $150,000 for a project period of up to 2 years. Available at www.nbme.org; click on "Research," then "Stemmler Fund."

- *Donald W. Reynolds Foundation:* Program on Aging & Quality of Life grants are aimed at improving the training of physicians in geriatrics. Periodic requests for proposals (RFPs) may be announced; unsolicited proposals are not accepted. Available at www.dwreynolds.org; click on "Programs."
- *Retirement Research Foundation (RRF):* RRF's mission is to improve the quality of life for U.S. elders. One area for funding is professional education and training projects that have a regional or national impact for older Americans. Of particular interest are programs that:
  - increase the knowledge and skills of professionals and paraprofessionals who serve the elderly; and/or
  - expand the capacity and number of professionals and paraprofessionals prepared to meet the growing demands of an aging population.

  The range of grants has been ~$10,000 to $100,000. Available at www.rrf.org.
- *RGK Foundation:* Provides small grants (mostly in $10,000 to $50,000 range). The foundation's programmatic areas of interest have broadened over the years to include education, community, and health/medicine. The range of projects funded has been broad. Available at www.rgkfoundation.org.
- *Robert Wood Johnson Foundation (RWJF):* The foundation seeks to improve the health and health care of all Americans. It awards most grants through calls for proposals (CFPs) connected with its areas of focus. Areas of focus vary over time. Current areas include reversing childhood obesity; health care coverage for all, bridging health and health care; cost, quality, and value; healthy places and practices; equal opportunity; vulnerable populations; discover, explore, and learn (cutting-edge ideas to accelerate progress in health care; twenty-first-century leadership in health care; future of nursing; and health in its home state of New Jersey). RWJF also accepts unsolicited proposals for projects that suggest new and creative approaches to solving health and health care problems. It funds projects that involve service demonstrations, gathering and monitoring of health-related statistics, public education, training and fellowship programs, policy analysis, health services research, technical assistance, communications activities, and evaluation. Grants are highly competitive. Awards have ranged from $3,000 to $23 million, and time periods from 1 month to 5 years; most awards have ranged from $100,000 to $300,000 and run from 1 to 3 years. Available at www.rwjf.org.
- *Schwartz Center:* Mission is to ensure that all patients and families receive compassionate care. Schwartz Center Grants have supported a wide range of innovative programs to improve the patient-caregiver relationship, especially in the areas of communication between patients and caregivers, promoting compassion and empathy, spirituality and end-of-life care, empowering patients and families, cultural competence, and disseminating best practices. In 2013, the focus was on supporting innovations that contribute to the development of Patient Centered Medical Home practices that exemplify compassionate health care. Grant range was $25,000 to $75,000; grant period 1 to 2 years. No grant funding offered in 2015. Available at www.theschwartzcenter.org.

Other Funding Resources

- *Fees/tuition:* For curricula serving multiple institutions, a user or subscriber fee can be charged (5); DocCom is an online curriculum that charges a licensing fee (6). Charging tuition may be an option for faculty development programs (faculty often have tuition benefits).
- *Institutional grant programs:* Educational institutions often have small grant programs available internally. Readers should learn about grants offered by their own institution.
- *Professional organizations:* For specialty-oriented curricula, contact the relevant specialty organization. Below are just a few examples of professional organizations offering education-related grants. Use *Grant Forward* (see above) and enter "medical education" as keywords to locate numerous others.
    - The American College of Rheumatology's Rheumatology Research Foundation offers a Clinician Scholar Educator Award (up to $180,000 for 3 years). Available at www.rheumresearch.org.
    - The Association for Surgical Education (ASE) Foundation of the Association for Surgical Education (ASE) has Center for Excellence in Surgical Education, Research and Training (CESERT) grants available for 1- to 2-year proposals, maximum of $25,000. Priorities are listed on the website. Available at www.surgicaleducation.com/cesert-grants.
    - The Society for Academic Continuing Medical Education (SACME): Phil R. Manning SACME provides two sorts of grants: 1) the *Phil R. Manning Research Award* for original research related to physician lifelong learning and physician change; up to $50,000 for 2 years. One is awarded every other year. 2) *Research Support Grants* for innovative pilot or preliminary investigations that focus on one of the following areas: continuing medical education (CME)/continuing professional development (CPD) research that engages patients or the public; integration of research into CME/CPD practice; or balancing the individual and the team in practice-based learning. Three grants of $10,000 were awarded in 2013 for 3- to 6-month projects. Available at www.sacme.org/SACME_grants.

REFERENCES

1. Thomas PA, Kern DE. Internet resources for curriculum development in medical education: an annotated bibliography. *J Gen Intern Med.* 2004;19:598–604.
2. Tekian A, Harris I. Preparing health professions education leaders worldwide: a description of masters-level programs. *Med Teach.* 2012;34:52–58.
3. Reed DA, Cook DA, Beckman TJ, et al. Association between funding and quality of published medical education research. *JAMA.* 2007;298:1002–9.
4. Reed DA, Beckman TJ, Wright SM, et al. Predictive validity evidence for medical education research study quality instrument scores: quality of submission to JGIM's medical education supplement. *J Gen Intern Med.* 2008;23:903–7,
5. Sisson SD, Rastegar DA, Rice TN, Hughes MT. Multicenter implementation of a shared graduate medical education resource. *Arch Intern Med* 2007;167:2476–80.
6. American Academy on Communication in Healthcare. DocCom [Internet]. Available at www.aachonline.org.

Index